METHUEN'S
MANUALS OF PSYCHOLOGY

(Founder Editor C. A. Mace 1946–68)
General Editor H. J. Butcher

Obsessional States

Edited by

H. R. BEECH

METHUEN & CO LTD
11 New Fetter Lane London EC4

First published in 1974
by Methuen & Co Ltd, 11 New Fetter Lane, London EC4P 4EE
First published as a University Paperback in 1976
© 1974 Methuen & Co Ltd
Printed in Great Britain
by Butler & Tanner Ltd, Frome and London

ISBN 0 416 60340 8 (hardback edition)
ISBN 0 416 70500 6 (paperback edition)

Distributed in the USA by
HARPER & ROW PUBLISHERS, INC.
BARNES & NOBLE IMPORT DIVISION

Contents

Contributors

H. R. BEECH   Consultant Psychologist at Withington Hospital, West Didsbury, Manchester

ALAN BLACK   Consultant Psychiatrist, Long Grove Hospital, Epsom, Surrey; and Queen Mary's Hospital, Roehampton, London

ROBERT CAWLEY   Consultant Psychiatrist, Maudsley Hospital, Denmark Hill, London

FAY FRANSELLA   Senior Lecturer in Clinical Psychology, Royal Free Hospital School of Medicine, London

H. C. HOLLAND   Senior Lecturer in Psychology, Bethlem Royal Hospital, Beckenham, Kent

R. LEVY   Consultant Psychiatrist, Bethlem Royal and Maudsley Hospitals

ANDRÉE LIDDELL   Senior Lecturer in Psychology, North East London Polytechnic, London

V. MEYER   Reader in Clinical Psychology, Academic Department of Psychiatry, Middlesex Hospital, London

PETER G. MELLETT   Consultant Psychiatrist, Netherne and Horton Hospitals, Surrey

J. PERIGAULT   Research Assistant and British Council Scholar, Netherne Hospital, Surrey

A. SCHNURER   Assistant Professor of Psychiatry, School of Medicine, University of South California, Los Angeles

P. D. SLADE   Research Psychologist and Lecturer in Clinical Psychology, Royal Free Hospital School of Medicine, London

M. STERNBERG   Consultant Psychiatrist, The United Bristol Hospitals, Barrow Hospital and Frenchay Hospital Group, Bristol

JOHN D. TEASDALE   Principal Psychologist, University Hospital of Wales, Cardiff

PART ONE

Clinical and Psychometric Descriptions

I

H. R. Beech

Approaches to understanding obsessional states

Of all forms of psychological disturbances the obsessional state must constitute one of the most puzzling. To some extent this may be attributable to the apparent normality which characterizes certain areas of functioning and which serves to contrast so sharply with other behaviour of an unreasoning or even grotesque kind. Perhaps, again, the distinctive quality of the disorder is enhanced by the variability of reactions to conditions, so that in apparently similar circumstances the patient may behave on one occasion 'reasonably' and, on another, pathologically. It may also be that the enigmatic quality is heightened by a superficial impression of simplicity of mechanism.

Where this latter point is concerned one may recall endeavours to explain and control two other psychological phenomena of deceptive simplicity, writer's cramp and stuttering. It is not, of course, that one would see any necessary connection between the motor aspects of the three disturbances in question, although interesting parallels may be observed, but that it is certainly the case that the very obviousness of the manifestation seems to hold out the promise of easy explanation. It is also perhaps curious, in the light of lengthy and relatively unrewarding investigations of obsessional disorder, how very much our formalized descriptions of the behaviour of obsessionals has become detached from reality. This may well be true of other kinds of psychological disturbances which have become embalmed by their psychiatric labels, but the gulf between the phenomena to be observed and the classical textbook descriptions appears to be wider for obsessionals than for any other group.

There is no obvious reason why this should be so, although one might argue that the substantial differences between cases considered to be obsessional has been partly responsible.

It may be that difficulties arising from this source could be avoided simply by adopting more stringent criteria for classification. Lewis (1936), for example, indicates that not only does obsessional disorder imply '. . . contents of consciousness . . . accompanied by the experience of subjective compulsion . . .', but also the resistance to the compulsive act and thought which the patient shows. In fact three essential elements are underlined; a feeling of subjective compulsion, a resistance to it, and the preservation of insight. Furthermore, Lewis cautions against the dangers of associating any kind of repetitious activity or ceremonial with obsessionality.

But a more likely explanation, it seems, is the special problems attaching to the conventional data gathering method of the interview. While we are used to drawing some distinction between what a patient says on the one hand, and what he or she does on the other, we often find ourselves placing an undue dependence upon the former. Nothing is more salutary than to introduce some check upon the statements made, probably in all sincerity, by the obsessional patient. At least our experience of doing just this has left a lasting impression.

Occasionally such objective checks can have an immediate and dramatic impact upon our thinking. In our study of obsessional patients (Walker, 1967; Walker and Beech, 1969), we have noted, for example, that mood state can assume a role of primary significance in the production of rituals, and that ritualistic observances can be suspended under certain circumstances, so that the inflexibility of performance usually ascribed to such patients is not always to be seen. Perhaps the most dramatic discovery, although one should hesitate to employ this term to describe what any intelligent observer might note, was that a ritual can be terminated by external means with benefit to the patient, a finding which is in sharp contrast to the dire forebodings of the worsening of state uttered in so many clinical textbooks.

It is of considerable interest to see how this interference with ritualistic behaviour has become part of Meyer's successful therapeutic programme (see Chap. 10). Yet again the disparity between the clinical impression and the realities of the situation is exemplified by our observation that the obsessional patient may deliberately 'contaminate' himself and then engage in ritualistic behaviour, an observation quite at variance with the simpler view that such confrontations with 'contamination' occur accidentally after careful and even desperate avoidance of such contact has marked the patient's behaviour. Often, from a perusal of textbook descriptions of the disordered obsessional or compulsive, it seems that the notions put forward by way of description, presumably to serve as the basis of identification and categorization, fall far short of ordinary standards of accuracy, and these descriptions appear only to serve the purpose of recording some private and irrelevant fiction about the nature of the disorder.

For example, Marks (1970) attempts to differentiate obsessive phobias from other phobias as being, among other features, '... beyond voluntary control'. While, superficially, this may appear to be the case, there is no doubt at all that obsessionals can 'decide' not to perform a ritual, and can be induced to modify or eliminate a ritualistic observance simply at the request of the therapist. Frequently, indeed, the most important error committed in reviewing this pathological condition is to confound opinion with demonstrable fact. In a fairly recent general psychiatric textbook by Redlich and Freedman (1966), we find numerous statements which purport to be factual but which might more reasonably be called conjectural. For example, there is no experimental evidence which could lead one to join the authors in concluding that all obsessive symptoms are regarded by the patient as strange, disturbing and incompatible with conscious thought, feeling and striving. Indeed, it is difficult to know quite what to make of this statement without any more precise notion of the way in which the authors are using the term conscious. Again, the authors state unequivocally that there is continuity between the superstitions of the normal individual and the bizarre behaviour of the obsessed, while we still await objective confirmation of this idea. Yet another instance of confusion of hypothesis and fact stems from the claim that 'the aggressive and anal character of such speech (in obsessive patients) is unmistakable'.

Of course it may be that the nomenclature of psychiatric classification is partly or even largely responsible for any disagreement in opinion. Redlich and Freedman find that '. . . all patients with obsessive symptoms show an obsessive character structure', by which they seem to imply that obsessives are all found to be obstinate, orderly, perfectionist, overly punctual, meticulous, parsimonious, and frugal. My own impressions of numerous cases would be at variance with this conclusion, as would available evidence referred to elsewhere in this book. Finally, and rather characteristically for this kind of text, Redlich and Freedman appear to capitulate to the extravagances of Freudian and neo-Freudian theories in which a connection is perceived between 'the battle of the chamberpot' and the fastidious housewife's attention to her duties, thus resurrecting that scientifically impotent concept of reaction formation to account for observations which flatly contradict theory. Furthermore, with a predictable disregard for evidence, it is argued that the ritual is a symbolic means to atonement. Cawley (Chap. 11 of this book) helps to clarify the scientific status of such statements.

Anyone who attempts to make sense of the behaviour observed in obsessional patients, taking these descriptions at their face value as their starting point, will clearly be in considerable difficulties.

Perhaps it is unfair to single out any one text for special comment, particularly where the faults described can be attributed to many different authors in many different books. Certainly the particular form of error shows some degree of variability from text to text, but uniformly they appear to represent the inability of authors to distinguish between opinion, interpretation, casual uncontrolled observation and established fact. What all agree upon, however, and about which there can be little room for doubt, is that what are called obsessional ruminative compulsive disorders are quite frequently severely incapacitating and the outlook can be very grim indeed (see Chap. 2).

Mayer-Gross, Slater and Roth (1955) conclude that, in their opinion, the prognosis in these patients '. . . whose illness has run an undeviating course, the outlook is at best status quo (but) more usually decline downhill'. Furthermore, in what they regard (somewhat obscurely in the context of their brief discussion) as 'true' obsessional state, the apparent irrelevance of 'social and environmental factors' make such disturbances less amenable to therapeutic attack.

Apart from the problems concerning observable and observed phenomena of obsessional disorder there are difficulties which we encounter in the models which have been put forward by various theorists.

We can, for example, agree with Solyom *et al.* (1971) that model experiments (Maier, 1949; Haslerud, Bradbard and Johnston, 1954) only suggest how obsessive behaviour *might* be acquired, but fail to establish that this is, in fact, how they came about. There is, as these authors point out, '. . . no evidence that such motor responses resemble obsessive symptoms any more than they resemble stereotyped or perseverative behaviour'.

A common assumption in such models is that rituals have a basis in anxiety-reduction (Rachman, Hodgson and Marzillier, 1970), although several authors have indicated the limitations of their view. For example, Kanner (1957), Walton (1960), Haslam (1965), Walker and Beech (1969), and Reed (1968), have observed that obsessive activities, contrary to what might have been expected from a displacement theory, may increase rather than decrease experienced anxiety. Indeed, Solyom *et al.* (1971) reported that almost 40 per cent of 'obsessive experiences' were found to be anxiety-provoking among their sample of patients. This formulation is examined in several chapters of this book.

Most frequently quoted, not surprisingly, is Sigmund Freud whose thinking appears to obtrude particularly in connection with this type of disorder. In fact much of what Freud said bears the hallmarks of shrewd and accurate observation, a quality often lost when his views are quoted. Concerning the predisposition to obsessional neurosis, for example (*Collected Papers*, Vol. 2, Chap. 11), his view of causes being divided between 'those which the individual brings with him into life, and those which life brings to him' is frequently abrogated, and the sole emphasis is placed upon early psychological trauma. Indeed, Freud goes on to conclude that such a view as his own imposes some limitations upon the psychoanalytic viewpoint and method.

In other regards Freud provides his usual diet of speculation and astute observation, the latter quality being nowhere more in evidence than in pointing to the discrepancies in behaviour and attitude exhibited by particular patients. Fastidiousness in matters of cleanliness are often accompanied, as Freud noted, by singularly dirty habits as judged by any ordinary standards. In this particular Freud argues that the contradictory behaviour must be determined by powerful instincts of a satisfying kind.

Whatever the explanation for these discrepant behaviours, they have the appearance of importance and they are often ignored in the clinical descriptions purveyed by many psychiatrists. Where Freud's explanations are concerned, however, it would be reasonable to say that his account falls short of what should be acceptable and involves considerable speculation in the absence of properly collected evidence. For example, his account of the ritualistic behaviour of an 11-year-old boy going to bed is contradictory, speculative and untested. (Freud claimed to have traced the boy's peculiar activities to sexual abuse by a servant girl some years before.)

In yet another case he argues that the pathology lay in the persistence of an emotional state and an idea associated with and appropriate to the original one. As such the case itself concerned a young man addicted to masturbation who reproached himself with all kinds of immoral acts including murder, rape and arson. But it is not at all easy to see from Freud's account how the ideas which the young man entertained were related to masturbation. Nor is it easy to see how the ideas could be regarded as defensive, as Freud alleged, for they would appear to be crimes of an infinitely worse character than the original sin. Furthermore, the ordinary investigator may well derive some puzzlement from Freud's apparent facility in discovering important clues as to the pathology with which he is confronted. For example, one patient suffering from obsessional disorder reported that in a dream a girl appeared 'in front of him with two patches of dung instead of eyes'. Freud declares that 'no one who understands the language of dreams will find much difficulty in translating this one'. Apparently the dream declared that he was marrying the girl not for her 'beaux yeux' but for her money.

Sometimes Freud's ideas bear a close resemblance to contemporary conditioning accounts. For example, when describing the substitution of one idea by another, or where an act is substituted for an idea, the substitute serves as a means of obtaining relief or protection. For instance in a case of arithmomania which he quotes, counting serves to distract from the ideas of temptation, and the impulse to count has replaced the original obsession. In the case of washing the hands in a ritualistic fashion, Freud relates the story of Lady Macbeth for whom the washing served the purpose of obtaining moral purity which had been lost as the result of some physical act of impurity. The purpose in substitution is that of protecting the ego but, so long as the substitution continues, so will the accompanying pathological emotional state.

This kind of theorizing is not far removed from the conditioning drive-reduction model, which is often postulated by the behaviour therapist, and in which the ritualistic activity affords relief from anxiety by some means or other and its continuance is ensured by its success in diminishing drive.

It is characteristic of Freud that he is perceptive of the numerous possible relationships which exist between the phenomena of obsessional disorder and the characteristic traits of behaviour which might be exhibited by the normal individual. An interesting example of this attempt at connection-forming occurs in his 1907 paper where he relates obsessive acts and religious practices. The ceremonials of a religious rite are similar, in his opinion, to a neurotic ceremony in three respects. In the first place there are pangs of conscience which are experienced after the omission of a ceremony; secondly there is conscientious attention paid to the details of carrying out the ceremonial; and, thirdly, there is the experienced need for isolation from other activity so that, for example, one may not be disturbed during the performance of some ritualistic behaviour.

According to Freud the differences are also threefold. In the first place religious rites are stereotyped, while the neurotic ceremonial may be quite varied; secondly, while religious rites tend to be public in character, the neurotic ceremonial tends to be conducted in private; and, finally, while the religious ceremony is full of obvious symbolism the neurotic ceremonies appear to be silly and meaningless, although this is not really the case. At the basis of these ritualistic behaviours of a neurotic kind there is guilt, which is unconscious, and the ceremony acts as the protective measure. In this sense it is comparable, according to Freud, to the protestations of the pious that they know they are miserable sinners. While at first petty and trivial, the symbolic ceremony becomes urgent and vital. Similarly, says Freud, in religious practices sometimes the original significance of the practices of rituals is lost and the rite itself becomes the important thing, and for this reason religions are subject to reforms to try to re-establish original meaning and value.

Freudian theory in respect of obsessionals is, as always, rich, full of significance and characterized by the astute clinical insight which we have come to recognize in all Freud's writings. Furthermore he continually displays a willingness to change and modify his ideas as a result of coming across some piece of conflicting and contradictory evidence in his clinical practice (see Chap. 11). However, these theoretical notions seldom achieve the coherence which we would now think of as being necessary, nor are they based upon evidence which carries any serious degree of conviction. Indeed, more often than not, the evidence is flimsy and insubstantial and may well be, because of the method of its gathering, inaccurate. Furthermore even Freud's often valuable tendency to abandon or modify theoretical formulations, can appear as a serious demerit when such abandonment occurs in the context of evidence equally flimsy to that which led Freud to the development of the original elaborate formulation. In no case is there a coherent unequivocal scrutiny of the ideas put forward and we must regard this theoretical framework as essentially speculative, unconfirmed and difficult to assess.

Pavlov's attempt at the crude formulation of a theoretical framework for evaluating obsessional neurosis also appears to suffer from certain important deficiencies. He begins his theorizing by remarking upon the finding that in some dogs there are peculiar and puzzling reactions of a pathological kind. For example a continuing tendency to turn towards the source of one c.s. even when other c.s.'s from other sources are substituted. Such pathological tendencies, he observes, may be corrected by bromide, and the notion is advanced that the cause of disturbance has been an abnormal balance between excitatory and inhibitory processes, with the former showing an exaggerated pre-dominance over the latter. Indeed, as the c.s. which first elicits the disturbance is essentially weak, but yet produces an unusual arousal in the animal, the overstrain of excitatory process appears to be implicated. In other experiments, attempts were made which were at first apparently successful, to transform stimuli provoking positive reactions into ones which provoked inhibitory process, and vice versa. However, it was noted that the reactions of animals sooner or later reverted to those found in the original pre-transformation period. These experiments suggested that the responsibility for the outcome was a continuing stability of the excitatory process while at the same time there was a weakening of inhibitory process. This morbid condition was given the name 'pathological inertness' by Pavlov.

He felt that stereotypy and perseveration in humans represented 'pathological inertness' of the motor area of the cortex and that this state could also apply to cortical cells related to sensations, feelings and conceptions. He noted that such states occurred in several types of disorder including hysteria and catatonic schizophrenia, and remarked upon the similarities which exist between obsessions and paranoid delusions, quoting from Janet and Kretschmer to support this conten-tion. Such pathology he regarded as more likely in his 'weak types' and in the 'strong but unbalanced types', just as is the case for experimental neurosis. The fundamental cause he believed to be some trauma of a physical or psychological kind producing 'overstrain' (excessive excitation) of cortical cells, although he also felt that conflict, arising out of life's vicissitudes, was another element also strongly implicated in studies of experimental neurosis.

None of the case illustrations which he provides, however, carries any degree of conviction for the reader. Certainly he offers a means of relating experimental evidence from the laboratory to human experi-ence and also indicates an integration of psychological forces and ner-vous process. But the result appears to be contrived and patchy, leaving so many gaps that we are left with suggestions rather than coherent ideas. In short, there is discontinuity between the simple theoretical notion and the complexity of human circumstances, as well as an inadequate consideration of the complexity of the characteristics of the obsessional condition.

Nevertheless, as in Freud's account, there is the recognition of one peculiar and striking phenomenon of the disorder, an isolated pathology involving cortical elements, with much else involved in the individual's functioning remaining intact. It remains open as to whether pathological inertness and the special conditioning phenomena brought into focus by Pavlov, are of relevance. There is the recognition, furthermore, that such conditions represent an unusual pathology not related in any detailed way to other clinical states although having some superficial resemblance to them (e.g. phobias). Such understanding as Pavlov provides, albeit primitive and inadequate, at least goes beyond the kind of gross over-simplification which sometimes characterizes published accounts. It seems unlikely now that one could endorse Wolpe's contention that the reciprocal inhibition model and desensitization treatment apply in a straightforward way to obsessionals. It seems unlikely, as Hussain has reported in 1964, that there could be a 92 per cent recovery rate for patients among whom were included a number of obsessionals. It seems probable that we would want to qualify the contention of Eysenck and Rachman (1965) that phobias and obsessions may be looked on as being similar in that they are 'persistent, unadaptive and surplus response patterns'. Similarly, there is no recent confirmation of Lazarus' contention (1963) that there is no essential difference between the outcome obtained with phobics (59 per cent improvement) and obsessional compulsive (55 per cent improvement). Nor would there be any serious support for the contention that reciprocal inhibition is a useful strategy in treating obsessional patients (Walton and Mather, 1964). Furthermore, Eysenck and Rachman (1965) have also argued that relapse should 'hardly ever' occur in dysthymic patients and have made special mention of obsessive compulsive reactions as an example of such disorders which consist of conditioned sympathetic reactions; here the use of antagonistic reactions in 'reconditioning treatment' will 'weaken and finally extinguish them'. More recent evidence serves to erode our confidence in the theoretical model as well as the empirical outcome of applying simple conditioning strategies.

What in fact is required in the way of theoretical formulations is a model which will embrace all the complexities of obsessional behaviour and which takes account of the often paradoxical nature of this kind of disturbance. It is generally believed that obsessions or compulsions comprise some act or thought which is repetitive, irrational and outside voluntary control and that it is unchanging and unmodified throughout its repetition, this latter state being called stereotypy. Furthermore, it is argued that the distinguishing feature of such disorders is the internal resistance (Mayer-Gross, Slater and Roth, 1955) to carrying out the act or thought, so that the pathological behaviour, whether of action or thought, appears to be against the will of the patient, and often seems to have the quality of disgust or repulsion; this urge to do something, yet to be repelled by it, is said to be a singular characteristic of the obsessional state. Other experience, both experimental and clinical, would suggest that these qualities are certainly not always found among such patients, nor, when they are found, do they appear in any unequivocal way.

Nevertheless, the identification of such qualities or characteristics, which at the moment we may regard as being purely hypothetical, enable us to make a start upon the experimentation which is necessary. Some of the experimental work which appears to be particularly relevant has a fairly lengthy history, such as that having to do with attempts to produce compulsive behaviour which is then interpreted as being 'perseverative' or 'fixated' behaviour of an unadaptive kind. In animal studies examples of such experiments have been provided by Maier (1949), Maier, Glaser and Klee (1940), and Feldman (1953). (See also Chaps. 7 and 9 in this book.) Among human studies of a similar kind are those by Marquart and Arnold (1952), Jones (1954), Hamilton and Krechevsky (1933), and Farber (1948). What such experiments suggest is that, in the presence of an insoluble problem, both rats and humans sometimes show stereotypy which persists even when the problem situation is altered so that a solution *is* possible. Two other factors also seem to be relevant, the first being that where the pressure to respond to the insoluble situation is great, there is an increased probability of stereotypy of response and, secondly, that the introduction of some emotionally arousing condition or cue appears to assist in the fixation of behaviour. Some theorists, like Wolpe (1953), suggest that stereotypy is obtained by the reduction of intense anxiety (see Chap. 9), and to some extent it seems that a high general drive level might help to promote fixations (Elliott, 1934). This latter idea would certainly be quite compatible with the theoretical model put forward by Beech and Perigault (see Chap. 5) and, in clinical practice, the author has found attempts to lower general drive levels of some value in dealing with obsessional patients for example, by advising more frequent sexual contacts with the partner (although this, in itself, is often a problem for the obsessional patient).

While escape from insoluble and intolerable conflict may activate response perseveration there seems, nevertheless, to be a considerable gap between the demonstrations which have concerned laboratory animals and normal human subjects on the one hand, and the hand-washing of obsessional patients on the other. In the first place the nature of the insoluble problem is not obvious in the case of the obsessional and, secondly, it is not apparent why certain rituals should be chosen out of the vast repertoire of available 'fixations', a matter which is discussed in later sections of this book.

Relatively modest advances have been made in the successful treatment of these states particularly where they have achieved a degree of severity. Certain methods appeared to hold considerable promise, one such being the methods which Meyer and his colleague have developed at the Middlesex Hospital (see Chap. 10). But for the most part the results of attempting treatment and modification strongly implicate the need for a good deal more research to be conducted before we can provide any comprehensive account of obsessional disorder together with a reliable method of treatment.

To the extent to which animal studies provide a useful guide the findings of Maier and Klee (1945) offer interesting possibilities showing that the 'guidance' of the experimenter facilitates the abandonment of adaptive behaviour whereas trial and error do not. In this connection it is interesting to note that Maier advances a two-stage hypothesis concerning the transition from stereotypy to adaptive behaviour. The first consisting of eliminating the fixation and the second comprising the acquisition of new and adaptive responses. One would suspect that this kind of formulation has wide applicability in connection with the learning theory models of psychological aberrations, and one such application has been suggested by Beech (1969) in connection with effecting changes in persons of deviant sexual orientation. Numerous other methods of treatment, electrical, chemical and psychological, have their adherents and have some limited claim to efficacy (see Chap. 12). However, as this book is intended to demonstrate, there is much to learn of the nature and implications of obsessions before a truly effective treatment can be devised.

It may be anticipated, from the foregoing, that the degree to which this type of psychological abnormality is characterized by evidence or information of a dependable and extensive kind is limited. Indeed, any ordinary perusal of the existing literature leaves one with a pervading impression of uncertainty and vagueness and, in consequence, prompts an attempt at compilation of such facts and ideas as are available. The editor's personal research interest in this area over the past twelve years certainly gave impetus to the task of gathering together and evaluating work in this field.

Accordingly, this book was planned to afford a useful coverage of the clinical, research and experimental, and treatment approaches to obsessional/compulsive states. The inclusion of material under these three headings may appear to readers to have a certain arbitrariness, for it proved difficult for contributors to be completely restrictive in their chapters, particularly where authors saw the need to provide a background against which their ideas or experimental data could be properly viewed.

Furthermore, recognizing the paucity of available studies and the problem of reconciling discrepant reports, the editor urged contributors to be speculative within the limits of whatever information of a hard kind was available to them. In this way it was hoped that clinicians might derive new and possibly useful ways of conceptualizing these problems, and that the researcher would find a source of valuable suggestions and hypotheses.

To attempt to summarize these contributions made by the authors, and to draw out their clinical and research implications, is a difficult but perhaps useful way of introducing the book.

A suitable beginning may be made by calling attention to Black's salutary comment that, while it is convenient to use the term 'obsessional', we remain unclear and divided in our views on many aspects of the problem. He goes on to remind us that, bedevilled by a dearth of systematic studies of this comparatively uncommon disorder, we have little knowledge of genetic and other possible causal influences, the part which 'personality' plays, or even sound ideas about the course and development of the disorder – if, indeed, only one disorder is all with which we have to deal. That it is a serious form of abnormality, often marked by great handicap, is undoubted, although prognosis is still a difficult matter in our present state of knowledge.

In the second chapter Mellett has brought out, in a clear and unequivocal way, the clinical picture which has come to be regarded as typical, but alerts us to some of the especially puzzling features found among these patients and which seldom receive adequate attention in widely used texts. Among these, and conveying important research implications, is Mellett's observation of the disparity which may exist between a patient's anxiety in certain situations and a degree of indifference when such situations are contrived by the therapist, leaving the latter with the '. . . uncanny feeling of treating symptoms which did not exist'. Especially striking too is Mellett's argument for the existence of a special mechanism in obsessional states which both 'imprints' behaviour patterns and which, subsequently, becomes a means by which such patterns are re-evoked. The need for such a model is a frequently recurring theme in this book.

Slade, in his contribution to the introductory section, in which he reviews a part of the psychometric evidence, draws important conclusions for both the clinician and the researcher. Among these are that, while psychological measurement studies suggest the independence of obsessional symptoms and obsessional personality traits, clinical studies do not. Furthermore, that, whereas there is strong evidence to suggest that obsessionals may be accurately characterized as neurotic introverts, the evidence is much weaker for personality traits such as inflexibility, and little support is found for the concept of the 'anal character' of obsessionals. Finally, Slade feels that the evidence argues the need for a multiple classificatory system to describe obsessionals and that, in all probability, this will imply a need for different therapeutic methods.

In the second section of the book Beech and Perigault have attempted to provide a model which integrates some of the salient features found among obsessionals. The emphasis in this theory is placed upon unusual disturbances in state as being characteristic of such patients, which allows for the development of pathological ideas and reactions to certain environmental events. They offer some account of the experimental background upon which the theory draws as well as information deriving from their own recently conducted studies.

In the following chapter, Beech and Liddell review the experimental evidence for links between mood state, decision-making, and the ritualistic behaviour of obsessional patients. Certain parts of this evidence are encouraging and help to clarify the nature of the abnormalities, although ambiguities and discrepancies still abound, not least of which is the controversy involved in the anxiety-reduction model of ritualistic behaviour.

The value of alternative approaches to understanding the phenomena of obsessional disorder is also well illustrated in the chapters by Holland and Fransella. Holland advances the view, based upon a systematic and comprehensive review of animal studies, that obsessional behaviour is a direct form of displacement and that, in order to obtain a clearer understanding of obsessionality, experimental inquiry into the mechanisms of displacement would be rewarding. Fransella, on the other hand, making use of Construct Theory in deriving her model of pathological thinking among obsessionals, argues that the construing system of such patients eventually leaves the patient with meaningfulness only in his obsessions while '. . . outside this area . . . all is vagueness and confusion'. She neatly relates this aberration of construing to what others have called 'decision-making'; in the context of her theoretical conception this abnormality is described as the avoidance of opportunities for validating predictions so as to eliminate invalidational experiences, for the latter would threaten the collapse of the entire construct system. While admittedly speculative, such a model offers interesting links with alternative approaches and, as Fransella points out, alerts us to new therapeutic possibilities. It may be, for example, that any success attending the treatment regime described in Chapter 10 could be seen as the result of contriving invalidation experiences to the point where a new and 'healthy' construct system is forced upon the patient.

The final chapter in this section, by Teasdale, examines the value of learning models as explanations for the phenomena of obsessive/compulsive states. In this chapter it is especially notable how a behavioural orientation introduces a measure of clarity into a descriptive exercise, and this is especially evident where Teasdale distinguishes between phobics, who show 'passive' avoidance behaviour, and the rituals of obsessionals which can be characterized as 'active' avoidance.

This directness of approach is also shown in Teasdale's emphasis upon the need for an explanation for *differences* between 'obsessional' and 'normal' behaviours, and from which he assembles his hypotheses and suggests the means by which they could be tested. Especially interesting, in the light of empirical research findings, is his conclusion from the theoretical considerations that an avoidance/avoidance conflict model is a useful way of conceptualizing the 'ritual' situation. This suggestion, as well as that which he offers in respect of the non-ritualistic behaviours of obsessionals, closely parallels propositions advanced by Walker (1967), Beech and Perigault (see Chap. 5), and by Beech and Liddell (see Chap. 6). Indeed, one of the important outcomes of this book has been the degree to which integration of approaches and agreement upon conceptual frameworks has become viable.

A further example of this again arises from Teasdale's account in which he points to the problems presented by an over-simplified 'associationist' account of the origin of obsessional behaviour and, instead, advances a sensitization hypothesis of the kind put forward by Beech (1971) and, again, by Beech and Perigault (see Chap. 5). Yet another example is the way in which Teasdale's therapeutic suggestions, based upon theoretical considerations, find empirical confirmation in the behavioural treatments described by Meyer and his colleagues (see Chap. 10).

Meyer has in fact pointed out that, where treatment is concerned, we are largely dependent upon single case studies, using different strategies, different methods of evaluation, and with quite inadequate control data. In the main the emphasis has been placed upon anxiety-reduction techniques, and the therapy described in Chapter 10 constrasts with this tendency. The results of the treatment programme devised by Meyer *et al.*, combining response prevention, hierarchical presentation of stimulus situations, social reinforcement, and modelling, has yielded encouraging results to date, although these authors are careful to avoid excessive optimism.

Similarly Cawley, in Chapter 11, points out that psychotherapy is in no better position than any other treatment in terms of an assessment of its value for obsessionals. His conclusion, that there is no evidence either to support or refute the proposition that formal psychotherapy helps patients suffering from obsessional disorder, is a salutary comment upon the inadequacy of our current knowledge and expertise.

In contrast, in the final chapter, Sternberg focuses upon current clinical practice *vis-à-vis* physical methods of treatment, and attempts to arrive at a consensus of clinical opinion as to their efficacy. Again, he feels it important to indicate that there is little or nothing in the way of proper evaluation of these methods and that, without adequate research we are unlikely to advance our knowledge or therapeutic effectiveness.

One may hope that in some way these contributions will help clinicians and researchers alike to clarify their ideas about these puzzling abnormalities. Certainly, from the editor's personal viewpoint, the contributors have achieved an important objective in providing an essential overview of clinical aspects, research ideas and experimental data, and information about treatment strategies. It is unlikely, even in a topic area as neglected as this, that we have succeeded in being fully comprehensive in our account and, indeed, we have consciously elected to minimize our coverage of particular aspects.

The reader will no doubt remark upon the disregard of obsessional phenomena found among children which we, the contributors, agreed would divert us from the proper focus of attention in this book. Similarly, we have opted to ignore what we felt to be the separate problem area of obsessional symptomatology associated with organic conditions. Finally, we chose not to attempt more than brief reference to the psycho-dynamic viewpoint, feeling not only that the material presented should be, if possible, predicated upon experimental evidence and that, in any case, the psychoanalytic literature on this topic is generally well known and readily available elsewhere.

These and other omissions will no doubt make this book less acceptable to some readers. For the bulk of readers we hope the work of collecting and evaluating what is known and what remains to be known will be of some value.

2

Alan Black

The natural history of obsessional neurosis

The natural history of a condition is, simply, an account of its development in time, from beginning to end. However, this is an idealized
definition, which carries certain implicit assumptions. By successively
questioning, testing and modifying these assumptions, they are progressively revised until they approximate as closely as possible to the
observed data. A basic assumption in the above definition should be
clarified first: one cannot validly speak of the natural history of a
condition but only of a person manifesting certain symptoms and
signs – the so-called condition is an abstraction, a shorthand convention.
The definition then assumes that a group of people exhibiting these same
manifestations will behave alike in other relevant ways, and for present
purposes we are interested in the course and outcome of these manifestations. If we find that they are similar in this respect as well, further
support is provided for regarding the group as homogeneous. However,
should there be appreciable differences in course and outcome one
would be led to question certain assumptions. These may relate to the
individuals at or before the onset of illness (the antecedent assumptions)
and during the course of illness (the intercurrent assumptions). Thus one
may ask if the group was homogeneous in all possibly relevant ways
beforehand, for example with respect to age, sex, constitution, personality, social class; and whether any intercurrent factors were responsible for differentially affecting course and outcome, such as treatment,
changes of health or of life situation? In effect what one is trying to do
is to classify observations into meaningful patterns. One has therefore
to select from the available data those items which are considered
relevant according to some *a priori* hypothesis – the assumption – and
test its actual relevance in terms of that particular hypothesis. Far from
being a weakness, making and testing assumptions is an indispensable

step in organizing our observations. By following the progress of a set of people defined according to certain morbid criteria, a basis is laid for asking what factors affect onset, course and outcome. Such a body of knowledge is termed the natural history.

HISTORY AND DEFINITION

The concept of obsessional disorder has gradually evolved from the progressive synthesis of clinical observations made over the last hundred years. Although Esquirol probably described the first case report in 1838, the earliest use of the term 'obsession' is attributed to Morel (1866). Westphal (1878) gave the first comprehensive definition as ideas which come to consciousness in spite of, and contrary to the will of the patient – ideas which he is unable to suppress, although he recognizes them to be abnormal and not characteristic of himself (Rosenberg, 1968a). In Lewis's (1957) opinion, however, it was Janet (1903) who made the most authoritative attempt to delineate a syndrome. In addition to the general weariness and lack of perseverance, he stressed the indecision, checking, hesitancy, the tendency to introspection and to depersonalization. The definition given by Schneider (1925) is frequently used: obsessions are contents of consciousness which, when they occur, are accompanied by the experience of subjective compulsion, and which cannot be got rid of, though on quiet reflection they are recognized as senseless. However, the contents of obsession are not necessarily senseless, e.g. fears of contamination; and on the other hand, symptoms of other conditions, such as anxiety and depression, may also be recognized as senseless. As Lewis (1936) pointed out, this part of Schneider's definition is not an essential characteristic of obsessional illness. Nor does it include one feature of Westphal's definition, the occurrence of ideas 'in spite of and contrary to the will of the patient'. Lewis (1936) held that there should be mention of the feeling that one must resist the obsession and in 1957 he emphasized this as the cardinal feature: 'The essence of an obsession is the fruitless struggle against a disturbance. . . .' This resistance is experienced by the patient as that of his free will (Westphal, 1878; Lewis, 1936). Various defensive manœuvres – rituals and compulsions associated with the struggle – are regarded as secondary manifestations of this experience: 'They carry into effect the urge to ward off the painful and overwhelming obsessions . . . (but again) – it is misleading to consider such devices as essential' (Lewis, 1936).

These features are generally accepted as central to the syndrome, but views on its boundaries vary. Phobic disorders are not usually considered part of the syndrome, and when they are this is more as a matter of arbitrary decision (Kringlen, 1965) or opinion (Anderson, 1971) than as a result of systematic investigation. Obsessional symptoms may occur in several conditions and it is usual to define an obsessional neurosis as a condition in which the obsessional symptoms predominate and are not secondary to another disorder. Unsatisfactory as this nosological position may be, it is hard to dissent from Lewis's comment (1957) that 'psychiatric syndromes at present have only a provisional heuristic value. . . . It is therefore still convenient to speak of obsessional neurosis. The obsessional neurosis *qua* neurosis rests more on its occasional tendency to become stabilized and systematized than on its exhibiting a constant grouping of symptoms.'

INCIDENCE AND PREVALENCE

Obsessional neurosis is relatively uncommon. Reports of its incidence, ranging from 0·1 per cent to 4·6 per cent (Table 2.1), are based on psychiatric populations and refer to various proportions of patients

TABLE 2.1 *Incidence of obsessional neurosis in psychiatric practice*

Author	Percentage of		
	Out-patients	In-patients	In-patient neurotics
Pollitt (1957)		< 4·0	
Blacker & Gore (1955)	2·9	3·1	
Kringlen (1965)		2·5	4·3
Eysenck (1947)		2·0	
Slater (1943)		1·0	
Ingram (1961b)		0·9	
Registrar-General (1953)		0·7	4·6
Registrar-General (1964)		0·6	3·5
Ross & Rice (1945)	0·3	0·2	
Lo (1967)	0·6	0·1	
Ray (1964)		2·0	

seen in out-patient clinics or admitted to hospital. These estimates should be accepted as rough indicators only: the figures are not necessarily comparable with each other because of differing diagnostic criteria and admission policies, and interests of particular doctors. Moreover, patients suffering from obsessional states tend to be more secretive about their condition than other neurotic patients and to postpone seeking medical help until later. It is therefore probable that those seen in psychiatric practice are relatively more severe cases and the incidence of their attendance does not reflect the actual figure in the community. Rüdin (1953) and Woodruff and Pitts (1964) estimated the prevalence in the general population as 0·05 per cent but published surveys of general practice patients do not include separate rates for obsessional illness.

Data for non-Western populations is meagre. Wittkower (1968) commented that obsessional neurosis is reported as rare in under-developed countries but cited only one paper, a comparative diagnostic study of psychiatric out-patients in Bombay and Topeka (Gaitande, 1958). The incidence given by Lo (1967) among Chinese patients attending the Hong Kong Mental Health Service over a fifteen-year period supported this view and is comparable with Western figures.

In a survey of 11,442 members of four aboriginal Formosan tribes representing different levels of social development, only 9 cases of psychoneuroses were found, and not a single example of obsessional neurosis (Rin and Lin, 1962; see also Lin, 1953).

GENETIC AND FAMILIAL ASPECTS

In the model suggested by Slater and Cowie (1971), the genetic contribution to neurotic illness may be made at two levels, predisposing to the development of various personality traits and independently, to the manifestation of particular stresses, including symptom formation. Because various personality traits will have varying degrees of association with varying kinds of neurotic symptomatology, the potential interrelationships will be highly complex, and attempts to measure the genetic contribution to neurotic manifestations will have to deal with very heterogeneous data.

In conditions which are probably determined by both polygenic and environmental factors, the study of concordance rates in twins at present offers one of the most sensitive ways of assessing the contribution of genetic factors. In order to compare the significance of any such findings, it is necessary to have a base line. Obsessional illness is the least common of the defined neuroses. No prevalence rates in the general population have been published, but both Rüdin (1953) and Woodruff and Pitts (1964) have estimated this as 0·05 per cent. Depending on the figure of identical twin frequency accepted (1 : 132 live births, Pearson, 1963; or 1 : 200 adults, Shields, 1962), the expected incidence in the general adult population of an index identical twin with obsessional neurosis is between 1 : 300,000 and 1 : 400,000; 0·05 per cent of these cases, between 1 : 600 million and 1 : 800 million, could be expected to be a co-twin with obsessional neurosis if concordance were only random. Thus, in the absence of common determinants, even one pair of identical twins concordant for obsessional illness would be highly improbable statistically. The existence of 20 such Caucasian pairs reported in the last thirty-five years might be held to exceed this chance expectation. Unfortunately the value of much of this material is vitiated by loose diagnostic criteria and failure to provide evidence of zygosity.

Rüdin (1953) found in the literature reports on 9 pairs of MZ twins with obsessional neurosis, to which she added one further pair; of these 10 pairs, 6 were considered as concordant. However, no specific data were given to confirm monozygosity and only scanty clinical descriptions were offered to support the diagnosis of obsessional illness.

Lewis (1936) refers to 3 sets of allegedly monozygotic twins: one set was concordant for obsessional illness and a second set, reared apart, for obsessional traits; the third set was discordant.

Tienari's (1963) study was the first to be based on a population survey, the material deriving from all Finnish-speaking male twins born in Finland between 1920 and 1929 and living in a defined geographical area; in addition he included findings from a psychiatrically screened sub-sample. 21 pairs were classified as neurosis cases with the tendency towards concordance being greatest in twins with phobic and obsessional symptoms. Tienari claims a concordance rate here of 91 per cent – 10 of 11 pairs. Accepting, as he points out, that the rate depends on the criteria of classification, it is nevertheless difficult to agree with the above claim from reading the case reports. Apart from including both phobic and obsessional features, traits and syndromes are poorly differentiated and it would often seem that the mere presence of a symptom or trait in common was sufficient to establish concordance. As far as could be ascertained, there is no support for the diagnosis of obsessional neurosis in a single case.

Woodruff and Pitts (1964) reported a pair of male twins whose monozygosity was supported by blood group data and the presence of glandular hypospadias. Both twins had post-natal grand mal seizures and suffered from migrainous headaches from $3\frac{1}{2}$ years which were relieved, following the demonstration at 13 years of minimal non-paroxysmal EEG activity, by diphenyldantoin. They showed similar manneristic behaviour disorders from $2\frac{1}{2}$ to $3\frac{1}{2}$ years and each developed similar pattern of obsessional behaviour from 6 years onward. Although the presence of mildly abnormal EEGs confounds the significance of genetic factors here, it is noteworthy that the father had marked obsessional traits and the paternal grandfather had phobic and obsessional symptoms.

No such familial history was present in the pair of identical twins reported by Marks *et al.* (1969), both of whom developed an obsessional illness at the age of 10. Although one of the twins was dominant over the other and the content of symptoms was probably influenced by mutual interaction, separation was not followed by improvement in the subordinate twin's condition.

Shields, in a personal communication cited by Marks *et al.* (1969), states that there were 6 cases of obsessional illness in the identical twin series documented by the Medical Research Council's Psychiatric Genetics Unit, 3 of which were probably concordant.

The conclusion that concordance in MZ twins is determined by genetic factors has not gone unchallenged. In arguing the importance of environmental factors as an explanation for identical twins both developing schizophrenia, Jackson (1960) laid considerable emphasis on two factors, a) their close identification, and b) the confusion of ego identities which is said to occur in identical twins. Whether or not the latter consideration is of aetiological significance for schizophrenia, there is no evidence of its relevance for obsessional neurosis. The contribution of mutual identification to this condition was examined by Parker (1964). From a series of 29 neurotic twins studied by the Medical Research Council's Psychiatric Genetics Unit, he selected two sets in which the identification of one twin and another was most marked, and confirmed monozygosity from blood groups and other physical features. (One set was one of the three discordant pairs mentioned by Shields, cited by Marks *et al.*, 1969.) Despite the presence of a marked identification, in both instances only one of the twins developed a severe obsessional illness. This finding is presented as a significant item of evidence against the theory that the high concordance rate for psychiatric disorder in MZ twins can be attributed to mutual identification. It is not, of course, evidence against a genetic contribution on the one hand or the effects of environmental factors on the other. Moreover, the existence of strong mutual identification does not exclude differences in other life experiences or of personality, as Parker demonstrated. He points out that, like other twin studies, his examples show how personalities of similar endowment develop differently as a result of special experiences and stresses.

In addition to these European and American cases, there are reports of two Japanese studies. Inouye (1965) considered 8 of 10 pairs of MZ twins to be concordant for obsessive–compulsive reaction, but he acknowledged that the diagnostic classification was arbitrary 'because it is not easy to determine whether or not they were or had been suffering from any type of neurosis'. In only 4 of these 8 pairs was the index twin regarded as having a typical obsessive–compulsive neurosis and judging from the case reports the co-twin of one pair may well have had an obsessional personality only. More significantly, one of these 4 index twins is described as suffering from multiple motor tics and loud utterances including coprolalia, starting from the age of nine, features which are pathognomonic, not of obsessive–compulsive neurosis, but of Gilles de la Tourette's syndrome (Fernando, 1967). Moreover the co-twin was a deaf mute who began making indistinct noises at the onset of the index twin's symptoms. (This case is also of more general interest because it seems to be the first, albeit inadvertent report of Gilles de la Tourette's syndrome outside of America and Europe, the only other ones being described in 1970 (Prabhakaran, 1970; Beg & Hasan, 1970).) Diagnostic confounding is also apparent in the study reported by Ihda (1965): although 10 of 20 MZ twins were claimed to be concordant for obsessional neurosis, these include index and co-twins with mild obsessional traits and the actual concordance rate is uncertain.

Despite the extensive and painstaking work involved in collecting these data, there would seem to be only three published instances of identical twins with obsessional neurosis in which both zygosity and diagnosis have been reliably determined (Woodruff and Pitts, 1964; Parker, 1964; Marks *et al.*, 1969). Even if one includes the 6 pairs (3 concordant, 3 discordant) documented by the Medical Research Council Psychiatric Genetics Unit, the information available is still quite insufficient to assess the contribution of genetic factors to the development of obsessional neurosis in identical twins.

FAMILY INFLUENCE

A more feasible but less direct and informative method of studying the possible influence of heredity is to examine the frequency and type of psychopathology in the close relatives of obsessional neurotics. More than in the twin studies, assessing the results of such investigations is fraught with difficulties, largely because of difference in sampling and diagnostic procedures and the absence of control data. Although several authors (Lewis, 1936; Brown, 1942; Rüdin, 1953; Müller, 1953;

B

Kringlen, 1965) refer to a raised incidence of neurotic personality traits and mental illness among first degree relatives of obsessional neurotics, it is difficult to know what is meant by this claim without further qualification. Only Brown (1942) provides data which allow comparisons between families of various neurotic groups and controls. Taking as his sample 63 cases of anxiety state, 21 cases of hysteria, 20 obsessionals and 31 medical in-patients controls, he investigated the nature and incidence of mental disorders in their parents and siblings aged over 15 years (Table 2.2a).

Compared with the controls, the parents of obsessional patients had a significantly higher incidence of obsessional neurosis (8 per cent), as did their siblings (7 per cent), of manic-depressive psychosis (8 per cent) and of anxious personality (33 per cent). The frequency of these conditions was also higher among first degree relatives of the obsessional patients than in those of patients with anxiety states and hysteria. However, the incidence of all mental disorders was no greater in the relatives of obsessionals (40 per cent) than in the relatives of anxiety state patients (43 per cent) and the overall incidence of neurosis was smaller in the relatives of obsessionals (10 per cent). Obsessional neurosis apart, only in respect of anxious personality did the relatives of obsessionals show an appreciably higher frequency (26 per cent) than those of the anxiety state (17 per cent) and hysteria groups (9 per cent), and this was largely accounted for by the almost twofold rate in their parents.

The only other available data which could be compared with Brown's are the findings on neurotic patients reported by Greer and Cawley (1966) (Table 2.2b), although these are based on a presumably more highly selected and severely ill in-patient sample from the Maudsley Hospital. Patients with obsessive–compulsive reaction had the highest incidence of family mental illness (not otherwise differentiated) – 53 per cent – but this was not significantly greater than patients with hysterical reactions who had the lowest incidence – 25 per cent – or of all non-obsessional patients – 36 per cent.

The remaining studies confine their observations to the relatives of obsessional patients. Investigating 547 first degree relatives of 144 in-patient cases of obsessional neurosis, Rosenberg (1967b) found that 51 (9·3 per cent) had received psychiatric treatment, mainly for anxiety and phobic states, depression and schizophrenia. Lewis (1936) reported the incidence of psychiatric disorders in the 100 parents and 206 siblings of 50 obsessional neurotics. His findings that 37 per cent of the parents and 21 per cent of the siblings had obsessional traits far exceeds the incidence of this category in any other study. Lo (1967) analysed in a similar manner data on Chinese patients attending the Hong Kong Mental Health Service. Accepting his use of broader criteria in defining obsessional neurosis and his reliance on relatives' reports on their

TABLE 2.2 *Incidence of mental disorder in first degree relatives of patients with certain neurotic states*

a) *Adapted from Brown (1942)*

Diagnosis in relatives	N's:	Obs. pts. P	S	Anx. St. pts P	S	Hyst. pts P	S	Controls P	S
		40	56	120	228	42	65	62	123
NEUROSES:									
obsessional		8	7	0	1	0	0	0	0
anxiety		0	5	21	10	10	5	0	0
hysterical		0	0	2	2	19	6	2	1
Total P + S		10		18		18		1	
PSYCHOSES:									
manic-depressive		8	2	6	1	0	0	0	0
schizophrenic		0	0	1	0	0	2	0	0
unspecified		0	0	1	0	0	0	2	0
Totals P + S		4		3		1		1	
ANXIOUS PERSON-ALITY		33	20	18	17	14	6	13	9
Total P + S		26		17		9		10	
PSYCHOPATHIC PER-SONALITY		0	0	2	4	10	0	2	1
Totals P + S		0		3		4		1	
ALCOHOLISM		0	0	2	1	7	0	2	0
Totals P + S		0		1		3		1	
All mental disorder		40		43		35		14	

b) *Greer and Cawley (1966)*

	N's:	P + S 19	P + S 44	P + S 16
All mental disorder		53	43	25

mental history, he found very different indices of mental disorder in first degree relatives. Despite the variety of cultural and methodological differences, he nevertheless felt it was difficult to explain the differences between his and Lewis's results.

Lo's finding that 9 per cent of parents of obsessional neurotics had pronounced obsessional traits is comparable with those reported by Rüdin (1953), Kringlen (1965) and Luxenburger (1930) – 5 per cent, 10 per cent and 11 per cent respectively. The incidence in the siblings was 5 per cent; Rüdin (1953) found it to be 2 per cent, and Luxenburger (1930), 14 per cent. Unequivocal data on the frequency of obsessional neurosis in relatives is even more meagre. It is perhaps surprising that in a sample with such a high level of obsessional traits, Lewis (1936) did not report any cases of obsessional neurosis in the relatives of his obsessional patients; possibly the obsessional trait figures might be thought to include a certain number of such cases if judged by different criteria. Neither did Kringlen (1965) mention any relatives suffering from obsessional neurosis as such, although his use of the term 'obsessive' makes it difficult to know whether this refers to personality or neurosis. The incidence in Rosenberg's study was 0·4 per cent. Appreciably raised rates of obsessional neurosis in parents and sibs have been reported only by Brown – 7·5 per cent and 7·1 per cent – and Rüdin (1953) – 4·6 per cent and 2·3 per cent.

Results of the two reports (Brown, 1942; Greer and Cawley, 1966) which allow the relevant comparisons to be made provide only tenuous support for the assertion that first degree relatives of obsessional neurotics have a high incidence of neurotic personality traits and mental illness, at least compared with the families of other neurotic sub-groups.

The evidence for an increased incidence of obsessional traits or symptoms in the families of obsessional neurotics would seem to be somewhat stronger but the significance of the observations is difficult to assess in the absence of agreed operational definitions and of control data. If the prevalence rate of obsessional neurosis in the general population is accepted as 0·05 per cent (Rüdin, 1953; Woodruff and Pitts, 1964) it is clear that the incidence of this condition in first degree relatives reported by Brown (1942), Rüdin (1953) and even Rosenberg (1967b) must be regarded as substantially raised. The key question, however, is whether this can be considered as evidence for a genetical predisposition to obsessional neurosis, bearing in mind that one can also interpret the findings in terms of behavioural patterns learned in a family setting. In the absence of studies of the offspring of obsessional parents reared apart from childhood by non-obsessional foster parents, it is not possible to distinguish between these alternative explanations. And to the extent that a case is otherwise made for a genetical contribution to obsessional neurosis, one would have to accept, on Brown's evidence, that the influence of hereditary factors is equally as strong as the case of patients with hysterical reaction and more than twice as marked for patients with anxiety states. Although both Brown (1942) and Rosenberg (1967b) considered that their findings did not support the existence of a specific obsessional predisposition, Slater (1964) disagreed with Brown's conclusion. Basing his opinion on the work of Luxenburger (1930), Lewis (1934), Brown (1942) and Rüdin (1953), Slater concluded that 'of all the neurotic syndromes, the evidence relating to genetical predisposition is best in the case of obsessional neurosis'. Whether or not one agrees with this particular conclusion, it is considered that the studies reviewed here do not provide sufficient evidence of a genetical contribution to obsessional neurosis.

SEX RATIO

The reported proportions of men to women suffering from obsessional disorders range from 8 per cent to 73 per cent. In addition to random variations of sampling, more specific factors probably account for these observed differences. For example, the relatively low proportion of women, 27 per cent, reported by Lo (1967) may be due to different referral patterns in a Chinese community. In Western series there is a tendency for the ratio of women to men to be even higher among out-patients than in-patients – 59 per cent and 54 per cent respectively in seven studies covering 751 patients. Exceptions to this trend suggest the influence of special factors – for instance the larger number of female beds available accounts for the higher proportion of women in the series reported by Ingram (1961b) – 62 per cent – and by Pollitt (1957; – 74 per cent. If one assumes no sex differences in predisposition, the more equal proportions among in-patients otherwise noted above may reflect the application of more careful diagnostic criteria to patients admitted to hospital. Ingram (1961a) noted that the larger the group the nearer does the sex ratio approach unity. A tabulation of eleven studies (Pollitt, 1957; Registrar-General, 1953; Rüdin, 1953; Müller, 1953a; Blacker and Gore, 1955; Ingram 1961b; Greer and Cawley, 1966; Lo, 1967; Kringlen, 1965; Ray, 1964; Noreik, 1970) shows a total of 651 men and 685 women, a ratio of 49 : 51. This finding confirms Ingram's view and justifies his conclusion that 'on the available evidence there is no reason to suppose that women are more disposed to obsessional disorders than men'.

SOCIAL CLASS

It is commonly thought that obsessional states are more frequently seen in upper- and middle-class patients. Evidence on the point is limited (Rüdin, 1953; Hollingshead and Redlich, 1958; Ingram, 1961b; Ray, 1964; Greer and Cawley, 1966) but tends to support this view. However, in the Chinese sample described by Lo (1967) only 23/88 were 'higher' social class, and Kringlen (1965) found no significant difference in this respect between obsessional and control patients. Because of variation or lack of data about sampling and controls, direct comparison and interpretation of these findings should be made with caution. Moreover, social class cannot be considered apart from factors such as intelligence and educational level which may themselves be related to manifestation of symptoms and case identification.

MARITAL STATUS

The few papers reporting the prevalence of marriage in obsessional patients agree that there is an unusually high celibacy rate of 40 per cent to 50 per cent. (Kringlen, 1965; Rüdin, 1953; Blacker and Gore, 1955; Ingram, 1961b). In the latter report significantly more obsessional patients (51 per cent) than anxiety neurotics (27 per cent) were single, and Blacker and Gore found that more obsessional men were single than in other neurotic disorders. Both these papers note a substantially higher celibacy rate in men, 68 per cent and 53 per cent respectively, compared with 40 per cent and 37 per cent for women – and in Ingram's group of 'nuclear' obsessional patients 9 of the 10 men were single, a finding which he takes to reflect 'the social incapacity caused by severe obsessional illness'. Although Kringlen found a relatively low male celibacy rate of 40 per cent (women 39 per cent), his observations were recorded at an unusually long follow-up averaging thirty years from the time of onset. His findings may thus reflect gradual improvement in some patients and a longer 'at-risk' period for marriage – factors which may differentially increase a man's likelihood of marrying if it is assumed that a woman's eligibility for marriage is more reduced by age than a man's. Nevertheless, even in the 35 patients who were married the marital relationship was regarded as bad or extremely bad in 25, within acceptable limits in 29 and good only in one case.

INTELLIGENCE

Kraepelin (1921) considered that obsessionals tend to be of high intelligence and Pollitt (1960) cites support for the general view that they 'are more likely to be found amongst more gifted, more intelligent and more energetic folk'. As with preceding characteristics, these conclusions are mostly based on clinical impressions. In the most recent paper (Noreik, 1970) intelligence was assessed clinically: 15 of 69 non-obsessional neurotics were 'assumed to be backward' and none of the 12 obsessional patients. In Lo (1967) assessment of intelligence was also made clinically and found to be significantly higher than in schizophrenic controls. Although Kringlen (1965) pointed out the paucity of systematic studies in this area, his own findings (statistically not significant) that obsessional and phobic patients seemed to be more intelligent and did better at school than other neurotics were again based on clinical assessment, and an admittedly unsatisfactory control group; similar methodological comments can be made of other work (Greenacre, 1923; Rüdin, 1953; Judd, 1965). Such criticism is not directed at the value of clinical judgment *per se* but to the unsatisfactory nature of such assessments in an area in which, more than in any other, objective standardized tests already exist. Nevertheless, these clinical assessments are supported by perhaps the two most reliable studies. Slater (1945) found that obsessional neurotics had higher scores on Raven's Matrices and Cattell's 2A and 2B tests of intelligence than anxiety neurotics and hysterics, with no difference between these two groups. These results were confirmed by Ingram (1961b), who reported that on both verbal and non-verbal tests, obsessional patients scored significantly more highly than anxiety neurotics and hysterics, again with no difference between the latter groups.

Lewis (1936) may have had in mind the need for a more rigorous methodological approach when he implicitly questioned the assumed relation between obsessional neurosis and intelligence: 'Critical appraisal of the obsession and recognition that it is absurd represents a defensive intellectual effort. . . . Perhaps it is emphasis on this criterion that has in the past led to the belief that intelligent people are more prone than stupid ones to obsessional neurosis.' Although the subsequent weight of evidence goes some way to resolving the matter, methodological shortcomings still permit such conclusions as, 'Intelligent people are likely to be more capable of thinking at the abstract level than unintelligent people, and abstract thinking predisposes to rumination and obsession' (Lo, 1967). Rather should we accept Ingram's (1961b) tentative conclusion: 'It is difficult to explain this consistent finding [of higher intelligence] in obsessional patients and to separate social class and intelligence, although the latter seems more important. Whether the link is a genetic one, or whether leisure or training and practice in abstract thinking predispose to rumination and obsession is uncertain.'

PRE-MORBID PERSONALITY

It is generally held that obsessional illness occurs more frequently in patients with particular personality traits which are often associated and constitute a characteristic obsessional personality. Janet (1903) gave an excellent description of this personality syndrome and sub-sequent writers have expanded it. The literature is extensive: in his monograph on the relation of personality to obsessional disorder Skoog (1959) details the evolution and complexity of these ideas which reflect the development of psychiatric and psychological concepts and theories more generally over the last hundred years.

The traits usually included are 'excessive cleanliness, orderliness, pedantry, conscientiousness, uncertainty, inconclusive ways of thinking and acting; perhaps also a fondness for collecting things, including money; sexual disturbances, though not of any characteristic sort, are common' (Lewis, 1938). Rigidity, inflexibility and lack of adaptability are stressed by Mayer-Gross et al. (1954), together with lack of internal security; they also point out the high ethical and social values that are placed on the corollaries of these traits, e.g. dependability, punctuality, precision, scrupulosity in matters of morals, capacity for self-effacement. Freud's (1908) formulation of the anal-erotic character, with its triad of orderliness, parsimony and obstinacy, has held an important position in psychoanalytic theory. Although it invokes particular aetiological assumptions Ingram (1961c), using a comparative matching technique, showed that descriptively it differed little from the above picture save in emphasis on the patients' adjustment and insight.

Considering the wealth of clinical detail in the literature, there are relatively few systematic studies of the obsessional patient's pre-morbid personality. Slater (1943) correlated personality traits and type of symptom in 400 neurotic patients and found the highest correlation (0·76) was between obsessional traits and symptoms. The majority of subsequent authors are concerned mainly to assess the extent of obsessional traits in obsessional patients before their onset of illness. These findings are summarized in Table 2.3a which shows that on average marked obsessional traits were reported in 31 per cent of 254 patients, moderate traits in 54 per cent of 166 patients, moderate to marked traits in 71 per cent of 383 patients, and no pre-morbid obsessional traits in 29 per cent of 451 obsessional patients.

The criteria for assessing obsessional personality traits in these papers vary widely and for this and other methodological reasons, direct comparisons are often not justified. Nevertheless the spread of

TABLE 2.3a *Incidence of obsessional personality traits in obsessional patients before illness*

Author	Marked n	Marked %	Moderate n	Moderate %	Moderate to marked n	Moderate to marked %	None n	None %	Total no. of patients
Lo (1967	41	47							88
Ingram (1961a)	24	31	41	53	65	84	12	16	77
Kringlen (1965)	15	17	49	55	64	72	25	28	89
Rüdin (1953)					78	72	31	28	109
Balslev-Olesen & Geert-Jørgensen (1959)					39	64	22	36	61
Rosenberg (1968c)					25	53			47
Pollitt (1960)							39	34	115
	80	31							254
Total n's and			90	54					166
mean percentages					271	71			383
							129	29	451

TABLE 2.3b *Incidence of obsessional personality traits in Kringlen's (1965) series of non-obsessional controls*

n	%	n	%	n	%	n	%	N
5	6	38	47	43	53	38	47	81

results does not seem greatly different from that expected from multiple sampling and the mean is perhaps not too inappropriate a parameter here.

The results in Table 2.3a also indicate that by no means all obsessional patients show obsessional traits before illness, their absence being noted in 16 per cent to 36 per cent of cases.

Other methods of personality description have also been used. Lewis (1957) refers to the study of Kaila (1949), who found that among 85 patients with obsessional neurosis there were remarkable differences in personality – 23 were schizothymes, 3 were cyclothymes in Kretsch-mer's typology, and the remaining 59 were rather nondescript. Skoog (1959) in an exhaustive controlled study of 285 anancastic patients, found a significantly higher proportion with marked asthenic (40 per cent vs. 19 per cent) and psycho-infantile (42 per cent vs. 18 per cent) pre-morbid personality features, but no significant difference in the incidence of marked hysteroid, syntonic and schizothymic attitudes. However, asthenic features were absent in 20 per cent and psycho-infantile features in 40 per cent of the anancastic patients. Rosenberg (1967c) confirmed the frequency of immature personality traits but found relatively more patients of schizoid type.

Skoog and others have documented the long-standing problem of whether or not there is a unitary relationship between personality and obsessional illness. In the context of this historical controversy Lewis (1936) postulated 'that to the "nuclear" group of chronic severe obsessionals . . . there correspond two types of personality, the one obstinate, morose, irritable, the other vacillating, uncertain of himself, submissive'. He later (1957) refers to the contrasting temperaments of Dr Johnson and Amiel to exemplify these two types of personality, the anancastic and the psychasthenic. In an attempt to validate this typology Ingram (1961a) rated the pre-morbid personality of 77 obsessional in-patients, on the basis of Lewis's (1938) list of obses-sional traits (see Table 2.3a) and attempted to fit the individual profiles to the personality types proposed by Lewis. Ingram found this pos-sible for 30/77 patients (39 per cent) but in the remaining 47 cases (61 per cent) the trait patterns were not applicable.

The positive findings so far reviewed – an average of 71 per cent of patients with pre-morbid obsessional personalities, and the high incidence of immature personality traits – must be balanced against the negative results – the absence of discernible obsessional traits in an average of 29 per cent of patients, the inconclusive findings of Kaila, and the doubts raised by some of Skoog's results and by Kringlen's control data (see Table 2.3b) about the specificity of the personality–illness relationship. Such considerations point up the paradox voiced by Lewis (1957): 'In no psychiatric condition is there a more obvious and specific association between illness and preceding personality than here, yet we meet people with severe obsessional symptoms whose previous personality revealed no hint of predisposition; and we meet people with pronounced unmistakeable anancastic personality who never become mentally ill, in that way or any other.' In discussing the relation between anal-erotic character and obsessional illness in 1936,

Lewis had already questioned two of the assumptions that may partly underlie the apparent paradox: 'But in any case it is not sufficient for the character-trait, in so far as it is not itself an obsessional symptom, to show a connexion with the neurosis that is essential and understandable in the light of a special theory; it is necessary that it shall be at least significantly more frequent in those who show obsessional neurosis than in others.'

In order to answer a question based on *a priori* data and to draw valid conclusions, certain requirements must be met. Essentially these comprise a testable hypothesis capable of refutation using an experimental design appropriate to the relevant statistical considerations. It is necessary to ensure at least an empirical definition and specification of the independent and dependent variables, a valid and reliable method of assessing them, and a satisfactory sampling of test and control populations.

Despite the enormous amount of time, effort and clinical acumen involved, it is unfortunate that these requirements are seldom met and it is therefore not surprising that the findings are so often conflicting, ambiguous or paradoxical. Without embarking on what would be a presumptuous critique, it may be salutory to illustrate two of the points raised. In the above quotations Lewis (1936) refers to the possible failure to differentiate and to define obsessional traits and obsessional symptoms – which are usually regarded as the independent and dependent variables. Whether they should be so depends on the hypothesis being tested, and this is seldom made explicit. Indeed the retrospective nature of the investigations precluded asking, even implicitly, whether people with obsessional traits are more likely to develop obsessional neurosis than other conditions, or whether they are more likely to develop it than people with other personalities. As Pollitt (1960) has pointed out, obsessional personality is also associated with a number of other psychiatric and psychosomatic conditions such as depressive illness (Lewis, 1934, 1936), anxiety states, the unreality syndrome (Shorvon, 1946), anorexia nervosa (Palmer and Jones, 1939), migraine (Elkington, 1946) and duodenal ulceration (Gainsborough and Slater, 1946). Retrospective inquiries of personality also rely heavily on the patient's self-assessment and this is only partly mitigated by obtaining information from relatives. Errors arising from this source may be further compounded in obsessional patients: often they do not come to medical attention until several years after the onset of the main illness and precursory symptoms may have started even five to ten years earlier than that – conditions which increase the risk of confounding early symptoms and traits. Skoog (1965) comments that obsessional patients remember the onset of symptoms with almost pathognomonic exactitude (indeed his findings here concerning the onset of anancastic conditions hinge on this assumption) but he admits that the retrospective method requires 'semantic alertness and critical evaluation of the patient's report'.

As a second example of the problems involved in interpreting some of the reported observations let us return to the last part of the above citation from Lewis's 1936 paper, which refers to the necessity for controls. In the absence of an appropriate comparison group the validity of any conclusion is very limited – and few of the studies listed in Table 2.3a are adequately controlled. Rather than pursue these, however, we can examine some effects of including a control group even though, in the opinion of the author concerned, it is not an entirely satisfactory one. The incidence of moderate to marked obsessional traits in Kringlen's (1965) patients – 72 per cent – is of the same order as in the other series listed. However, the clinical significance of this figure assumes a different perspective when it is seen that these features are also shown by 53 per cent of his non-obsessional control patients (see Table 2.3b). Although the difference is statistically significant it is evident that the personality–illness relationship here is less than specific and that personality can be no more than one factor associated with the development of obsessional illness. While the control data show on the one hand that the relationship is more attenuated than might otherwise be thought, on the other hand further analysis indicates that the relationship is nevertheless a consistent one. Kringlen reports only a significant overall chi-square for his data but partitioning of this value reveals that the proportions of obsessional and control patients showing marked, moderate and no obsessional traits each differ significantly. Provision of a control group thus enables the findings to be interpreted meaningfully but sets limits on what can justifiably be inferred from them.

COURSE OF THE ILLNESS

Precursory symptoms

Defining the onset of illness is an arbitrary process. Even accepting that obsessional patients can usually date the onset of their symptoms fairly accurately, this is not necessarily tantamount to the onset of the disease *per se* and in obsessional states, as in other conditions, precursory phenomena tend to blur the picture (Skoog, 1965). Whether or not neurotic symptoms in childhood should be considered as specifically precursory, they figure frequently in the anamnesis of obsessional patients (Rüdin, 1953; Pollitt, 1957; Ingram, 1961a; Kringlen, 1965, 1970; Lo, 1967). Of course mild phobic and ritual behaviour is shown by most children at some stage of their development and to that extent is to be regarded as normal. Berman (1942) considered that of 62 children showing obsessional phenomena in the broadest sense, only 4 were suffering from a true obsessional neurosis. The value of a comparison group is nicely demonstrated in the study by Greenacre (1923, cited by Ingram, 1961b): 64 of 86 obsessional patients had a history of ritual behaviour before puberty – and so did 29 of 30 normal controls. Kringlen (1965) also found most of the patients in both his groups were nervous as children – 83 per cent of the obsessional and 72 per cent of the controls. More neurotic but not necessarily specific precursory symptoms were noted during puberty or early adolescence in 35 per cent of obsessional patients by Rüdin (1953) and in 33 per cent by Lo (1967). Ingram (1961b) found similarly 36 per cent of his obsessional patients to have had neurotic symptoms before the age of fourteen and only 18·5 per cent in the control group of hysteria and anxiety neurotics. However if the 22 obsessional and 4 control patients who had phobias and rituals during this period are excluded, the proportions showing other neurotic symptoms fall to 11 per cent and 17 per cent respectively. Kringlen (1965) points out that the initial picture frequently includes symptoms other than obsessional or phobic ones: pain in the head, chest and abdomen, and hypochondriacal and neurasthenic symptoms are not infrequent – more than a quarter of his patients also had anxiety, and about a fifth, depressive symptoms. Skoog (1965) agrees: 'in many anancastic states specific precursory symptoms – perseverative, depressive, anxious – are common'. Perseverative prodromal states had also been noted previously (Janet, 1903; Friedmann, 1914; Kretschmer, 1950), as had affective ones (Janet, 1903).

Age of onset

On average, the first symptoms of obsessional illness appear in the early twenties – Lo (1967) found the mean age of onset to be 23·1 years, and Ingram (1961b) 24·7 years (compared with 32·3 years for hysteria and 32·2 years for anxiety states); the mean age in Pollitt's (1957) series was rather earlier, with virtually no difference between men – 20·2 years – and women – 21·6 years. However, the age distribution, shown in

Figure 2.1, is skewed: the highest incidence of first symptoms occurs between the ages of 10 and 15 years, by which time the illness has started in nearly a third of cases; by the age of 25 over half of the patients have symptoms and by 30 nearly three-quarters.

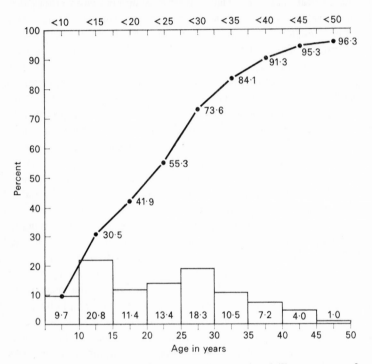

Fig. 2.1 Age of onset of first symptoms in obsessional illness, expressed as percentage distribution and cumulative frequencies. ($N = 357–667$)[1]

Precipitating factors

Defining and identifying precipitating factors depend on the particular criteria used. Taking 'definite evidence of adverse change in the physical state or environment of the patient within six weeks of onset of key illness' as their yardstick, Greer and Cawley (1966) reported precipitating factors in 30 per cent of 23 patients with obsessive–compulsive reactions, compared with 55 per cent of 162 patients with other neurotic illnesses. Defined as events considered significant within six months of

[1] Data based on cumulative figures from Rüdin (1953), Pollitt (1960), Ingram (1961b), Ray (1964), Kringlen (1965), Skoog (1965), Lo (1967), Noreik (1970). Percentage distribution frequencies calculated from cumulative percentages.

onset, Lo (1967) noted precipitants in 56 per cent of 88 patients, while Ingram (1961b), extending this period to a year, found them in 69 per cent of 89 cases. The incidence in Ingram's controls was 46 per cent. Rüdin (1953) considered precipitating factors to be significant in 58 per cent of 130 cases, Pollitt (1957) in 66 per cent of 141 cases, and Kringlen (1965) in 59 per cent of 91 cases.

The kinds of precipitants considered to be important varies from author to author and there is little overall consistency. Müller (1953) and Pollitt (1957) agree that sexual and marital difficulties are most frequent and the preponderance of sexual factors in Pollitt's obsessionals, 30 per cent of all precipitating factors in this group, was significantly greater than that in his controls – 3 per cent. Ingram (1961b) however found the incidence of sexual or marital precipitants in his obsessional and control patients to be little different – 19 per cent and 23 per cent. Pregnancy and delivery, on the other hand, were the most frequent in Ingram's study, occurring in 24 per cent of his cases and 10 per cent of the controls; the incidence was particularly high in the 19 married women, 9 of whose obsessional illnesses were precipitated by these factors. Nevertheless, in Pollitt's patients, pregnancy and delivery were only modestly represented, in 11 per cent of obsessionals and 10 per cent of controls, and were also found to be unimportant factors by Lo (1967) and Balslev-Olesen and Geert-Jørgensen (1959). Müller (1953) and Pollitt (1957) noted that illness or death of a near relative often seemed to provoke the onset of obsessional illness. Pollitt found these to account for 15 per cent of all precipitating factors in the obsessional patients, compared with 2 per cent in controls. Ingram (1961b) observed a similar incidence, 18 per cent, but in his study this was matched by 25 per cent of controls. The most frequent precipitants in Lo's (1967) series were frustrations and overwork; these constituted 32 per cent of all precipitating factors and might be thought to represent the particular cultural and socio-economic stresses to which many Chinese in Hong Kong are exposed.

Mode of onset

Although naturally occurring variations in the course of the illness are to be expected, the use of differing criteria to define the onset may explain some of the reported differences in the early clinical picture. Skoog (1965) found 47 per cent of his 251 anancastic patients had an acute onset (compared with 11 per cent of controls); in 62 per cent of these the acute symptoms had been preceded by slowly developing ones.

Obsessional States

Müller (1953) found the majority of his patients had an insidious onset and Pollitt (1969) agreed that many patients have a continuous train of symptoms starting from childhood, but pointed out that others have episodes which resolve completely before the onset of the main illness. 50 of his 150 patients, however, had no such episodes beforehand (Pollitt, 1957) but very few recalled a sudden onset (Pollitt, 1960). Ray (1964) noted previous attacks in 20 per cent of his obsessionals. Kringlen (1970) concluded that the initial course is usually episodic. In some cases there is complete disappearance of symptoms but later there are fewer remissions and improvements.

Four types of initial course were recognized by Ingram (1961b): constant, with progressive worsening; constant and static; fluctuating but

TABLE 2.4 *Percentage distribution of cases according to initial course of illness, as classified by Ingram (1961b)*

Type of course	N's:	Ingram (1961b) 89	Ray (1964) 42	Lo (1967) 88
Constant { Worsening		39	33	
Constant {		54	61	58
Constant { Static		15	28	
Fluctuating		33	24	31
Phasic		13	14	11

never completely symptom-free; and phasic, with one or more remissions. These categories were also used by Ray (1964) and Lo (1967): as can be seen from Table 2.4 the distribution of cases in these English, Indian and Chinese samples is strikingly similar. The proportion of patients running a phasic course agrees with Rüdin's (1953) finding of less than 15 per cent in this category. Ingram's figures refer to all his obsessional patients; of the 37 suffering from nuclear obsessional neurosis, 8 per cent showed a phasic course, compared with 17 per cent of the remainder. Although he suggests that 'the more typical and severe the symptoms, the less phasic the course', the proportions in his sample do not differ significantly.

A hundred patients in Pollitt's (1957) series reported previous episodes: 82 had sought medical advice at the time and were known to have suffered 162 attacks of obsessional illness before the onset of the main illness. Twenty-eight per cent of these attacks occurred between the ages of 11, and 15, 23 per cent between 16 and 20, and 17 per cent between 21 and 25. In most cases the attacks lasted less than a year: 27 per cent were over within three months, 46 per cent within six months and 79 per cent within twelve months.

The main illness, defined as the unremitting train of obsessional symptoms for which the patient ultimately seeks psychiatric advice (Pollitt, 1957; Lo, 1967), usually manifests itself in the mid-twenties but psychiatric contact may not be made until many years later. Half of Pollitt's patients began their main illness between 16 and 30, the mean age being 28 years; half of all patients made psychiatric contact within two years of onset of the main illness but almost a quarter were only seen after ten years of suffering; the average duration between onset and attending was 7·5 years. In Lo's series the mean age of onset of main illness is almost identical, 29 years, as is the distribution of age groups. The proportion seen within a year of onset is not dissimilar – 38 per cent (Pollitt – 31 per cent) – although only one in 20 patients delayed seeking advice for ten years or more. Pollitt's and Lo's series include in-patients and out-patients. The average age of patients admitted to hospital was 33 years (Blacker and Gore, 1955), comparable to the 34 years for men and 36 years for women reported by Kringlen (1965). In Ingram's (1961b) study the mean age was 36 years, somewhat younger than for his patients with hysteria – 39 years – and anxiety neurosis – 41 years. However, 54 per cent of the obsessionals were not admitted until five years after the onset of illness, compared with 37 per cent of the anxiety neurotics and 32 per cent of the hysterics.

In summary, the evidence suggests that of patients who are developing an obsessional illness, about a third will give a history of neurotic symptoms in puberty or early adolescence, but this incidence may be no higher than in patients who develop other neurotic illnesses; persistent phobic, ritual or perseverative features are perhaps the only precursory ones more specific to obsessional disorder. The illness most often begins between the ages of 10 and 15 years and by the age of 25 it has started in over half the cases; only one person in twenty becomes ill for the first time after the age of 40. Significant changes in the life events are associated with the onset of illness in a third to two-thirds of cases but again these frequencies may be no different from those found in other neurotic conditions. The type of precipitating factors most commonly described are sexual and marital difficulties, pregnancy and delivery, and illness or death of a near relative, but there is little agreement on the absolute or relative importance of these. In most patients the initial illness follows a slowly progressive course, sometimes punctuated by exacerbations; in others the onset is acute and continuous, or presents with discrete phasic attacks. The main illness – persisting symptoms eventually leading the patient to seek psychiatric help – usually develops in the mid-twenties, with a mean age of 28 years. About half the patients will not come to psychiatric attention for two years or more and in an appreciable minority of cases this delay may be more than ten years. If admission to hospital becomes necessary this tends to occur in the mid-thirties.

Development of the illness

Seen retrospectively during the course of follow-up, obsessional disorders present various patterns of development. In an unusually long follow-up – a mean of 30 years after onset and 17 years after first admission to hospital – Kringlen (1965) found on personal examination of 91 patients that 31 per cent were unchanged throughout; a further 27 per cent showed no change for some years, then gradually improved, while another 6 per cent made a continuous improvement; 28 per cent ran a fluctuating course, with or without periods of complete remission; and 8 per cent showed continued worsening.

Some of these variations in the pattern and severity of symptoms may be due to influence of intercurrent factors. Improvement may occur when tension is reduced or when the patient has to deal with new external difficulties (Pollitt, 1957). The beneficial effects of religion were pointed out by Müller (1953); these are not confined to Western patients: in a study carried out in New Delhi, Ray (1964) found that in patients with strong religious tendencies, dramatic improvement followed pilgrimages involving the performance of some expiatory rites. The disappearance or reduction of symptoms during a patient's war service, only to return afterwards, has been noted by writers from Janet (1903, 1925) onwards, an improvement attributed by Lewis (1936) to the routine and lack of responsibility. Perhaps for similar reasons, remission of phobic symptoms was seen among patients in concentration camps (Kral, 1952). Aggravation of symptoms may follow increased responsibility, fatigue, recurrence of situations originally precipitating the illness, and any circumstances which increase tension (Pollitt, 1969).

Some authors have examined whether the tendency to improve begins at any particular time, and whether the outcome as observed may reflect the duration of observation. Compared with patients followed up over four to five years, the improvement rate in those followed up under four to five years was higher in two studies (Ingram, 1961b; Grimshaw, 1965) and lower in another two (Lo, 1967; Kringlen, 1965).

Outcome

Assessment and comparison of patients' condition on follow-up is again confounded by the differences already mentioned – essentially those in sampling and assessment – to which is added here differences in length of follow-up. With the exception of leucotomy, no treatment has been shown to influence long-term outcome of obsessional illness, so fortunately, in this respect, the influence of different therapies can be discounted. Table 2·5 sets out the condition of patients at follow-up in sixteen studies, grouped according to whether they are based on in-patient, out-patient, or mixed samples. Outcomes are graded mainly in terms of symptom change; more comprehensive ratings, based on symptom change and social adjustment, are used in four studies (Müller, 1953; Pollitt, 1957; Ingram, 1961b; Lo, 1967).

The average overall improvement rate of out-patients assessed one to fourteen years later is 60 per cent, that of mixed in-patients and out-patients is slightly lower, 57 per cent, and is lowest of all for in-patients, 46 per cent, the average length of follow-up in these two groups being appreciably longer. Since there is no evidence of a consistent relationship between outcome and length of follow-up, it is possible that the outcome of these three groups reflects differences in initial severity of illness.

Not only symptomatic change but level of social adaptation appears to parallel severity of illness. At follow-up, out-patients had maintained or recovered their former adjustment in 77 per cent of cases (Grimshaw, 1965), although 13 per cent of them were symptomatically unchanged or worse. However, Kringlen (1965) found nearly 40 per cent of in-patients were living without any normal contact with friends or relatives and less than 20 per cent led an apparently normal social life. Concerning employment, only 28 per cent had never shown any reduction in their ability to work because of symptoms; 65 per cent had been impaired to some extent and 7 per cent severely impaired at some time during the follow-up period. At the time of follow-up 50 per cent felt their work capacity was good while 19 per cent were severely disabled. Among out-patients samples, on the other hand, two-thirds of patients were working at follow-up (Ingram, 1961b; Ray, 1964). These findings lend support to Lewis's (1936) observations on the capacity of all but the most severely obsessional patients to continue work.

TABLE 2.5 Outcome in follow-up studies. (Includes only patients for whom information was available and who were alive and not leucotomized at time of follow-up)

Author	N	Years of follow-up	Condition at follow-up – numbers and (per cent)			
			Asymptomatic/Much improved	Improved	Slight/No change	Worse
OP ONLY						
Grimshaw (1965)	99	1–14	40 (40)	24 (24)	29 (29)	6 (6)
Luff et al. (1935)*	49	3	19 (39)	13 (27)		17 (34)
Ray (1964)	42	1→4	18 (43)			24 (57)
All	190	1–14		114 (60)	76 (40)	
OP + IP MIXED						
Rüdin (1953)	130	2–26	16 (12)	34 (26)	42 (32)	38 (29)
Lo (1967)	84	1–14	18 (21)	44 (52)	12 (14)	10 (12)
Balslev-Olesen et al. (1959)	52	0–8	3 (6)	30 (57)	17 (33)	2 (4)
Pollitt (1957)	65	0–15	16 (25)	24 (37)	8 (12)	17 (26)
Lewis (1936)	50	>5	23 (46)	10 (20)	17 (34)	
All	381	0–26	76 (20)	218 (57) / 142 (37)	79 (24) / 163 (43)	67 (20)
IP ONLY						
Kringlen (1965)	82	13–20	21 (25)		55 (68)	6 (7)
Ingram (1961b)	46	1–11	4 (9)	14 (30)	12 (26)	16 (35)
Greer & Cawley (1966)	21	4–6	3 (14)	5 (24)	5 (24)	8 (38)
Noreik (1970)	6	>5		2 (33)	4 (67)	0 (0)
Müller (1953a)	57	15–35	16 (28)	12 (21)	29 (51)	
Hastings (1958)*	23	6–12	3 (13)	9 (40)	11 (47)	
Langfeldt (1938)*	27	1–11	7 (26)	11 (41)	9 (33)	
Rennie (1953)*	47	20	17 (36)	18 (38)	12 (26)	
All	309	1–20	71 (23)	142 (46) / 69 (23)	167 (54)	30 (19)

* Results taken from Goodwin et al. (1969).

Prognostic indicators

There are relatively few studies which have tried to relate outcome to antecedent factors in the patient's history or clinical state, and few of the findings which have been reported are consistent.

Factors indicating a good prognosis

1. Pre-morbid personality. Müller (1953) considered that a normal previous personality was a favourable influence. An obsessional pre-morbid personality was found to be significantly associated with improvement by Lo (1967) while Pollitt (1957) noted a similar association among patients with moderate obsessional traits (in contrast to those who had either many or none). However, other evidence on this point is contradictory (Kringlen, 1965; Langfeldt, 1938), while Ingram (1961b) found no significant relation between obsessional personality and outcome.

2. Episodic course. Both Müller (1953) and Pollit (1969) regarded an episodic or phasic course as prognostically favourable; although such a course indicates that remissions are more likely, so are recurrences. No significant association was found by Ingram (1961b).

3. Precipitating factors were significantly related to improvement in one study (Lo, 1967) but not in another (Ingram, 1961b).

4. Atypical symptoms such as prominent anxiety and depression tend to favour improvement (Ingram, 1961b) and patients with predominant phobic and ruminative symptoms had a significantly better prognosis than those with a nuclear illness and (in contrast with Ingram's findings) those with marked affective features (Lo, 1967). However, Kringlen (1965) found that type of symptoms – predominantly obsessional, phobic, mixed or atypical – had no influence on outcome.

5. Duration of symptoms before key illness. Ingram (1961b) and Pollitt (1960) both found that patients who improved had significantly shorter illnesses before first being seen, the mean duration of symptoms in the symptom-free or improved and the unimproved cases being 3·7 years and 12·4 years, and 3·0 years and 8·1 years respectively. Similar trends had been noted earlier (Strauss, 1948; Gutheil, 1950) but were not found by Lo (1967). The association is an interesting one, having also been observed on long-term follow-up of neurotic in-patients (Noreik, 1970) and out-patients (Giel *et al.*, 1964).

Factors indicating a poor prognosis

Like Langfeldt (1938), Kringlen (1965) found obsessional pre-morbid personality to be significantly associated with a poor prognosis, as was a severe clinical picture on admission. Also associated with a poor prognosis but not to a statistically significant extent, was unmarried status and nervousness in childhood. Obsessional symptoms in childhood, however, were significantly related to poor outcome in Ingram's (1961b) series, as was the presence of obsessional motor symptoms. Like Strauss (1948), Ingram considered there was a possible association between early age of onset and poor prognosis, but further evidence is inconclusive.

Factors unrelated to prognosis

In addition to the qualifying reports already mentioned, consideration of the following factors has failed to reveal any significant association with prognosis: positive family history (Ingram, 1961b; Lo, 1967), childhood symptoms (Lo, 1967), sex and intelligence (Ingram, 1961b; Lo, 1967), unmarried status (Ingram, 1961b), acute versus insidious onset (Kringlen, 1965) and previous attacks (Pollitt, 1960).

It is perhaps not surprising that so many of these findings are inconsistent, especially because none of the studies concerned was planned as a prospective inquiry and it was therefore unlikely that systematic efforts were made to ensure the reliability of the data collected. Failure to demonstrate a relationship does not of course mean that such a relationship does not exist. Nevertheless in only a few instances is there statistically significant and uncontradicted support for a prognostic indicator – favourable for cases with phobic-ruminative symptoms, precipitating factors and short duration of symptoms before the main illness, and unfavourable for those with childhood symptoms, a severe clinical state on admission, and with motor symptoms.

COMPLICATIONS

The term complication refers to new symptoms apparently related to but not part of the original clinical picture. According to Rosenberg's (1968b) criteria, the symptoms should be of sufficient severity to warrant a) a second diagnosis and/or b) treatment in their own right. Depression is probably the commonest major condition associated with obsessional illness – but then it is itself a common condition. Evidence for there being a specific relationship with depression and with schizophrenia is considered below.

Depression

A relationship with depression has often been claimed because of the frequency with which obsessional symptoms occur in depressive illness and depressive symptoms in obsessional illness; obsessional attacks may also sometimes occur periodically without external precipitation. As Lewis (1957) pointed out, the safest indication of an underlying identity is a greater frequency of one syndrome in families of patients showing the other syndrome than would occur by chance. In the earliest such study Brown (1942) reported the incidence of manic-depressive psychosis in the families of 20 obsessional neurotic patients to be 7·5 per cent in the parents and 1·8 per cent in the siblings, compared with 3·0 per cent of parents and 0·2 per cent of siblings of non-obsessional neurotics and controls; these differences are not statistically significant. More extensive data were provided by Rüdin (1953): in her series of 130 obsessional patients, manic-depressive psychosis was no more frequent in the sibs than in the average population; the incidence was higher in the parents, grandparents, aunts and uncles – possibly reflecting their greater period at risk compared with the siblings. The frequency of suicide was also somewhat greater in relatives than in the population at large. Lewis comments that one cannot use Rüdin's figures to argue a genetic factor common to both disorders since a) schizophrenia is also more common in relatives of obsessional patients than in the general population, and b) the raised percentage of manic-depressive illness – and schizophrenia – in relatives of obsessionals is still lower than the percentage of such affected relatives in families of manic-depressive and schizophrenic patients. In a recent investigation of a Japanese population, Sakai (1967) found 10·8 per cent of 65 obsessional patients had at least one member of their families affected by depression whereas only 5·6 per cent of non-obsessional neurotic patients had a relative so affected; the proportions do not differ significantly. Although these three familial studies are suggestive of a link, none conclusively supports the notion of a specific association between obsessional and depressive illness.

An alternative, though less satisfactory method of seeing if a connection exists is to ascertain whether patients with obsessional neurosis are more likely to become depressed than patients with non-obsessional neurotic disorders. Rosenberg (1968b) compared the frequency of depression supervening within ten years of the onset of illness in 144 obsessional and 144 anxiety neurotics: 49 (34·0 per cent) obsessionals and 37 (25·7 per cent) anxiety neurotics had received treatment for moderately severe depressive illness. Neither these nor the proportions of each group attempting or committing suicide are significantly different.

Because depression itself is so much more common, the relationship with obsessions is more readily studied in cases of depressive illness. The largest and most systematic study was reported by Gittleson in a series of papers (1966a, b, c, d). He examined the case notes of 398 patients with depressive psychosis admitted to the Professorial Unit of the Maudsley Hospital over a four-year period and who met defined criteria. Fifty-two patients (13.1 per cent) had shown frank obsessions before the onset of depressive illness. Compared with the others, they were younger, more frequently showed depersonalization, delusions of cancer, blockage and poverty, and had made fewer suicidal attempts. Thirteen of them lost their obsessions during the depression. This is almost the same proportion (24.6 per cent) of patients with no pre-morbid obsessions who developed obsessions while depressed. In all, 124 patients (31.2 per cent) showed obsessional symptoms during depression and in 51 per cent of these the content was suicidal, homicidal, or both. The actual suicidal attempt rate of the obsessional neurotics (13·5 per cent) was under half that of the other depressives (29·8 per cent); and that of depressives with obsessions (5·7 per cent) was six and a half times less frequent than that of depressives without obsessions (37·6 per cent). The suicidal attempt rate was unrelated to whether or not suicidal/homicidal ideas formed the content of the obsessions. Among the 124 depressed patients with obsessions the incidence of pre-morbid obsessional personality was twice as great, and frank obsessions, ten times as great, as the depressed patients without obsessions. They were also more likely to show self-reproach, depersonalization and diurnal variation of symptoms. Transition of the obsession to a delusion occurred in 21 patients (5.3 per cent), a small but, as will be seen below, theoretically important group. Persistent worsening of the obsession after remission of the depression was found in 13.5 per cent of patients with, and 2·8 per cent of patients without pre-morbid obsessions.

Gittleson concluded that obsessions are common in the course of depressive psychosis and that they are based on the activation of pre-morbid traits. They appear to have a marked protective effect against suicidal attempts and this effect depends on the obsessions being phenomenologically an obsession. In the obsession–delusion transition group the suicidal attempt rate was 38·1 per cent, similar to that of depressives without obsessions (37·6 per cent). Conversely the low rate

5·1 per cent, in the obsessional neurotics who retained obsessional symptoms while depressed was similar to the 5·9 per cent of depressives who first showed obsessions during their depression. The pre-existing obsessional neurosis itself seemed responsible for the younger age of onset of depression and the greater incidence of obsessions in the depression. On the other hand the greater incidence of depersonalization and the lower rate of suicide in the depressed obsessional neurotic was due to their having obsessions in their depression three times as often as other depressives, and not to the existence of the obsessional neurosis *per se*.

Finally one should mention a rare group of patients with recurrent endogenous obsessional neurosis. Mayer-Gross *et al.* (1960) comment that although any depression 'may appear entirely secondary . . . nevertheless these illnesses remit and relapse in much the same way as cyclothymic illnesses, may show just as much regularity of timing, and are probably to be included, from the aetiological point of view, in the manic-depressive disorders'. Although this may be a necessary basis, it does not at present seem a sufficient one for so classifying them. If it were, by the same token one would also have to include in the manic-depressive disorders a variety of other periodic illnesses.

Schizophrenia

There is little doubt that an obsessional condition can change into a psychotic one. As mentioned above, Gittleson found an obsessional-delusional transition in 5·3 per cent of his obsessional series. However, such delusional or psychotic syndromes are not necessarily schizophrenic ones. The problem in classifying these cases demonstrates how ill-defined our boundaries may be (Anderson, 1971) and Lewis (1957) and Roth (1959) suggest that they are more appropriately regarded as examples of a mixed psychosis. As Lewis (1936) commented: 'The surprising thing is not that some obsessionals become schizophrenic, but that only a few do so. It must be a very short step, one might suppose, from feeling that one must struggle against thoughts that are not one's own, to believing that they are forced upon one by an external agency. The actual projection, however, is rarely made . . .' Views on whether there is a specific relationship are conflicting. Some, including Kraepelin, deny any intrinsic connection. The majority, led by Bleuler, consider obsessional neurosis as a mutant variant or prodrome of schizophrenia. What evidence is there on the matter ?

As part of his study mentioned earlier, Sakai (1967) investigated the incidence of schizophrenia in first and second degree relatives of 65 obsessive–compulsive patients. The sample excluded patients who later turned out to be schizophrenic. The calculated morbidity risk of schizophrenia among sibs and parents, 1·0 per cent and 1·7 per cent respectively, was slightly higher than that of the Japanese general population – 0·7 per cent. It was exceeded among sibs and parents of cases of hypochondriasis – 1·4 per cent and 0·9 per cent, anxiety reactions – 4·1 per cent and 2·3 per cent, depersonalization – 4·9 per cent and 0·0 per cent and oversensitivity – 5·7 per cent and 9·3 per cent (Mitsuda *et al.*, 1967). In order to examine possible effects of heterogeneity, Sakai divided his obsessional patients into a simple group and a complicated one – in which the condition was associated with symptoms such as depersonalization, anxiety and hypersensitivity. Three and a half times as many patients in the complicated group (37·9 per cent) had at least one first or second degree relative affected by schizophrenia as did patients with a simple obsessional illness (11·1 per cent) (p < 0·01). Sakai considered his results supported the view that obsessive–compulsive neurosis was not uniform, either clinically or genetically, and that it consists not only of a neurosis as a normal variation based on the polygene but in some cases as a pathological variant founded on major genes responsible for other conditions, including schizophrenia. The differences between the simple and complicated groups are of considerable significance, both statistically and theoretically. However, it is a pity that the differences in morbidity risks of schizophrenia among relatives of all the various diagnostic groups of patients was not more critically assessed. As it is, one wonders if the risk in sibs and parents of obsessional patients is significantly greater than one would expect by chance; and certainly by comparison with the risk of relatives of oversensitive patients and those with anxiety reactions and depersonalization the risk appears to be modest and far from specific. This conclusion is in keeping with the results of Brown's (1942) investigation of the incidence of psychoses in parents and sibs of 20 obsessional patients and 115 other psychoneurotic patients and controls. No case of schizophrenia was found in relatives of the obsessionals; the incidence in the families of the anxiety neurotics was 0·6 per cent and of the hysterics 0·9 per cent.

The development of schizophrenia in obsessional patients is reported in a number of follow-up studies (Table 2.6.).

In a majority of studies the incidence is no higher than about 3 per cent. As emphasized earlier, consideration of these findings raises problems of sampling and comparability. Much of the uncertainty hinges on differences of diagnostic criteria, either of the initial diagnosis (Ingram, 1961b; Kringlen, 1965; Rosenberg, 1968b) or that of the subsequent psychosis (Müller, 1953; Rüdin, 1953; Bratfos, 1970).

In Ingram's series the only 4 cases of schizophrenia in non-leuco-tomized patients were found in the 15 obsessionals (not included in Table 2.6) who were initially classified in the doubtful schizophrenic group. On retrospective assessment of their samples, the initial diag-nosis was considered to be schizophrenia in 3 cases by Kringlen, and in 4 cases by Rosenberg. In 6 other cases of Rosenberg's the patients

TABLE 2.6 *Subsequent incidence of schizophrenia in patients with obsessional neurosis*

	Years of follow-up	N	Incidence of schizophrenia n	%
OP ONLY				
Ray (1964)	1–4	42	1	2·4
OP AND IP MIXED				
Lo (1967)	1–14	88	2	2·3
Pollitt (1957)	0–15	67	1	1·5
Rüdin (1953)	2–26	130	13	10·0
IP ONLY				
Müller (1953b)	15–34	57	7	12·3
Kringlen (1965)	13–20	91	3	3·3
Bratfos (1970)	12–22	126	0	0·0
Ingram (1961b)	1–11	49	0	0·0
Rosenberg (1968b)	1–28	144	0	0·0

showed periods of apparent loss of resistance and insight but neverthe-less were not regarded as psychotic. Such a diagnostic difficulty appears to arise in patients with a schizoid pre-morbid personality (Skoog, 1959). No cases of schizophrenia at all were found on a lengthy follow-up (mean 16·8 years) by Bratfos but 8 patients (6.3 per cent) developed reactive psychoses. Cases were identified by the Central Register for Psychoses which records all such admissions in Norway. In reactive psychosis the underlying cause is considered to be an interplay between personality and environment; the symptomatic picture is usually marked by depression or paranoid–hallucinatory experiences and prognosis is good. However, it should be noted that the initial diagnosis of reactive psychosis is not infrequently changed on later admissions to schizo-phrenia or manic-depressive psychosis (Ödegård, 1966) and when alternative diagnoses of psychosis were present, Bratfos used the first one. Moreover, as Bratfos mentions, not all cases of psychosis, even initially, are admitted to hospital. For both these reasons the absence of schizophrenia reported here may not represent the actual incidence.

Rosenberg and Bratfos also report the incidence of subsequent schizophrenia in other neurotic groups. Together with his 144 obsessionals, Rosenberg followed up 144 cases of anxiety neurosis: one such patient was found to be schizophrenic. Accepting the above limitations which are equally applicable here, Bratfos reported the incidence of schizophrenia in 321 anxiety neurotics to be 1·3 per cent, and of reactive psychosis, 3·1 per cent; in other types of neurosis the incidence of schizophrenia ranged from 1·2 per cent to 2·3 per cent, and of reactive psychosis, from 3·6 per cent to 5·8 per cent; these variations are not significant.

The third type of evidence concerning a relationship, comes from retrospective studies of obsessional phenomena in schizophrenic patients (Jahrreis, 1926; Stengel, 1945; Müller, 1953). In a review of all 848 schizophrenic patients admitted to the Bethlem Royal and Maudsley Hospitals over a four-year period, Rosen (1957) found 30 (3·5 per cent) in whom obsessional symptoms had been noted at some time. In every case, obsessional symptoms had preceded or accompanied the emergence of schizophrenic ones; in none had they begun after schizophrenic symptoms had appeared. In 23 patients the obsessions continued largely unchanged in content and severity after the onset of schizophrenia; 6 showed a transition from obsessions to delusions. Depressive and paranoid symptoms predominated in most cases, a prevalence to which Stengel (1945) had drawn attention. Stengel also observed that obsessive–compulsive symptoms tended to prevent or retard disintegration of personality in schizophrenia, and the longer their duration before the emergence of psychosis, the more benign the course. These findings were confirmed by Müller (1953) and by Rosen (1957), who also found that patients with the more elaborated and varied obsessional symptoms had the less severe schizophrenic illnesses.

A variety of relationships between obsessional illness and schizophrenia have been postulated (Mayer-Gross, 1932; Stengel, 1945, 1948; Rosen, 1957; Lo, 1967). Several studies (Stengel, 1948; Müller, 1953; Rosen, 1957) confirm the apparent inhibitory influence of obsessional symptoms on the severity of a subsequent schizophrenic illness. The predominance of depressive and paranoid symptomatology in such cases has also been noted. Taken together, the observations tend to support the view that in at least some of these cases one is dealing with a mixed or reactive psychosis rather than schizophrenia.

Another interpretation relates to the good prognosis carried in schizophrenia by marked affective features. The possible influence of these on the psychoses of obsessional patients has been discussed by Roth (1959), although he does not go as far as Maudsley (1895) who felt that obsessional illness was itself a latent affective psychosis. However, concerning the substantive question, on the basis of the reported risk of schizophrenia in obsessional patients and their families, one must conclude with Rüdin (1953), as Lewis (1957) did, that 'there is no close affinity between obsessional neurosis and schizophrenia or manic depressive psychosis'.

CHILDHOOD OBSESSIONAL DISORDER

The existence of normal compulsive and ritual behaviour in children is well documented (Piaget, 1954; Gesell, 1940) and the criteria by which one distinguishes this from symptoms of obsessive compulsive neurosis in childhood are similar to those in adults. As distinct from individual case reports and psychological interpretations, the amount of systematically collected information is scanty. Judd (1965) reviewed the literature and found much of it contradictory and inconclusive: diagnostic problems and paucity of validated cases are some obvious reasons. Of 3050 patients admitted to the Children's Service of Bellevue Hospital, 62 had been diagnosed as suffering from obsessive compulsive disorder, but closer scrutiny of these revealed only 6 true cases (Berman, 1942). Judd screened 405 children under the age of 12 who had been seen in Los Angeles as in-patients or out-patients; a diagnosis of obsessive compulsive disorder had been made in 34 cases but only 5 met strict diagnostic criteria, most of those excluded being schizophrenic. Even among the slightly older patients in an adolescent unit, only about 10 per cent of one follow-up series showed a definite obsessive compulsive state although over half had become ill before the age of 10 (Warren, 1960). By the time obsessional patients are seen as adults, the proportion of cases whose illnesses began in their first decade was only 5 per cent (Pollitt, 1956). The average age of onset in Judd's study was 7·5 years, somewhat younger than previously reported. All five children showed high intelligence, an initially rigid moral code and sudden onset of illness; they had an active fantasy life, and persistent guilt about their thoughts and actions. Four were excessively ambivalent and aggressive to their parents and there was a family history of psychopathy, often with marked obsessional features, characteristics also found in previous studies. Judd was unable to confirm the reported difficulties in toilet training, and the sudden onset was an unusual finding.

Results on follow-up were reported by Berman after three to five years, and by Warren after seven years. Berman found that 2 children showed early signs of schizophrenia, 1 had persistent obsessions, and 3 were mildly disturbed but symptom free. Of Warren's 15 adolescents, 1 had been leucotomized and 4 were severely handicapped by obsessional symptoms; only 2 were regarded as quite normal. In the light of what is known from retrospective studies about the episodic nature of many obsessional illnesses it is difficult to evaluate the significance of these findings, but considering that among Pollitt's (1957) 150 patients, 22 per cent had had obsessional symptoms, as distinct from the present illness in adulthood, before the age of 10, Warren's results, based on the longer follow-up in older children, 11 of whom became ill under the age of 10, is not encouraging.

OBSESSIONAL DISORDERS IN OLD AGE

Perhaps surprisingly in view of possible connections between obsessional disorders and organic cerebral impairment (see Grimshaw, 1964), few elderly patients develop true obsessional symptoms in the setting of an organic psychosis. Benaim (1956) reviewed 46 patients over 60 with marked obsessional phenomena and found only 4 cases. The remaining patients fell into two groups:

1. Primarily obsessional illnesses that had mainly begun by early adult life, with features similar to those described earlier.
2. Primarily affective illnesses with obsessional symptoms in patients who only rarely had experienced such symptoms (as against personality traits) before middle age. Primary obsessional symptoms usually improved and secondary ones often disappeared after the depression had remitted.

According to Post (1965) obsessional symptoms, even strictly defined, are encountered quite frequently in the elderly. He confirmed Benaim's findings that most of these patients also show affective symptoms, adding that in his experience obsessional patients in late life do not come for psychiatric advice unless they are also depressed.

3
Peter G. Mellett
The clinical problem

DEFINITION

Obsessional patients feel reluctantly compelled to do and/or think certain things so frequently and repetitively that their happiness and efficiency are impaired. As most authors rightly emphasize, obsessional patients feel 'resistance' to their compulsive activity, which is recognized as, in some way, alien and seemingly beyond their control. They differ from phobic patients. While phobics have irrational fears, the fears are only evoked by the fear-producing situation (e.g. being out-of-doors, being near birds, etc.). The obsessional similarly says he 'fears' situations but additionally spends much time scanning his environment and monitoring his own thoughts seeking the very features which are alarming to him in his environment or thoughts. He may claim to 'fear' dirt and feel compelled to check his clothing for its absence, but he will go on *thinking of* and *looking* for dirt in the cleanest possible situation, when the bird-phobic patient will rest content in an ordinarily bird-free house.

The obsessional patient is therefore more often distressed and presents greater distress to his family, friends and doctor. He may become totally incapacitated at work and so unbearably disturbing to all around him, that hospital admission is sought. As there is no standard treatment for the condition, his situation may be improved only in that more and better-informed people share his distress in circumstances in which they need not themselves become overwhelmed.

A 'SALVAGE GROUP' AS AN OBSERVATION MILIEU

Such obsessional patients among those with other conditions were taken from time to time into an experimental in-patient 'salvage' group in a mental hospital. It was intended in the group to study and try to help patients who were suffering from chronic neurotic illnesses, which had necessitated long-term admission and where conventional treatments had failed. They were to be given any treatment or combination of treatments, which might appear potentially valuable.

The group of seven or eight patients of either sex was 'open', in that it could be left or joined by individuals at any time agreed by the doctor in charge. It was based upon both short-stay wards and a long-term rehabilitation ward for both sexes. A small room in one or other ward was available for meetings and activities. Otherwise no special facilities were reserved for the group. The doctor had other responsibilities in the wards and in other parts of the hospital. In spite of various changes of staff and ward arrangements, the special group continued, with appropriate modifications and gradual changes of patient membership, for three years. No patient remained in it for more than fifteen months.

Lack of planned special facilities was no handicap in a hospital itself liberally and realistically conceived as an arena, in which patients might encounter all manner of treatments and approaches, some of which might be appropriate for them (Freudenberg, 1966). The philosophy behind the activities of the staff serving the group was that of a guerilla force rather than a regular army with an 'establishment' of numbers, a circumscribed field of activity and a restrictive hierarchical communication and command system. With this agreeably ill-defined background and much good-will, the staff strength during the period here studied amounted most of the time to:

  1 psychiatrist with special interest in psychotherapy and behaviour
    therapy – half-time. (Occasional assistance from other doctors.)
  1 occupational therapist – approx. half-time.
  1 occupational therapy helper – approx. half-time.
  1 physiotherapist – for two half-hour relaxation sessions weekly.
  1 potter, who took special interest in patients from the group.

These workers met weekly as a staff-group for one hour to pool information, plan treatment strategies and share difficulties. Meanwhile, the ward nursing staffs gave all possible help, short of that which might have been interpreted as favouritism by ward patients, who were not members of the group. From time to time other wards and occupational therapy departments were used for brief periods (e.g. close observation of a patient in bed or in a work situation), and their staffs, perhaps inspired by the novel situation and the enthusiastic interest of the group staff, readily assisted with observations and the application of schedules of activity.

Occasionally, when the staff members were away carrying out special treatments (e.g. behaviour therapy in the field), patient members of the group monitored the behaviour of each other. Usually the group staff or experienced nurses kept observations according to a twenty-four-hour rota. Round-the-clock observation of all patients was thus made possible and detailed records kept. The freedom of the staff to use any hospital facilities and invent others allowed for multiple 'interventions' and the observation of patients' reactions to them.

Every patient, on entering the group, was interviewed by the psychiatrist on several occasions in a semi-structured way. A formal history was thus built up, though patients were free to present material in their own way, to pursue side-issues or digress into immediately current matters. Meanwhile the group met regularly for two one-hour periods per week of psychotherapy, in which interpretation of behaviour, mutual support and freedom for catharsis of anger etc. appeared important. The rest of the time was spent in ordinary activities (e.g. shopping, going out to tea), occupational or behaviour therapy.

Spouses and parents of patients were seen by the psychiatrist separately, minimally on one or two occasions each and in a one-hour weekly evening 'relations group' intended to enable them to share and discuss difficulties. Notes were made relating to their own personalities and reactions and their own observations regarding the patients.

The special 'salvage' group therefore allowed for thorough observation of the characteristics of all its members in changing situations.

VALUE OF OBSERVATIONS

From the start it was realized that observations on very small numbers of patients could not be the basis of all-embracing conclusions. Nevertheless, medical ignorance as to the cause and treatment of obsessional neurosis was such that a return to direct examination of histories and detailed observation of a few patients seemed desirable as a basis for speculation and the planning of wider studies.

OBSERVATIONS ON INDIVIDUAL PATIENTS

(The descriptions of individual patients have been altered sufficiently to preserve their anonymity, but not in such a way as to facilitate any new explanatory concepts or to hamper the formulation of psychodynamic or other explanatory concepts.)

c

Four patients treated in the salvage group and followed up for periods of five to eight years are described below in detail.

Rose Newcombe

Rose Newcombe was a 32-year-old housewife, formerly a calculating-machine operator and copy-typist. Since the birth of her third child three years previously she had had recurrent thoughts that, through her negligence, safety-pins might be lost in her baby's vagina, that she might drop a duster into a lavatory pan and use it, thus smearing furniture, that she might touch the genitals of men who were strangers, that she might say 'VD' in ordinary conversation and that she might push children in perambulators in front of traffic. Her anxiety had become such that she would telephone her husband, a stockbroker, to come home from his work twenty miles away or even drag at his coat begging him to stay at home, when he was about to go to work. She regarded herself as depressed on account of her fears, which limited her life and made her much-loved husband unhappy. Unless questioned, however, she rarely complained of depression. All her spontaneous talk and innumerable notes, check lists, etc., written for herself and her husband, nurses and doctor, related to her search for reassurance that she had not allowed the things, of which she recurrently thought, to happen. She longed to go back 'before all this started' – i.e. before the end of her third pregnancy, through which she had felt very happy. She often seemed to picture her fears and compulsions as due to some 'outside force' which was not part of her normal personality; this was not truly an 'idea of influence'.

The patient's mother had been quarrelsome, untruthful and emotionally unstable. Sometimes she had been considerate and sometimes enraged over trivial matters. She had been excessively fussy over cleanliness and tidiness, shutting doors to the family once a room was clean. She had never been known to make anything – even a simple article of clothing. She had spent a great deal of time polishing her rings, of which she had several, and cleaning her teeth. She never actually wore any ring apart from her wedding ring.

The patient's father had been a coach-builder and died of stomach cancer three years before the birth of the third child. Usually placid and kind, he had been enraged occasionally to the point of physical violence by the mother's tantrums. The patient, who hated rows, had sometimes as a child pulled her parents apart.

Rose had been born and brought up in a small cottage in Tunbridge

Wells. Her first memory (when aged about 4) was of being invited to use a chamber pot, while at the home of a neighbour, while her mother was out. For some reason the neighbour became angry with her, when she used it, and she recalled saying 'You said I could'.

This memory evoked another memory in the same interview. She had been working in an office several years previously. She had thought of passing urine, then wondered whether the content of a lavatory pan was in the teapot on the office desk. (This preceded the present illness by several years). In the interview she went on to say that she was frightened lest she had 'lifted her skirt and forgotten herself' in the ward kitchen. She was worried lest she had messed up lavatories in the hospital and forgotten that she had been in them. She recalled seeing a biro pen during the last group meeting and thinking of a man. 'I am so ashamed', she said. This had been followed by the thought, while washing-up in the kitchen, that she must not go into the larder or the broom cupboard. The last point had worried her at home. It had occurred to her that she should try to stop these recurrent worries by knitting but she had checked her notebook of the day's activities and got involved again, worrying if she had made a mess anywhere. She had only been helped by concentrating on typing in the occupational therapy department as she 'knew she must not make a mistake'.

She was able to recall another disturbing early memory of her mother pushing her away in her push-chair on the promenade at the seaside and allowing it to run for several yards before catching it up again. She had felt 'lost and angry'.

She recalled a row between her parents, when she was aged about 4, at the end of which her mother had taken something from a drawer and thrown it in the fire. She associated this with going to a chemist's shop a few days later with her mother, who bought something, the assistant asking the mother whether the patient was a very knowing little girl. She had some notion at the time that there was something secret and exciting going on. In adult life she had realized the object was a 'Dutch cap' contraceptive.

Another memory (when she was aged about 6) was of going to a library with her mother, who obtained a book for each of them. She was unable to read properly but sat at home running her finger along the lines as if reading; it was a bore and she continually looked up at her mother fearing some criticism. She was only allowed to have two friends to tea on one occasion (aged 8); one friend spilled some honey on the tablecloth. The patient's mother made faces at her behind this friend's back.

At about this time the patient had also once been left by the mother in a department store with her father. She had been terrified lest her mother would be lost.

Her school days were happy. She began at a County Council Infants' School and, when aged 8, moved to a Church of England School attached to a 'High' Church. She made good progress but worried a lot and often fainted, when standing or sitting still. Her Confirmation was carried out 'very properly – mother was good about that'.

She recalled being sent to a different class for special tuition in arithmetic. She was advised not to tell her mother, who might punish her on this account. She feared one of the aggressive teachers, who threw the board duster about the class. Sometimes her mother connived with her, so that she could stay away from that teacher's lessons, and took her to the pictures instead.

She had some worries over the school lavatories. Other girls bustled in and out and she seemed to stick there a long time.

When aged 14 she had a bladder infection. In the interview she was reminded that, in talking of illness, she always feared she would say VD. She associated this with lavatories. She began her first job when aged 15. This involved some typing and she feared she would type VD in the middle of a letter. This fear became so great that she left the job 'to get over it at home', telling her boss, with her mother's agreement, that her mother wanted her there. He had asked whether she would always be tied to her mother's apron strings and unavailingly offered her more money. She appeared to have some fears that, by starting work, she might lose much of her mother's concern.

After a few months at home she had obtained another job. She had three posts for long periods. She was eventually taught the operation of a calculating machine by a firm, for which she worked for a long period in London.

Rose recalled some excitement over boys from infancy. When aged 8 she had played nurses and doctors with a little boy neighbour, in the course of which they had inspected each other's genitals. The episode had been interrupted by the arrival of the boy's father, who sent the boy away with a threat but questioned her about the behaviour and as to how she was different from boys. He had touched her hand, making her excited and afraid. She asked to go. At this point in her interview, she asked for assurance that she had not that morning spoken to a single man in the ward lavatory. An interpretation of her fear and of this immediate association was given in terms of the conflict between need for instinctual satisfaction and fear of the consequences. She appeared to accept the interpretation as meaningful to her but followed it with several more requests for reassurance as to her earlier behaviour that day.

Menstruation had begun when the patient was 15. She had learned all about it from other girls and had wondered why it had not started. Her periods were regular and normal in every way.

She had had her first boyfriend when aged 14 to be in the fashion with other girls. She had not fancied kissing and had broken-off with him with some difficulty. When aged 17, a man in her office, who praised her work, asked if he might look between her legs while she was typing. He had offered her a very pretty musical cigarette box as a reward. She felt sorry for him as he had a withered hand. In the interview she went on to wonder whether she had been asking men for cigarettes in the occupational therapy department that day.

After one or two superficial friendships with other men, one of whom exposed himself to her whilst saying goodnight, she had a serious boy-friend when aged 19. Her mother pressed her to write to him and break off the friendship while he was having a difficult time in the army. A few months later her mother again persuaded her to give up her boyfriend.

She had met her husband in the train on the way to work when aged 22. Her mother had been fairly reasonable about this attachment but had flown into a temper when she became engaged because, in her opinion, the engagement ring had not a big enough stone. Her mother had been helpful in seeing that the wedding was very properly conducted. The marriage had been very happy. Both partners had been delighted with their first two children – a girl and a boy. The patient had 'found it difficult to get pregnant again' and had been delighted when this was achieved. She was in no way ill until after the birth of this child.

She enjoyed sexual intercourse about two to three times weekly but never achieved orgasm without manual stimulation by her husband after full intercourse. She thought he was considerate and kind over this but often wished he would be brutal in intercourse and had fantasies of pleasurable rape.

Since her admission to hospital, her husband had continued to be kind and helpful. He disliked her long repetitive requests for reassurance and she believed he held the phone away from his ear saying, after a few minutes, 'Have you finished?' On some occasions she had told him she was about to go home and he had ordered her to do as he said whilst in hospital. On one occasion, uncharacteristically, she had explosively told him 'not to be so bloody pig-headed' which led to his laughing and asking where she had learned this language.

Inquiries of the patient and her husband showed that she had previously been an affectionate, placid person, easy-going with the children, but a bit fussy over locking doors, switching off lights, etc. She had been a good mother and devoutly religious. She smoked moderately – much more so since the beginning of the present illness. She drank only small amounts of alcohol occasionally.

Examination showed her to be a very cooperative, over-compliant woman with a worried expression, which sometimes in appropriate circumstances gave way to a warm and genuine smile. She usually walked with short steps and a slightly bowed posture which, with her childlike manner of speech, gave the impression of a subdued infant. Her affective state was of wistful sadness. There was no intellectual deficit and no evidence of psychosis. Her facial expression and posture contrasted sharply with that shown in numerous photographs, taken over the few years preceding her present illness, in which she appeared to be a cheerful, confident, pretty and sexually attractive woman.

The patient's husband was interviewed privately on several occasions and was a fairly regular attender at the evening group for relations of patients. He was a pleasant, kindly, very active man, who was extremely alert to all the implications of his wife's illness and the methods of treatment proposed. He was evidently industrious but not a hard task-master. He showed no obsessional or other obvious neurotic traits. He completely confirmed his wife's account of her family and upbringing. He showed an appropriate degree of exasperation with his wife's more irritating conduct and seemed to gain a little comfort from hearing the similar experiences of other relations of patients.

In the group and about the hospital she was regarded as essentially kind and considerate. Meanwhile she irritated patients and some members of staff, whom she knew well, with her continual requests for reassurance that she had not carried out the sort of misdemeanours described above. On a country walk with an occupational therapist and other members of the group she exasperated one patient (who suffered from social anxiety) with constant chatter about her symptoms whilst the group were clustered around an ice-cream van. In fact reassurances gave no relief but led only to more elaborate requests and even to her seeking signatures on check lists of things she thought she might conceivably have done.

In group therapy sessions (like the other obsessional patients) she showed little interaction with others, occasionally addressing accounts of her preoccupations directly to the doctor alone. She tended to be very frank and, although her tone was of shame or self-depreciation, from the earliest meetings she spoke of such things as 'a feeling of rejection' when the occupational therapist was away. If the doctor had been monitoring activities late the previous evening, her thoughts would be 'He's not getting a break'. If he was not available, she would think 'He's let me down'. On one occasion when the doctor had uncharacteristically left a meeting, without stating the time at which he intended to return, she thought 'you filthy rotten pig'.

Amongst other pastimes in the hospital setting, she had found that painting to some extent relieved her anxious ruminations. Her paintings all consisted of crude repetitive patterns giving an impression of a wallpaper design rather than a realistic or abstract portrayal of an object, scene or thought.

In common with the other obsessional patients and phobic patients in the group, Mrs Newcombe was taught a standard system of progressive relaxation. A hierarchy of situations, progressively more likely to arouse severe anxiety, was devised. At one end were such items as seeing an advertisement for a perambulator in a magazine and at the other such items as waiting to enter a telephone box, in which a man was already present, or bumping into a perambulator in a busy street with much traffic. In a relaxed state the patient was presented with progressively more disturbing imaginary situations and later, after initial periods of relaxation, she was taken to face potentially disturbing real situations (e.g. walking past rows of doors into what might have been small rooms or cupboards, walking slowly past lavatories or walking on promenades, where there were many perambulators, immediately adjacent to busy main roads). The general principles of desensitization by reciprocal inhibition were followed, whereby, following a relaxation procedure, in both imagined and real situations the patient was invited to signal any feeling of anxiety, whereupon the imagined or real noxious stimulus was removed and familiar phrases associated with relaxation were repeated. In fact she gave no sign of increased anxiety in the course of these procedures. Following 'field work' she would, however, refer back to various episodes, for example asking for reassurance that she did not, in fact, touch any of the prams which she had passed.

She appeared able to face any of the allegedly disturbing situations without difficulty in the company of familiar therapists. She could, for example, talk or paint quite calmly in the presence of a therapist, even though many safety-pins were displayed on a nearby table and on the floor. Meanwhile if, by chance, she saw a safety-pin on the floor in the absence of her therapist, she would soon be seeking reassurance that there had not been another, which she might have picked up and lost on or in her own person, without remembering that she had done so.

It was evident that she was not responding to the association of anxiety-relieving stimuli with 'anxiety-provoking' situations in the manner which was usually quite easily achieved with a phobic patient. The impression was given that the patient's anxious ruminations went on in an autonomous fashion and were quite unaffected by the various learning situations, even though she would often spontaneously say how much safer she felt in the presence of her familiar therapists. (No 'thought-stopping' or 'operant-conditioning' techniques were used at that time.)

During her period of treatment in the special group, this patient was given Trifluoperazine, 5 mgms three times daily, as this seemed to relieve her distress to some extent. In the fifth month she was also given Haloperidol in doses of 1·5–3 mgms three times daily on account of increased distress, which was not satisfactorily explained. It may have related to the increasing anxiety on the part of the patient and her husband because the treatment, though apparently intensive, was unsuccessful. By the sixth month, the patient complained of depression, was sleeping less well and often cried when alone or with one other person, with whom she was very familiar. ECT was given – six times in all – with improvement in her mood to about the same level as that shown on her admission.

Although treatment with various Monoamine Oxidase Inhibitors and tricyclic anti-depressants and ECT had produced little improvement over the two years preceding the patient's admission to the special group, it was decided that she should have a period of several weeks' continuous 'modified' narcosis combined with treatment with Monoamine Oxidase Inhibitor and tricyclic anti-depressants and ECT. 'Modified' narcosis implied calculation of sedative drug dosage and timing such that the patient was rousable for meals.

Following this treatment the patient showed a remarkable recovery, being regarded by herself and her husband as in every way the person she was before her third pregnancy. Treatment with Monoamine Oxidase Inhibitors and tricyclic compounds was continued for several years.

Shirley Fleetway

Shirley Fleetway was a 38-year-old housewife with a bright smile and a brisk manner. She was married to a moderately well-paid instrument inspector employed by an electronic company. They had three children: girls aged 17 and 16, and a boy aged 11.

She had found herself somewhat depressed and jittery following the birth of her son and five years later consulted her General Practitioner because she was 'in a tizzy, found it difficult to get through a day's work and worried a lot'. She denied any real sources of worry but admitted to epigastric and left chest pain for which no organic cause was found. Her doctor thought she was depressed and withdrawn but she refused tablets as 'she could never swallow pills'.

She was referred to a psychiatrist for possible ECT. This was eventually given, though at first her condition did not appear serious enough to justify this. After two out-patient treatments she ceased to attend for more.

Six years later she was referred to another psychiatrist as she was finding it difficult to eat at home on account of 'a strange feeling that, if she or anyone ate food cooked by her, they would die or go blind'. She could eat at friends' homes and in restaurants without difficulty and 'apart from all this, felt cheerful and normal'. An essentially depressive illness was suspected and Phenelzine 15 mgms three times daily was prescribed. She managed to take only one tablet daily, showed no improvement after one month and completely gave up cooking for the family, leaving this to the others and feeling depressed about it at meal times. She refused further out-patient ECT but reluctantly agreed to be admitted to a ward for patients with acute psychiatric illness.

In an unhurried interview in hospital she said she had an irresistible belief that, if food had been touched by others to her direct knowledge, it might be harmful. In such a circumstance she would buy more – and then from trusted small shopkeepers, not from supermarkets even if their prices were lower. She again said that, if she cooked food, she believed that those eating it would become blind or drop dead. The fact that members of her family had eaten food cooked by her in the past without harm did not alter this conviction. Food that had been in the house at the time of a row or even of someone dropping something was dangerous and must be replaced.

Exclusively when being driven by her husband in his car, she felt compelled to add up the numbers of various manufacturers' cars which they passed. If she failed to note the make of the car, she would feel greatly concerned that she would never be able to find it. Seeing ambulances and fire-engines on the road 'was a bad omen' and made her feel worried. (When referring to her husband she cried. Otherwise her expression and manner were bland as she recounted these symptoms.)

Her father, now aged 69, had been a research chemist employed by an oil company. He was also a pianist, chorister and amateur choir conductor of considerable ability. He was said to have had a 'nervous breakdown' when the patient was an infant. He had certain odd ways – for example never putting on his hat until he was outside the house, even if he had much to carry. The patient was fond of him though he was 'retiring and distant'. When she was 13 and doing a lot of cooking at home, which pleased him, he had developed a retinal detachment and become blind in one eye.

Her mother had been a quiet, capable, likeable person, who played the violin, to whom the patient felt very close and for whom she would do anything until her death from pneumonia (aged 61) two months before the birth of the patient's third child.

Her one sister, two years older than herself, had become a missionary in Bengal. The whole family had led a rather quiet isolated life, with few friends or relations ever calling at the house. Anger was never openly expressed and the atmosphere was happy though controlled.

Shirley had been born and brought up in a rambling old house set apart from the others in a Kentish village. Her first memory, when aged 4, was of eating raspberries with her sister in the garden and suddenly being afraid that her parents had gone out. As a child she was shy and afraid of dogs, mice and unfamiliar tradesmen who might come to the house.

She liked school, though she continued to be shy. Academically she was undistinguished but she was good at netball and tennis and represented her small local grammar school in these games. On leaving, after taking the School Certificate Examination (aged 16), she helped her mother at home for nearly a year before taking up general office work locally.

Her future husband later joined the same firm for a time and she met him when aged 22, marrying him one year later. She was not sure that she had really loved him but he had been very persistent and she eventually 'gave in'. He was four years older than herself. She had no previous boyfriends and no very close girl-friends. She gave up her job at the time of her marriage.

When first married she and her husband had lived in an unattractive house rented by his mother. The patient had a good deal of friction with her. Frequently her husband took her part against his mother, but the patient did not feel better for this. Her first two children were born and spent their infancy at this house. The patient often felt her mother-in-law was stealing the little girls away, when she kept them in her own room upstairs, although she knew it was time for them to come down for a meal. Two years before the patient's son was born, the mother-in-law became chronically ill, usually staying in her room. One day the patient gave her a cake she had made specially for her but omitted to look in on her before going to bed at night, as was her usual custom. In the morning the old lady was found dead in bed – presumably of a heart-attack. The patient blamed herself for not having seen her mother-in-law the night before.

The family moved to a more agreeable house. Just over a year later the patient was displeased to find herself pregnant. There had been a contraceptive mishap, for which she blamed her husband.

From that time onwards, she felt antagonistic towards sexual inter-course. She had not been pleased to have another child. She did not know if his being male affected her attitude. Later she realized he was bright like his sisters and became fond of him, being especially pro-tective if his father hit him or reprimanded him, which he, having become chronically irritable, often did.

After five years of feeling that her life was limited and unexciting, she developed the symptoms described above, which gradually became more marked, though she told her General Practitioner and first psychiatrist only of her anxiety, difficulty in coping with the house-work and 'not wanting to eat much'. (This last symptom was described by her doctors as anorexia, no account of the patient's special reasons for not eating having been given to them.)

Over the five years preceding her admission to hospital, she had enjoyed a part-time job in the research department of a canned food factory. Before her illness she had been a cool, controlled, 'reserved' person who could leave nothing unfinished or out of order. She was fond of needlework and gardening. She had liked tennis and dancing but had pursued these activities very little as her husband had not accompanied her. She had always had a vivid imagination (sometimes evident in letters though it was not often evident in her rather inhibited conversation). In general she had been fond of her children and easy-going with them. She could relax and talk with them though she was otherwise uncommunicative. This had been so even with her mother, to whom she had felt close. While she was able to talk of agreeable happenings, she could not express her troubles. She was a confirmed member of the Church of England but not a church-goer.

Examination showed a healthy-looking, smallish, slightly greying, round-faced woman, who moved softly and delicately, sat without fidgeting, often looking thoughtful but never withdrawn, and was, in fact, very observant of all that occurred around her. She smiled readily in appropriate situations and rarely showed distress, weeping only when talking of her husband's failure to provide excitement in her life or of his alleged ill-temper.

The husband was a regular attender at the relations' group, in which his attitude was friendly and warm and his conversation often witty. He was clearly a fairly exacting person but not 'obsessional' outside normal limits. He showed considerable concern for his wife and appeared genuinely to wish for her recovery for her own sake. He appeared to gain support from the companionship in misfortune offered by other members of this group. He had remarkably readily accepted part of his wife's role in the household, being an efficient and expert cook. He was a quick-tempered man but he could talk with good humour of angry episodes in retrospect.

In the psychotherapy group she was usually completely silent but it was evident from the earliest days of her membership that she was well liked by her fellows, who spoke of her as 'unworried, always having a smile and always ready to listen or to help' in ordinary situations about the ward.

Her behaviour to the nurses was impeccable and her craft work in the occupational therapy department skilful and industriously carried out.

Though forthcoming in the earlier individual interviews, where a definite history was being obtained, she offered no 'asides' or associations with the events of the immediate present as did Rose. In later interviews with no programme, she would often sit silent for periods of 20–30 minutes, though eventually an interpretation of her posture (which might for example be expressing obvious weariness or withdrawal, in that her head drooped and she was slightly turned away from a conversational position) often evoked some comment expressed with relief, as though she had long wanted to say something. It was to take many months before she could even occasionally speak freely for a few minutes, write a letter (usually interesting and colourful) as to what she would have liked to have said or call back after an interview to apologize for saying nothing. Challenged on her frequent silences, she would repeat that she always came hoping that one day something useful would come up.

In behaviour therapy, she was taught relaxation and taken through a hierarchy of disturbing situations, from seeing a cushion displaced in the sitting-room to having a row with her husband, without any sign or report of anxiety.

Though she was no better when allowed home for weekend leave, her strong wish to return was granted. She attended on a daily basis, fitting in treatment activities with her part-time job and appeared happier doing this.

Meanwhile she was taken through another hierarchy of real situations – of eating eggs cooked in front of her husband and herself by the doctor in an occupational therapy kitchen, cooking them herself and having the doctor and her husband eat them and of doing this in an atmosphere of disturbance, with objects being dropped and angry swear words used. In all of these situations she showed and reported no anxiety whatsoever and the therapist had an uncanny feeling of treating symptoms which did not exist, though patient and husband never questioned the reasonableness of the procedure. Eventually instructions were followed to make a cake at home and to leave it where it would eventually be eaten by the family, though the patient would not be told when this took place. This also was accomplished without difficulty.

Meanwhile the husband had settled down to doing the cooking at home. From time to time (more so, if there had been any overt expression of anger in the household) he was told various foods could not be used. Initially he bought more but soon began routinely to pretend that he had discarded food and bought more, when, in fact, he had simply brought back the 'discarded' food. He had little doubt that his wife saw through this wholly understandable and economically essential subterfuge but believed she preferred to pretend not to know.

No conspicuous advance was made in persuading the patient that she could safely cook for her family, though she was able to arrange some cocktail snacks for a Christmas reception in her home for the neighbours without anxiety.

In view of the demands of her job and her failure to participate actively in the therapeutic group, the patient was allowed after a few months to attend for individual evening interviews until it was evident that she had confidence in her therapist. With her knowledge her husband was also separately interviewed for a few weeks, after which she was regularly seen for half an hour before her husband joined her and her therapist. A major object of this work was to confront the couple with what had appeared to be a provocative (though often ambiguous) situation to the patient in the preceding week and to facilitate their discussing their interpretations of it and their intentions and feelings at the time.

To some extent this procedure appeared to lessen hostility between the two. The collecting of car numbers became a less prominent symptom but the fear about preparation of food remained.

Some months later the patient became markedly depressed for no clear reasons. She refused to come into hospital, asserting that her husband had long wanted to 'put her away'. She talked of taking a room and living apart. Eventually, as her distress became greater and her symptoms (of condemning food as unacceptable and sometimes begging her family not to eat a dish because of a minor disturbance, such as the dropping of an object, while it was being prepared) became more florid, she agreed to enter hospital, where she was treated with several weeks' continuous narcosis, Monoamine Oxidase Inhibitors, tricyclic anti-depressants and ECT twice weekly.

This treatment produced a remarkable improvement in mood and the symptoms relating to food became markedly less obvious. Much more disturbance in the household was tolerated. The principal intractable symptom was, however, that the patient did not dare to cook in her house for the family. Treatment with tricyclic anti-depressants was discontinued on account of giddiness but MAOI treatment was continued.

Nine months later a further exacerbation of depression occurred, with much weeping, feelings of hopelessness and increased concern over the possible ill-effects of food in the house. Tablets were refused as these also were regarded as dangerous like the food in the house. Hospital admission was readily accepted. A three-week period of modified narcosis, ECT and MAOI and tricyclic anti-depressants was again successful.

Following this, further admissions for about three weeks were required on two successive occasions but the patient's condition improved rapidly with no specific treatment. The hospital itself appeared to be a haven, which relieved the patient's symptoms. Consequently she was allowed to attend subsequently for many months as a day-patient once or twice a week, usually spending her time in a craft department.

Whilst her symptoms varied in intensity with episodes of depression, they did not disappear completely until about three years after her first joining the special group. The circumstances of her 'cure' were extraordinary. She had been extremely worried for several weeks by the serious illness of her son and had lost much sleep over this. He eventually recovered. During his stay in hospital the patient came to know a visiting clergyman very well. As a consequence of this contact, she attended a faith-healing service in a Non-Conformist church. Following special prayers and the 'laying on of hands', she 'felt as if a great weight had been lifted from her'. Her obsessional ruminations and 'fears' about food completely disappeared.

Valerie Scott

Valerie Scott was a 33-year-old housewife suffering from compulsive hand-washing and ritualistic cleaning of her clothing. She was also grossly abnormally fastidious about washing-up crockery, which she did strictly according to a standard system.

Her mother, aged 60, dominated the family. Her personality was markedly obsessional and there was abundant evidence that she had been extremely punitive in the toilet training of the patient and her sister.

Her 60-year-old father was a retired printer. He had always worried excessively, had a rigid but not forceful personality and for many years had had a chronic duodenal ulcer.

The patient's 25-year-old sister had no particular obsessional traits, had never been very 'close' to the patient, and had lived away from home for several years.

The patient recalled that the home atmosphere in her childhood had been over-regulated and lacking in warmth. Some of her earliest memories were of her mother screaming at her that she was 'the filthiest girl in the world' or 'the most evil girl in the world'. The patient believed these and other things said by her mother absolutely.

Probably her earliest memory, when aged 3, was of cuddling a ginger kitten in the garden.

She had been bright at school, getting along well with the teachers and other pupils. Nevertheless she had been so frightened of asking to be excused from the class that she quite often wetted herself. Subsequently she would go to great trouble to hide this happening from her mother. In her school days she was particularly fond of telling stories to young children and of caring for other neighbours' children.

She began work in the drawing office of a large engineering firm when aged 16. She was rapidly promoted, being placed in charge of a large office and entrusted with particularly exacting work. She had continued to hold this post up to the time of her admission to hospital, her employers looking forward to her eventual return.

Her periods had begun when she was aged 15 and had presented no problems. She had had a few boyfriends after leaving school and became closely attached to a 21-year-old man, when aged 19. They had intended to marry. For no clear reason her mother had been antagonistic to him. She had upset the patient's arrangements to spend a Christmas holiday with her boyfriend's family and subsequently pressed the patient to abandon the attachment. Shortly after the break-up of this love-affair the patient's obsessional symptoms had begun. Seven years later she had married a mechanical engineer, ten years older than herself. A previous wife had deserted him and subsequently died. The husband, himself, had an obsessional personality and suffered from a recurrent duodenal ulcer which kept him off work for periods of several weeks. He frequently showed exasperation over his wife's symptoms. It was noteworthy that she tended to become depressed following his episodes of acute illness, through which she nursed him devotedly.

Her symptoms had begun with excessive fussiness over the cleanliness of paper at work. This had led to her destroying large quantities of paper, which she regarded as imperfect. At the same time she had felt compelled to wash her hands repeatedly and for long periods for no good reason. Some months later she became increasingly fussy about her clothing, checking it for dirt and developing a ritualistic procedure in which she wiped over the whole outer surface of a garment with paper tissues before putting it on. As far as she could remember there had been some mild fluctuation in her symptoms. A period of intensive psychotherapy for one year from a psychoanalyst before her marriage produced no improvement. Following her marriage, exacerbations of her symptoms and increased hand-washing occurred concurrently with episodes of depression, which usually followed her husband's attacks of physical illness.

In-patient treatment with ECT five years after her marriage produced improvement in her mood but little change in her obsessional symptoms. A few months later she became moderately depressed and, after further successful treatment of her depression, was so bothered by her intractable obsessional symptoms that she readily accepted bilateral rostral leucotomy. Following this she showed anger much more readily than before. On some occasions nurses, who had been instructed to re-train her not to wash excessively, forcibly prevented her washing, provoking violently angry responses. On the other hand both before and after operation it was noted that she could postpone washing indefinitely when in the company of a trusted therapist. Three months after operation the patient joined the special group.

An account of the patient's personality before the onset of her symptoms, based on her own evidence and that of her mother, showed that she had always been fussy over tidiness and cleanliness and set herself extremely high standards of neatness at work. She could be stubborn but rarely showed overt anger. She expected high standards of reliability in others as well as herself. Her particular interests had been dress-making and music. She tended to underestimate her abilities. Though not a regular church-goer, she believed in some sort of God.

Examination showed her to be a neat smartly dressed young woman, who tended to look directly at the person to whom she was talking, for very long periods at a time; her facial expression was relatively fixed. She spoke very frankly and gave a clear account of herself in a controlled manner, rarely showing great variation of emotion though rapport was good. Occasionally she made angry remarks. She very rarely showed obvious sadness even at times when she stated convincingly that she felt very depressed.

Her husband, who regularly attended the relations' group, made no secret of his own liking for tidiness and for everything 'being just so'. He talked readily and helpfully to other members. He frequently appeared mildly angry and related this largely to the difficulties imposed upon him by his wife's illness.

In subsequent individual and group psychotherapy, interpretations were offered of the patient's behaviour as an attempt to placate the tyrannical mother, who appeared to have had such power over her, and to disprove her filthiness and the evil character attributed to her by the mother. It was also suggested that the energy expended in her rituals arose from her intense murderous anger, which was deflected into her compulsive actions. These views were accepted as plausible but did not appear to be incorporated into the patient's outlook, though she did increasingly complain of the harm her mother had done to her.

As with the other obsessional members of the group, transference phenomena were never very obvious. There were some signs of the patient's positive regard for her therapists but no transference of negative feeling ever became apparent.

Desensitization by reciprocal inhibition to imaginal and *in vivo* stimuli (e.g. urine, which was alleged to be the unbearable contaminant) was unsuccessful. Though the patient 'learned' to bathe her hands in urine, sit for hours and finally eat without subsequent washing, when left alone she washed excessively as before.

A new strategy was then adopted. The patient 'felt really safe' and free of compulsions only when in bed. She was therefore put to bed in

a ward with a well-instructed friendly nursing staff. She was allowed
to wash briefly in bed and allowed up for periods increasing from ten
minutes to eight hours. It was agreed that feelings of unbearable compulsion would be met by a return to the safe but neutral bed. In the
early stages this was sometimes necessary. For her periods up she was
always accompanied by a cheerful, interesting occupational therapy
helper, whom she liked. They spent the time in entirely normal
activities in the country or town. The compulsive symptoms disappeared and the patient's mood became buoyant.

She was discharged very well but relapsed rapidly at home, where her
husband was irritable over a business failure.

Over the following seven years her symptoms fluctuated with variations in her marital relationship and her husband's work situation.
Recently both have improved and the patient's compulsive symptoms
have decreased but not, by any means, been extinguished.

Grace Hargreaves

Grace Hargreaves was a 30-year-old single physiotherapist. She complained of fears that she would be contaminated by faeces – her own,
other people's and that of animals. She avoided muck of all kinds and
checked her clothes elaborately for periods of $\frac{1}{2}$–1 hour after using a
lavatory.

She had been born in Ireland in comfortable middle-class circumstances. Her mother had died suddenly of a sub-arachnoid haemorrhage
(aged 24) whilst pregnant, the patient being aged 3. She had been
excessively fussy over the toilet training of the patient. The father, now
aged 54, a bank manager and a kindly worrier, had married again two
years after his first wife's death. The second wife, a widow, was also
strict and fussy. (These parental characteristics were verified by interviews with various members of the family.)

The patient's first memory, when aged 5, was of playing happily in
the garden at home, then being told of the death of an uncle in a car
accident. So far as she recalled it, her childhood was not unhappy,
though at times she resented her stepmother's strictness. She was sent
to a boarding school when aged 10 and was fairly happy there. Academically she was moderately good. She played two school games well.
She played the violin very well. She had one particularly close girl-
friend. She was never a leader. She was always fussy over her clothes
and tidiness. Her periods began when she was aged 13 and presented
no particular problem. When aged 14 she felt herself in love with an

older girl, without her knowledge, and became firmly attached to a Christian sect after attending meetings of a travelling Evangelist.

She left school when aged 16 to reside and study at a Nursery Nursing School, where she missed her old friend. She hated cleaning the infants and giving pots. She began washing her hands excessively. Her work consequently became slow and she asked to leave after one year.

She returned home, became more cheerful, ceased to wash excessively and, after a period serving soap and toiletries in a chemist's shop, became a student physiotherapist when aged 18. She lived at her training hospital.

Throughout her student years she had a close friendship with a fellow girl student. She became depressed when the other girl was, for a time, less interested in her. At this point she became increasingly concerned regarding her personal cleanliness, often getting up in the night to check over her clothing.

After treatment in a private hospital with ECT, she passed her final examination and took a job in another hospital. She again made a single close friendship with a female colleague and felt sad when she left. She considered going out with men but never did and 'sometimes found them frightening'.

On one occasion she was scornfully accused of failing to be available for a weekend duty, there being some confusion over a rota. She immediately became progressively depressed and again had private in-patient ECT. She seemed to improve, but soon after reaching home, saw horse dung in the road near her house. The thought haunted her and she became markedly depressed. She checked her clothes for dirt and especially faecal staining for long periods. This soon led to admission to a National Health Service psychiatric hospital. Treatment with ECT and anti-depressant drugs produced improvements of mood at times, though, over a period of two years, frequent relapses occurred and her compulsive checking of her clothes continued. She became dull and weary in appearance, was unable to work and, after a further depressive swing, was re-admitted to hospital and designated by one psychiatrist as 'very chronic'.

On examination the patient was noted to be a plump sad-looking young woman, who answered questions readily but had little or no spontaneous conversation. She showed little variation of facial expression but, confronted with an amusing situation, would give a curiously secretive smile. She showed no intellectual impairment or psychotic features.

Her life was relatively isolated and very restricted. She usually had one close friend amongst the patients, in particular a depressed hysterical woman of her own age and later a depressed manipulative schizophrenic, for whom she felt very sorry. She retained her rigid religious convictions, sometimes played the violin very well, was listlessly resentful of occupational therapy activities and talked almost exclusively of her symptoms.

In the special group, these patterns were repeated. At meetings she would show no reaction to other patients' problems but occasionally say directly to the doctor that her checking was getting worse. All her activities lacked zest and, though she made a single friendship with a female member of the group, this was never apparent in meetings. Indeed she often appeared secretive, though she would talk fairly readily and frankly in private interviews.

She attributed her depressed state to her compulsive symptoms, her worries over cleanliness, her wearisome checking and her feeling that she must avoid all contact with faecal material anywhere. To this last-mentioned end she would suffer the discomfort of going to the lavatory as seldom as possible.

In the relations' group, her father gave an impression of being considerate and kind in a controlled, distant manner. Her stepmother was also genuinely concerned but strikingly objective in her comment and controlled in manner. Both had noted various details of the patient's behaviour, such as avoidance not only of muck but of walking near the doors of lavatories at home.

Interpretations of her faecal contamination avoidance behaviour, as infantile attempts to please her mother and avoid the punishment of being deprived of her, were accepted as plausible at a purely intellectual level and did not appear to be incorporated by the patient in her outlook. Ideas of gratification being involved in the delay of defaecation and urinating were regarded by the patient and, indeed, the whole group as valueless in the context of this sort of illness, though it was agreed such voluntary delay might be pleasurable. Around the time of these interpretations first being offered to the group, this patient often arrived late for personal interviews and 'hoped the doctor wouldn't mind' as she'd been 'checking', saying these things in a manner which implied at first fear of criticism then secretive amusement that the doctor had been made to wait. This notion was discussed and again accepted as plausible but appeared to produce no change. It may possibly have contributed to the very slow development of some warmth in the patient–doctor relationship over many months, the patient sometimes saying how much she appreciated the attempts made to help her.

Interpretations of the onset of depressive episodes as related to losses of much-loved female friends, echoing the loss of the mother in childhood, were accepted as appropriate and probably true. Nevertheless they appeared to have no therapeutic value.

Meanwhile the growth of new friendships, which were never mentioned to the doctor by the patient, and the restoration of waning friendships appeared always to produce improvements in mood state.

An attempt was made to relieve the patient's alleged fear of contamination by behaviour therapy based on reciprocal inhibition. The patient was taught a system of progressive relaxation and taken through a hierarchy of contamination situations as imagined in the office. These varied from using coloured as opposed to white towels up to walking through heaps of manure.

The patient showed a striking lack of anxiety during these supposedly de-conditioning procedures, though she might later say she did not like subsequently thinking of the situations presented. Following the imaginal 'desensitization', she was taken through a hierarchy of real situations including walking through uncleaned stables and cowsheds and deliberately treading in faecal material. Again the patient showed no anxiety. Left alone she continued to avoid any muck as before.

There was a distinct impression that something quite different from a phobia was involved in the patient's symptomatology – *not* a fearful situation but a fixed behaviour pattern occurring almost autonomously, if no therapist were present to take control, and *rationalized* as due to an anxiety by the patient in her attempt to convince herself that she had conscious control.

Following the loss of a particular friend amongst the other patients, this patient became much more markedly depressed and was treated with a period of six weeks' modified narcosis, ECT and MAOI and tricyclic anti-depressants. She showed considerable improvement in mood and very limited improvement of her compulsive symptoms. Shortly after this an unexpected opportunity arose to stay for a few weeks' holiday in the country with her old school friend. It appeared that she adopted a strongly disciplined approach towards the patient, showing much affection but refusing to allow any time to be wasted on checking etc. The patient returned to hospital in an extremely cheerful mood and showed marked reduction in her obsessional symptoms. There was a possibility of her staying permanently with the old friend. When, after a few weeks, this plan foundered as the friend had to go abroad with her firm, the patient rapidly relapsed into a relatively depressed state with her compulsive symptoms as before.

For several years subsequently she showed a fluctuating course, at times managing a few months' work as a hospital helper but continuing to be handicapped by periods of depression and the same compulsive symptoms.

The detailed descriptions above illustrate certain striking aspects of patients with obsessional states, some of which appear insufficiently to have been stressed in the past. Many of the important features of these patients occurred commonly amongst others, who passed through the 'salvage group' or were otherwise studied intensively on an in-patient and/or out-patient basis in five hospitals in central or suburban London over a ten-year period.

The outcome of these clinical observations is summarized in the following table and the succeeding commentary.

Pre-morbid obsessional traits (e.g. obstinacy, liking for order, tidiness, accuracy, fairness, etc. to a high degree but within normal limits) were characteristic of all these patients, whose illnesses had their onset within the second to the fourth decades. (Less exacting observations on elderly patients with early dementia not surprisingly show a similar trend.) These findings merely confirm those described by many others.

Somatic symptoms often associated with anxiety appeared in the complaints of only 4 patients. The symptoms particularly sought were: headaches, dizziness, blurring of vision, trembling, abnormal sweating, breathlessness, left sub-mammary pain, palpitations, 'indigestion', nausea, poor appetite, diarrhoea, frequency of micturition and disturbance of menstruation. Only one patient complained of constipation and she had deliberately avoided defaecation to escape the laborious ritual following it. In spite of their depression, only one male and two females complained of poor sleep.

Meanwhile of 20 patients matched for age and sex and suffering from phobias of such simple entities as enclosed spaces, open spaces, sexual intercourse, birds and spiders, 18 also complained of at least two of the above physical symptoms and 9 of three or more, excluding sleep disturbance and constipation, which also occurred in 8 and 4 respectively before any drug treatment had been commenced.

Of 20 patients with depression, without obsessional symptoms and also matched for age and sex, 16 complained of at least two of the physical symptoms and 6 of three or more, excluding sleep disturbance and constipation, which also occurred in 16 and 7 respectively, before any drug treatment had been commenced.

Whilst all twenty 'obsessional neurotics' recognized that they were depressed during at least part of the period of their observation and at

TABLE 3.1 *Clinical observations*
Total: 20 patients, 5 male, 15 female
Age at onset of symptoms ranged from 14 to 31 years

Characteristic	Female	Male	Total	% Female	% Male	% All
Pre-morbid obsessional traits	15	5	20	100	100	100
Somatic symptoms commonly associated with emotional stress	3	1	4	20	20	20
Feelings of 'generalized tension'	15	5	20	100	100	100
Unusually prone to depressive reactions	15	4	19	100	80	95
Unusually inclined to suppress anger	10	3	13	67	60	65
Onset of symptoms coincided with depression	15	5	20	100	100	100
Onset of symptoms also coincided with suppressed anger	11	3	14	73	60	70
Onset of symptoms also coincided with subjective feeling of powerlessness to deal with cause of anger	8	2	10	53	40	50
Compulsive activity or ruminations related to happening in past (in infancy or adult life) associated with intense sadness, guilt or anger – sometimes with additional sexual excitement	13	3	16	89	60	80
General 'indecisiveness' during illness	14	4	18	93	80	90
Schizophrenic symptoms or signs over average period of seven years	0	0	0	0	0	0

the onset of their symptoms, they therefore differed strikingly from phobics and non-obsessional depressives. (It is worth noting that they did not commonly have constipation, which has, in the past, been linked with 'anal fixation' or 'obsessional personality'.)

While phobics appeared to have unstable vegetative nervous systems and non-obsessional depressives also had multiple symptoms suggestive of autonomic instability, the obsessionals appeared clinically to show a relative *stability* of their autonomic functions – at least so far as the patients were aware of their manifestations.

Review of the 3 females and 1 male among the obsessionals, who complained of physical symptoms, showed that these patients were particularly inclined to use any symptoms, including their compulsive symptoms, to manipulate situations. While this observation may be insignificant in such a small number of patients, it might well be pursued in some larger prospective study.

Suffice it to say that these observations suggest that, far from being characterized by instability of the autonomic nervous system (which to some behaviour therapists, at least, is the keystone of 'neurosis') our patients were, *in this sense*, un-neurotic. Use of the time-honoured term 'neurotic' may possibly be justified, however, in that the obsessional's neuro-psychic system is certainly functioning abnormally and in general he is more clearly aware that something is amiss than most, but not all, psychotics, some of whom – particularly schizophrenics – are well aware of the malfunctions of their minds.

It may be said that symptomatically the majority of our obsessional patients show a relative fixity rather than instability of function of their autonomic nervous systems. This appears to reflect the fixity of their thinking and behaviour, which they experience as compulsive and appear unable to alter in a desirably adaptive manner, so long as their depression is untreated.

This observation may be crucial in explaining why it has been found difficult to classify the obsessional state along with abnormal states involving anxiety or its physical concomitants. It would, perhaps, be more satisfactory, if, apart from the functional psychoses, *anxiety states* (general and specific), *dissociation states*, and *'behavioural fixity'* states were clearly distinguished from each other rather than linked as 'neuroses'.

The behavioural fixity states would then most commonly appear to be a special reaction to depression (rather than anxiety) occurring in individuals, whose normal behaviour patterns and mental outlook were unusually, though not pathologically, ordered – possibly more because of the genetically determined structure of their central nervous systems than through the 'training' they received.

Feelings of 'generalized tension' were evident, if they were appropriately questioned, in all twenty obsessional patients. The tension was not synonymous with the sort of anxiety felt on waiting for an oral examination or running 'to catch the last train'. Patients described it as an exaggerated awareness that 'something not done must be done' or that they must do something or avoid some situation. *Compulsion* to thought or action of a certain kind was the underlying feature of the tension rather than *fear*.

Proneness to depression: the majority of the twenty patients appeared unusually prone to depressive reactions. As with Valerie Scott on her return to adversity at home or Grace Hargreaves, when she was separated from a friend or admonished, difficulties with which most healthy people could cope rapidly produced depressive states and exacerbations of compulsive behaviour. No specific scale of measurement of proneness to depression was used and no comparison made with any control group. Such a study would be desirable, completely to substantiate this clinical observation, which may be affected by observer bias. Nevertheless it is supported by the report of H. R. Beech (1971).

Suppression of anger: all the patients studied were clinically assessed as to their tendency to suppress anger abnormally by a) their own account of their behaviour in various real situations discussed in a series of interviews, b) by the overt display of affect observed in interviews and c) at least one – often several – other witnesses' accounts of the patient's behaviour (e.g. relations, nurses dealing with the patient, etc.). Over half appeared abnormally inclined to suppress anger.

On the evidence available it was impossible to say to what extent this was learned. It was not by any means true that all patients came from households where the overt expression of anger was discouraged. Nevertheless, at some stage in their development, the patients may have experienced reinforcement of a less obvious kind in the direction of suppressing anger. Alternatively it could be suggested that the failure to express an affect overtly might itself be another aspect of behavioural fixity. In this connection it may be noted that individuals with obsessional personalities, within normal limits, are characteristically controlled, avoiding extravagant expression of any emotion and rarely, for example, laughing uproariously. Meanwhile criticism, anger, approval, pleasure and sadness are often expressed tersely in wit, of which they are often masters. The audience may be greatly affected but the obsessional originator of the witticism may show little change in his own 'controlled' behaviour.

Onset of symptoms coinciding with depression: while it has been widely accepted that obsessional states often occur as a manifestation of a depressive illness, the regular association of these states has not been widely recognized. Attention has been drawn to this possibility by H. R. Beech (1971). Clinical experience suggests that patients so often stress their obsessional ruminations and compulsions, that depression is missed. Careful assessment of the patient's life situation at the time of onset of the symptoms will usually show potentially depressing factors. Adequate inquiry and observation – including observation of the affective tone at interview – will show that depression is present. Energetic treatment of depression alone will frequently relieve the obsessional symptoms. A stumbling-block is that many patients with obsessional states do not experience sleep disturbance or loss of appetite for food or sex, and attribute their depressed mood state, loss of self-esteem and impaired work performance to the intrusion of compulsive thinking or activity.

Thus Rose's symptoms began with post-puerperal depression. Shirley's began with puerperal depression, which became chronic and was reinforced by the death of an exasperating mother-in-law. Valerie's began with her mother's sabotage of an important love-affair. Grace's began with her separation from her stepmother, which was likely to be specially painful in view of the death of her true mother, when the patient was an infant.

Impressions based on clinical assessment of twenty patients suggest that depression is *always* present at the onset of obsessional symptoms, when these are of pathological degree.

The relative infrequency of the commonly observed full depressive syndrome with sleep and appetite disturbance can only be speculatively explained. It may be that just as, in these patients, the depressive affect appears to exaggerate fixity of thinking and behaviour, so also the normal behaviour patterns and underlying neurophysiological mechanisms of sleep and appetite tend to be fixed in relatively normal states rather than disturbed.

Onset of symptoms coinciding with suppressed anger appeared characteristic of 14 of 20 patients. Thus Shirley was angry about her pregnancy but did not show it and Valerie was furious with her mother for spoiling her romance, though she only expressed this years later. Depression has been conceptualized as anger turned upon the subject himself. Even without this concept, it is common experience in psychiatry that depression and anger are associated, particularly during the onset and recovery phases of depressive illness. Suppressed anger and depression may both be factors in intractable asthma (Mellett, 1970) and it would not be surprising if both these affective disturbances gave rise to profound disturbances of more general behaviour, as in obsessional states, just as they disturb breathing behaviour in certain patients, who are subject to asthma.

Feelings of powerlessness to deal with the cause of anger at the time of the event were elicited in 10 of the 20 patients studied. This was so with Valerie with regard to her mother and Shirley over her pregnancy. This may merely have reflected the tendency to suppress anger and a general tendency not to take violent action. It may have related to underestimation of personal rights to happiness, or to indecision. Certainly it would have made the healthy canalization of anger more difficult and still further increased its special pathological effect in these patients.

Compulsive activity or rumination related to past happenings associated with intense sadness, guilt or anger, sometimes associated with sexual excitement: in 16 of the 20 patients studied, the first few interviews led to the recall of past events, which appeared to explain the specific nature of the obsessional symptoms. Shirley, for example, associated the sudden death of her mother-in-law with her having given her a cake. At the time she was already depressed; the death of the mother-in-law, towards whom she felt much anger, left her feeling more guilty. It was reasonable to suppose that this experience led to a general concept that, if the patient were angered by anyone – even one of the family dropping something – then the food she cooked for them might have fatal effect. A further generalization made any food in the house at the time of any violent happenings or words equally dangerous. The father's development of partial blindness when being fed by his daughter, who resented his 'distant' manner, also meant that her food could cause blindness. Meanwhile the fatal food fear had been registered over five years before an increasingly hopeless, resentful, depressed mental state was reflected in the fear of harm, due to her food, befalling the family who depended on her. An even longer period had passed since her father became partially blind, when he ate her food but exasperated her. It seemed therefore that episodes associated with depression, anger or guilt feelings had been revived with more severe depression.

Rose, saddened and angered by her parents' rows, had picked up some notion that violence was associated with something – the Dutch cap – which went inside her mother and of which she must be rid to end an angry scene. There had been more violence after the replacement of the mysterious and exciting object. It may be inferred that her tyrannical, unpredictable and house-proud mother had been angry at the possibility of faecal smearing of furniture and there was the first memory (possibly screening another more disturbing event) of her being admonished for using a chamber pot in a living-room, when she thought it was all right.

She had been caught at the 'doctor-game' by the threatening father of her playmate, experiencing anger, excitement and possibly the sadness of facing the difference between herself and boys. She had been touched on her arm by the seductive father of the boy, feeling excitement and guilty fear.

She had felt rejected and lost as well as angry, when pushed away in a perambulator by the unpredictable mother, whom she so much feared to lose.

With her schooldays nearly over, she had had cystitis but thought of it as associated with venereal disease. Actually having left school and at work away from her mother, she had feared typing VD in the middle of a letter. This had cleared up when she spent some time at home with her mother again, presumably being relieved of the anxious depression over separation from her mother.

These events – all associated with mixed affects of pleasurable sexual excitement, guilt, rejection and murderous anger (as in pushing another baby away in its pram) – appeared to have been revived as ruminative symptoms, when the patient was depressed many years after their original occurrence.

With Valerie and Grace, the compulsion to wash or avoid muck could easily be associated with their mothers' well-authenticated punitive and exacting toilet training. It is reasonable to suppose that this would have made Valerie murderously resentful because of the excessive control and interference in her life. Yet, though in the group and private interviews, after her leucotomy, she could say with immense feeling 'I could murder that woman', she was preoccupied with the fixed idea that she was 'so dirty that, when she died, she should be burned to nothing', that her urine might harm others and that she must wash and wash to be cleansed of it. Equally crockery should be washed according to a fastidious ritual and clothing must be ritualistically checked over.

Grace, who was depressed at almost any loss of a friend or rebuke, somewhat differently appeared to be avoiding being soiled. This had no doubt been demanded of her to an infuriating degree. Meanwhile she had also suffered the depressing death of her infuriating mother and continued trying to placate her by cleanliness under the shadow of guilty sadness.

Separated again, when at the Nursery Nursing School, and given the evocative task of 'potting' the infants, her childhood avoidance of muck appeared to be revived against a background of depression then and at many times of separation thereafter.

Not all of the 4 hand-washing or contamination-avoiding obsessionals amongst the 20 patients studied had clear histories of punitive early toilet training.

One 22-year-old single female orchestral violinist, Sarah James, whose excessive hand-washing had begun on her first tour abroad in America, had no such history. On this account she was not included amongst those numbered in the table as having compulsive activity related to past experience. It is also likely that many children subjected to punitive early toilet training do not develop obsessional states, for many sibs of obsessional patients are free of such conditions. A predisposition to 'fix' a certain behaviour pattern, in a manner such that it will later be revived in an exaggerated fashion, must be postulated. If, as it is argued here, the affective state is important, it must also be postulated that some individuals react to the exasperation associated with toilet training with an exaggerated affective response.

A fourth patient in this category – a 20-year-old female hotel clerk, Prudence Stamp – washed her hands in excess only for a few weeks before returning to normal washing, whilst becoming increasingly fastidious about the cleanliness of her home environment, clothes, etc. to the point at which her mother could only move by prescribed routes and in fashions determined by the patient. If the mother refused to conform, the patient would scream wildly until the neighbours complained. While the psychopathology of her symptoms was never elucidated in any detail, she recovered steadily when removed from home and treated with anti-depressant drugs.

Other patients exhibited very clear-cut histories of the 'fixing' or (in a wider sense than that implied in ethology) 'imprinting' of their symptoms.

A 14-year-old, highly intelligent boy, Adrian Harmer, had outbursts of rage and ruminated compulsively for six months on the idea that the earth was about to explode. At times he felt compelled to repeat poetry to himself 'to be sure he had not forgotten it'. His mother had died suddenly of a cerebral haemorrhage three years earlier. Though fond of him, he found his father a burden as he was extremely 'nervous', having suffered badly as a prisoner of war. Recently the boy had been worrying about important school examinations. He recalled reading Jules Verne's *Journey to the Centre of the Earth* (in which a volcanic eruption occurs) around the time of his mother's death.

Psychotherapeutic interviews enabled him to mourn his mother's death and express his anger towards his stifling father. His rages and ruminations disappeared and he has remained symptom-free for eight years. In this exceptional case there was a shorter latent period than usual between the 'imprinting' at a time of intense sadness and the revival of the symptoms with a later depressive episode. The boy had probably been depressed since his mother died but became more disturbed on account of his father's behaviour and the stress of school examinations.

It may well be suggested that the explosion of the earth had a special symbolical significance, in that it represented the catastrophe which overtook the mother. The compulsion to repeat poetry for the reason given may also have symbolically implied a wish not to risk 'letting go' of an idealized love-object.

It is noteworthy that the interpretation of these symptoms in treatment appeared to be insignificant beside the relief obtained by the patient when he was persistently led to talk about his mother and her death. This led to a period of much more obvious sadness in therapy sessions but the disappearance of the obsessional symptoms within a period of nine months.

General indecisiveness during illness was very definitely evident in 18 of the 20 patients studied; but it was not measured in any systematic way and this would be desirable in future studies – comparisons possibly being made with patients with somatic illnesses, other neuroses or depression without obsessionality. The obsessional patients clinically appeared different from otherwise depressed patients, in that they seemed able usually to accept an unequivocal proposal, e.g. that the next appointment should be at a certain time and place, when a severely depressed patient might express immediate doubts about coming at all or being able to wait so long. On the other hand, given a choice of appointments, the obsessional would find it difficult to decide which to accept, expressing the 'pros and cons', while the severely depressed patient would appear to lack the drive to consider the choice at all.

Indecisiveness was also considered in connection with the termination of a compulsive activity or rumination. From the accounts elicited from patients, who were closely studied, and their observed behaviour, it appeared that they often became preoccupied with a detail (e.g. washing a particular area) then developed a renewed uncertainty as to whether other things (e.g. washing of adjacent areas) had been accomplished satisfactorily. The whole procedure was repeated until it had been accomplished with full attention; then the patient terminated it. An accidental interruption by someone else would act like a 'preoccupation' episode and lead to full repetition of a washing ritual. Meanwhile, a deliberate, firm but friendly instruction from a well-known nurse or therapist could easily lead to the almost immediate termination of a ritualistic activity.

If a patient were left alone, her actual washing or checking time was usually predictable in a standard setting (e.g. washing before breakfast). The patient knew the usual time taken within a minute or two but seemed unable to shorten it, e.g. from 40 to 30 minutes, in order to arrive at a meal at the correct time. Presumably the 'preoccupation episodes' occurred about as often in the same setting from one day to another if the mood state was constant. Increased depression lengthened the 'ritual' time; from several patients' accounts it increased 'preoccupation' or inattention. Improvement in concentration of attention, consequent upon the alleviation of depression, may have accounted for reductions in ritual activity times, which occurred in these circumstances.

Paradoxical results of preoccupation with rituals could occur as, for example, when an adolescent boy accidentally fell from a tree, while reaching out to touch a certain branch in a compulsive manner. This episode not only illustrates the poor 'survival value' of excessive obsessionality, but also the degree of preoccupation with a compulsively determined task, which so often precluded the full attention to a series of operations, which was required before a ritual could be terminated.

Schizophrenic symptoms or signs did not occur in any of the 20 patients who were followed up for periods averaging seven years. The concept of 'obsessional neurosis masking or leading to schizophrenia' is perhaps questionable. Certainly some schizophrenics show compulsive phenomena and, when questioned, will readily say that they make certain movements or say certain things because 'they just feel they must', i.e. they are compulsive but *not* felt to be ordered by an outside agency. Such compulsive phenomena may constitute signs of illness early in schizophrenia, though they do *not* precede other pathognomonic signs; perhaps it is for this reason that the notion of obsessional neurosis leading to schizophrenia exists.

Fixity of behaviour patterns is, again, common in schizophrenia,

some patients adopting fixed postures, or dressing in the same stereotyped manner, exhibiting bizarre fragmented residues of their old selves
and seeming to play a single role in the same way regardless of reason
or circumstance. This degree of behavioural fixity does not appear to
occur in 'obsessional neurosis'. Though some generalized behavioural
limitation may occur – as with Rose's regression to 'little girl' postures,
movement and speech (all suggestive of hysteria rather than schizophrenia) – obsessionals retain far greater flexibility. Their adaptation
to social situations remains appropriate even if restricted by their
specific compulsions.

Some miscellaneous items requiring comment are not covered by the
table of characteristics of the patients studied above.

The remarkable recovery of Shirley Fleetway cannot adequately be
explained by the glib comment that obsessionals think magically (which,
in a sense, they do) and are therefore receptive to a magical cure (which
cannot be logically inferred). At the time of her recovery, Shirley had
had a period of intense anxiety over her son, which, with associated
loss of sleep, may have produced a neurophysiological state described
as the 'ultra paradoxical' phase of brain activity by Pavlov and cited by
William Sargant (1957, p. 12). Possibly this facilitated the sudden
change in direction of her hitherto 'fixed' behaviour patterns. While
it cannot be said that the phenomenon is fully understood, it is reasonable to suppose that a sudden major reorganization of brain-activity
occurred. This is particularly reasonable when we note that our
obsessional patients, who are allegedly in the grip of an overwhelming
compulsion, can so readily switch it off, if attention is *agreeably* occupied
(e.g. by talking with an accepted kindly therapist).

The compulsive thought or behaviour could be conceived as a
response to commonly occurring stimuli, which does not become extinguished spontaneously and cannot be extinguished by 'desensitization' procedures alone.

The psychological phenomenon of *attention* and the neurophysiological phenomena of *arousal* and *central inhibition* might then be important to our understanding of obsessional states. Attention to interesting matters facilitated by circumstances producing an agreeable
affective state may inhibit other signals from the environment and
memory stores, blocking the obsessional response.

Meanwhile a massive input of signals in certain circumstances (e.g. of
extreme fatigue) may, like 'religious conversion', reverse a group of
reflex responses, which, it is suggested in these patients, are obsessional
behaviour patterns.

Apart from the rare patients, in which sudden cure occurs without the simultaneous use of physical methods of treatment, it is a common observation in obsessionals, including hand-washing patients, that total changes of environment produce temporary improvements, providing no particularly depressing or anger-producing events occur. Thus Valerie Scott, taking a weekend holiday in an hotel, would find herself much less 'compelled' to wash excessively. A *prolonged* stay in a different environment seemed, however, to lead to the gradual return of symptoms with the same intensity as before.

It may tentatively be suggested that the psychologically 'exciting' and physiologically 'new' signals from a totally fresh environment lead to such central inhibition of commonplace signals from the environment and 'association areas' in the brain, that the 'reflex' obsessional behaviour response does not receive its usual stimulus until habituation to the 'new' environment signals has occurred, when inhibition of commonplace signals is reduced and their force in eliciting the previous behavioural response is restored.

FURTHER INFERENCES

All the studies described above were made upon patients referred to hospital. It appears highly likely that many obsessional patients, such as Shirley's father, live out many years or a lifetime without referral to a specialist or consulting a doctor at all. There is clearly room for detailed study of such non-complaining patients in general practice populations – certainly as to their individual characteristics and perhaps from an epidemiological point of view.

Within their obvious limits, these studies illuminate certain important aspects of obsessional patients:

1. *An innate proneness to obsessional disorder* is likely in view of the frequency of pre-morbid obsessional traits. The effect purely of nurture is unlikely in view of the frequent occurrence of non-obsessional sibs. Genetic determination of the tendency appears likely, though some other mechanism, e.g. an immediately post-natal disturbance and modification of the central nervous system, cannot be ruled out.

2. *A tendency to rigidity rather than instability of the vegetative as well as the sensori-motor nervous systems* seen in these patients requires further controlled study on large groups.

3. *Unusual proneness to depressive reactions and an unusual tendency to suppress anger* appears so common as to demand further prospective study.

D

4. *An onset of symptoms at the time of depression, suppression of anger or exasperation as inability to deal with a cause of anger* appears to be the rule.

5. *Recall of happenings* (associated in the past with depression, suppressed anger or exasperation) *which could plausibly be seen as the basis for the specific symptoms* is found in many patients, if they are studied carefully enough. The exceptions were confined to those few predominantly concerned with dirt and hand-washing. Two of these had highly punitive toilet training. The others *may* conceivably have suffered the ill effects of excessively early training or developed their symptoms purely on account of an abnormality of neurophysiological and psychic make-up. In defence of this concept, it would appear likely that toilet training produces the earliest and most repetitive 'collisions' between infantile and maternal wishes. It may therefore be argued that preoccupations with cleanliness may be especially deeply 'imprinted' in association with the anger engendered by this training. It follows that not *all* obsessionals are 'anally fixated', but *some* may have symptoms related to faeces or urine because of the 'collisions' producing anger, exasperation or depression. Other obsessionals, meanwhile, have totally different symptoms determined by other, and usually much later events, associated with these affective states. Patients with obsessional symptoms associated with toilet training may not readily recall the 'imprinting' events purely because they were so early in their lives.

6. *Fixity of behaviour was associated, not surprisingly, with difficulty over choices, apparent as indecision.* This could be more specifically measured. The factor of 'preoccupation' (i.e. abnormal limitation of 'attention') may be important especially with regard to terminating rituals.

7. *Obsessional states did not appear to be 'defences' against schizophrenia or anxiety.* Schizophrenia did not occur. Anxiety was not produced by unaggressive prevention of compulsive behaviour. Anxiety was not apparent when alleged 'de-conditioning' to anxiety associated with certain situations was carried out. Meanwhile the treatment was ineffective.

8. *Relief of depression or anger tended to relieve obsessional symptoms.* Ruminations and some rituals learned later in life (e.g. walking by certain routes, manipulating or recording numbers, or repeating poetry) were more readily simply given up with improvement of mood.

9. *Some patients required special training after normal mood was restored.* Hand-washing tended to persist after the restoration of normal mood state. Experience with one patient, Valerie Scott, showed that a

programme, rewarding non-compulsive behaviour and offering relief, but not punishment or permission to wash, when the compulsion was felt strongly, could eliminate a hand-washing compulsion. This returned when the patient was re-stimulated to marked anger and depression after leaving hospital.

A more recent experience (with Sarah James) has suggested that the hand-washing obsessional must first be restored to normal mood, then re-trained by *reward for success* in not washing and by *relief* from tension borne alone (e.g. by conversation with an understanding nurse). Relatively brief follow-up (six months) suggests this procedure is successful as long as a cheerful mood state is maintained.

Earlier 'implosion therapy', in which garments were heavily 'contaminated' by handling in front of the patient in her home, had led to some apparent decrease of concern about this particular matter. Meanwhile the patient had become increasingly angry and depressed. Relief of the depression by physical methods of treatment (tricyclic antidepressants and ECT) had not altered the hand-washing compulsion.

Experience with Valerie Scott and the last-mentioned patient, Sarah James, showed that hand-washing compulsions may exist even when depression has disappeared. Nevertheless the contention that the behaviour pattern is both 'imprinted' and revived during episodes when depression or anger are marked is not, on this account, disproved. It would seem likely that the compulsive behaviour pattern simply continues in some patients until they are taught by measures, not themselves evocative of anger or depression, to give up the behaviour, which, in these particular people, is not spontaneously extinguished.

Given this concept, it is then possible to explain why some patients are regarded as having 'obsessional states with depression', others 'pure obsessional states' and others 'recurrent obsessional states'. All three may be, in fact, particularly vulnerable to depressive mood swings (and often inclined to suppress anger). All that distinguishes them may be the phase, in which they are seen by the psychiatrist: some with obvious depression, some in a phase of recovery without extinction of the fixed compulsive behaviour and some over a series of depressive phases with re-activation of obsessional behaviour.

Among the patients described, recurrences of obsessional behaviour never occurred without depression or suppressed anger and it is doubtful if such recurrences ever occur without such affective disturbance. This may be of very limited duration. At least three patients have been observed, who only had compulsive symptoms in the pre-menstrual and menstrual period (Alapin, 1972). Obsessional activity within normal limits (e.g. tidying up to an unusual degree for that person) is common-place in the pre-menstrual period and some women predict the onset of menstruation on experiencing a compulsion to tidy the house.

It is possible that compulsive symptoms sometimes occur wholly as a 'depressive equivalent', i.e. without any gross manifestation of depression but in circumstances where depression might have been expected. (This phenomenon is occasionally seen in asthmatics, who appear to have a series of attacks as a substitute for depression, which appears absent until very careful inquiry reveals some mild features. Many respond well to the treatment of depression – both physical and psychotherapeutic.) It may also be that the failure of extinction of symptoms in some patients, with *apparent* recovery of mood, implies that full recovery of mood has not occurred at a physiological level.

Certainly these clinical studies emphasize the importance of the affective states of depression and suppressed anger in the *psyche*, which, in the obsessional patient, presumably *physiologically* involve the limbic system in a 'locking' effect, both 'imprinting' behaviour patterns and reviving them when these affective states are induced by other circumstances.

The overwhelming importance of the depressive mood state in *all* obsessional patients, as is suggested here may explain the striking improvements in patients with obsessional states recently attributed to clomipramine ('Anafranil') even in the alleged absence of depression (Capstick, 1971).

Whilst not reporting 'ideas of influence', characteristic of schizophrenia, many patients describe their symptoms remarkably objectively and as if they were dissociated from conscious 'reasoning' or control. The compulsive behaviour or thinking pattern seemed to be conceptualized more as an autonomic reasponse. Patients might say 'my checking is getting worse' just as otherwise healthy people might say 'my palpitations come on more often'. There was therefore an objective and subjective loss of control and limitation of the *appropriate adaptation* of behaviour, which normally characterizes the higher animals.

Only when the hypothetical limbic 'lock' was broken by restoration of normal mood state, did it seem possible to restore flexibility of behaviour patterns and for useless patterns to be extinguished spontaneously or by training (involving both reward and avoidance of exasperation).

From the psychotherapeutic viewpoint, it appeared relatively unimportant to study the 'meanings' of symptoms, which were often quite readily apparent to patients. Useful psychotherapy appeared to be that directed towards the expression of depression, mourning, anger or exasperation in the individual or group situation, and that directed towards easier communication and the avoidance of anger-provoking misinterpretations of comment and behaviour within families. Symptoms so often limited the lives of spouses etc., that they could be used for 'secondary gain' and expressing retaliatory anger. The psychotherapeutic improvements of family relationships was therefore essential to eliminate this motive for retaining symptoms.

It is questioned whether some psychoanalytic failures in the treatment of obsessional patients have arisen because of excessive preoccupation with symptoms and the elaboration of their 'meaning' rather than analysis of the behaviour patterns leading to depression. Moreover, as it would appear that, even where depression is eliminated, specific re-training is required in some patients to obtain extinction of symptoms, something more than analysis alone may often be required.

In view of their peculiar proneness to depressive reactions, it would also seem possible that re-training, specifically directed to produce non-depressive reactions to the ordinary upsets of everyday life, might be necessary for these particular patients.

CONCLUSION

Studies of 20 obsessional patients referred to hospital, many of whom were admitted and studied in great detail, suggest that 'fixed' behaviour and thought patterns are 'imprinted' and evoked by depression or suppressed anger. These patients tend to show overall 'fixity' of neurophysiological function. Psychologically they show rigidity and a tendency to become depressed very easily. Anxiety does *not* appear to be of fundamental importance.

The brain may be conceived (in Heinz Wolff's terms, 1971a) as itself the 'target organ' of the pathological interaction between patient and environment, which gives rise to depression or undischarged anger. The restoration of the function of the brain to normal is essential before the 'imprinted' thought or behaviour patterns either disappear or are amenable to elimination by training. The return of higher control which facilitates flexibility and adaptation appears in some way contingent upon the restoration of normal affect.

Re-training has nothing to do with relief of anxiety. Reward but never punishment (which may provoke anger and reinforce symptoms) should be used. Operant conditioning methods may prove helpful.

These patients need protection from depression and chronic anger. Psychotherapy directed towards cartharsis and improved communication in families and especially between husbands and wives is often desirable.

4

P. D. Slade

Psychometric studies of obsessional illness and obsessional personality

INTRODUCTION

Lewis and Mapother (1941), on the basis of their clinical observations of obsessional patients, concluded that:

> Very many obsessional patients have for years before they became ill shown a rather characteristic mental constitution; they are extremely clean, orderly, and conscientious, sticklers for precision, they have inconclusive ways of thinking and acting; they are given to needless repetition. Those who have shown such traits since childhood are often morose, obstinate, irritable people; others are vacillating, uncertain of themselves and submissive.

In this brief extract a number of crucial issues concerning obsessionality are raised. Firstly, a distinction between obsessional illness or neurosis, on the one hand, and obsessional personality traits on the other, is suggested. Secondly, a particular type of relationship between the two is implied; namely that a particular set of personality characteristics is the common precursor of an obsessional neurosis. Other investigators, notably Foulds (1965), have argued that the relationship is neither a necessary nor a sufficient one. And thirdly, Lewis and Mapother suggest that there may be more than one kind of obsessional personality constellation. Related to this point, but not mentioned by Lewis and Mapother, is the possibility that there may be more than one form of obsessional neurosis. These issues are all amenable to empirical test by the psychometric method. The appropriate techniques would seem to be factor analysis and correlational analysis.

Two further issues which are open to psychometric investigation should be briefly mentioned. Firstly, the nature of obsessional personality characteristics and their correlates; and secondly, the relationship between cultural, social, and demographic variables and psychometric assessments of obsessionality. Group-difference and correlational studies would seem to be the preferred methods for such investigations.

In the following account an attempt will be made to summarize and evaluate evidence from a variety of psychometric studies in relation to the issues raised above.

OBSESSIONAL NEUROSIS AND OBSESSIONAL PERSONALITY

Foulds (1965), in line with his general thesis concerning classification, argues for the importance of distinguishing between 'symptoms and signs' of personal illness on the one hand, and personality 'traits and attitudes' on the other. Three criteria are suggested for making this distinction, namely:

1. Traits and attitudes are universal; symptoms and signs are not.
2. Traits and attitudes are relatively ego-syntonic; symptoms and signs are distressful, either to the patient or to his closest associates.
3. Traits and attitudes, particularly the former, are relatively enduring.

With respect to the problem of obsessionality, the second of Foulds' criteria has probably been the most widely used. Marks (1965), for example, distinguished between obsessional symptoms and traits on the basis of whether the particular behaviour helped the individual or hindered him. If it helped, it was a trait, if it hindered him, it became a symptom.

The experimental studies of Foulds and Caine (Foulds and Caine, 1958, 1959; Foulds, 1959) in distinguishing between obsessional illness and obsessional personality will be reviewed in the next section. Let us consider now evidence from factorial studies. Two points must be made about the techniques of factor analysis before proceeding further. Firstly, factor-analytic methods provide no more than a means of simplifying correlational data, of reducing a large matrix of inter-correlations to a smaller and more manageable set of cluster of correlations or factors. The factors themselves may have no basis in reality. Secondly, what emerges from a factor analysis is entirely dependent upon what is put into it. Leaving aside the thorny question of what precise technique to use (and there are many alternatives), selection of both items and subjects will have a large influence on the findings. Thus, if a sample of hospitalized psychoneurotic patients is rated simply on a set of *obsessional symptom* scales, one might expect to get out an *obsessional-symptom* factor, but not an *obsessional-trait* factor. Conversely, if a group of normal people were rated on a set of obsessional *trait* scales, one might expect to discover from the analysis an *obsessional-trait* factor but not an *obsessional-symptom* factor. The question of selection of both items and subjects would seem to be fundamental when evaluating the findings of factorial studies of obsessional symptoms and traits. For a more comprehensive discussion of factorial methodology, the reader is referred to Lawley and Maxwell (1963).

O'Connor (1953) carried out a factor analysis on 67 symptoms rated in a sample of 300 male psychoneurotic out-patients. Of the eight factors he identified in his final analysis, only one represented an obsessive–compulsive reaction. Lorr, Rubinstein and Jenkins (1953) obtained a similar result on a sample of 184 veteran patients receiving psychotherapy. However, in both these studies obsessional-trait items were not included in the final analysis. In a further study Lorr and Rubinstein (1956) carried out a factorial analysis of 50 of the 61 items of the MSRPP rated on a group of 215 non-psychotic World War II and Korean veteran patients. Of the ten first-order factors identified, one (a bipolar factor) was interpreted as representing a character trait of 'obsessive conscientiousness', while another was interpreted as the 'obsessive–compulsive' reaction factor previously identified. Two second-order factors emerged from the analysis: one is loosely describable as 'anxiety-tension' and the other as 'hostility-resentment'. Of interest is the fact that the obsessive–compulsive symptom items tended to load on the 'anxiety-tension' factor, while the obsessive trait items tended to load on the 'hostility-resentment' factor. This study, therefore, provides evidence not only for separate obsessive symptom and obsessive trait factors, but also for their relative independence. The two second-order factors would also seem to bear some resemblance to Lewis and Mapother's two 'obsessional personality' descriptions.

Sandler and Hazari (1960) analysed the responses of 100 patients (50 males, 50 females) to the Tavistock Self-Assessment Inventory (Sandler, 1954). They extracted from the data the patients' self-ratings on a set of 40 items relating to obsessional–compulsive character traits and symptoms and subjected them to a centroid factor analysis. Two orthogonal factors emerged (accounting for 14·95 per cent and 7·61 per cent of the total variance), which were then rotated through 45 degrees. The first factor was identifiable as representing 'obsessional character traits' while the second clearly represented 'obsessional symptoms'. On the basis of the factor loadings, Sandler and Hazari were able to give a clear description of the type of individual obtaining high scores on each of the two factors. Since the descriptions are of considerable interest they are presented in full below.

Factor A (obsessional character traits): Picture of an exceedingly systematic, methodical and thorough person, who likes a well-ordered mode of life, is consistent, punctual, and meticulous in his use of words. He dislikes half-done tasks, and finds interruptions irksome. He pays much attention to detail and has a strong aversion to dirt.

Factor B (obsessional symptoms): Person whose daily life is disturbed through the intrusion of unwanted thoughts and impulses into his conscious experience. Thus he is compelled to do things which his reason tells him are unnecessary, to perform certain rituals as part of his everyday behaviour, to memorize trivia, and to struggle with persistent 'bad' thoughts. He tends to worry over his past actions, to brood over ideas, and finds himself getting behind with things. He has difficulty in making up his mind, and he has inner resistance to commencing work.

It can be seen that the two descriptions fit quite well with Foulds' 'ego-syntonic distressful' criterion.

Cooper and Kelleher (1972) carried out a principal component analysis of the responses of normal subjects to the Leyton Obsessional Inventory (Cooper and McNeil, 1968; Cooper, 1970). This inventory consists of 69 self-assessed obsessional items, which are divided into 46 symptom and 23 trait items on the basis of their apparent 'ego-syntonic/distressful' nature. Four separate analyses were conducted on various combinations of the original criterion groups (Cooper, 1970) and the Irish and English subjects from Kelleher's study (Kelleher, 1970). The four subject groups were English men and women combined (N = 140); Irish men and women combined (N = 73); English and Irish men (N = 168); and English and Irish women (N = 134). Three components were common to all four analyses and were concerned with being 'clean and tidy', 'a feeling of incompleteness', and 'checking'. Two other components kept appearing in 'recognizably similar form' which, although more difficult to characterize, seem to be concerned with 'having unpleasant or gloomy thoughts' and 'being methodical'. Although Cooper and Kelleher rightly point out that these factors should be considered personality traits as the analyses were performed on 'psychiatrically normal' people, it is clear that at least two of the item-clusters resemble descriptions of obsessional symptoms in a milder form.

In contrast to the Lorr and Rubinstein and Sandler and Hazari studies, therefore, the Cooper and Kelleher study suggests the existence of more than one obsessional-trait factor and, perhaps, more than one obsessional-symptom factor. Two methodological differences may account for this discrepancy. In the first place, Cooper and Kelleher analysed data based on 69 obsessional items, while Sandler and Hazari used only 40 items relating to obsessionality, and only a proportion of Lorr and Rubinstein's 50 items were obsessional in nature. If the latter sets of investigators had included more items they might have found more than one 'trait' and one 'symptom' factor. The second major difference between the Cooper and Kelleher and the other studies concerns the statistical tool used. Cooper and Kelleher used principal component analysis which, while being very neat mathematically, does not take into account errors of measurement .With psychological variables which are especially vulnerable to error one must necessarily be cautious in interpreting the results. In contrast, the other investigators used factor-analytic methods which start with the assumption that error is involved. The reader is referred once again to Lawley and Maxwell (1963). However, in the present case, the different results are probably not due to difference in statistical technique, as Cooper and Kelleher have obtained almost identical solutions using factorial analysis.

To conclude, in both external rating and self-assessment studies in which both obsessional-trait and obsessional-symptom items have been included, factorial analysis suggests separate trait and symptom factors. Whether a single trait and a single symptom factor emerge, or a number of both, is probably dependent on the range of behaviour studied.

THE RELATION OF OBSESSIONAL SYMPTOMS TO OBSESSOID PERSONALITY TRAITS

Slater and Slater (1944), in an investigation of neurotic soldiers during the Second World War, found a correlation of +0·8 between clinically observed obsessional–compulsive symptoms and obsessoid personality traits; this correlation was substantially higher than that for any of the other corresponding pairs of symptoms and traits they studied. Likewise, Ingram (1961a), in a clinical study of 77 in-patients with severe obsessional states, found evidence of pre-morbid obsessional personality traits in 84 per cent of his group of patients. He therefore concluded that obsessional personality and illness are intimately connected.

Sandler and Hazari (1960), on the basis of their factor-analytic study previously described, argue for quite a different type of relationship. They suggest that their Factor A probably represents a set of person- ality characteristics which are quite independent of obsessional illness: that their Factor B, on the other hand, probably represents a continuum ranging from obsessional character (in its mildest form) to obsessional illness (in its severest form). It follows from this argument that the relationship between obsessional traits and symptoms will depend entirely on how the obsessional traits are defined.

Perhaps the largest body of evidence on the relationship between obsessional symptoms and obsessoid personality comes from the work of Foulds and Caine. In line with their central thesis concerning the necessity of a double classificatory scheme (i.e. illness and personality), Foulds and Caine (1958) gave a battery of tests and questionnaires to a group of 68 female neurotic patients, classified in respect to both psychiatric diagnosis (hysteric or dysthymic) and personality type (hysteroid or obsessoid). Their findings indicated that some of the measures differentiated between hysterics and dysthymics, regardless of personality type, while others differentiated between hysteroids and obsessoids regardless of diagnostic category. They noted that approxi- mately 50 per cent of the dysthymics were rated as having a hysteroid personality (however, only a small percentage of these were diagnosed as suffering from an obsessional illness). A similar general finding emerged from a second study by Foulds and Caine (1959) using a group of neurotic men, although the discriminating measures were different for this group. In another study Foulds (1959) attempted to test the proposition that, while diagnostic classification would tend to change over time, personality classification would not. NB. Foulds' third criterion for distinguishing between traits and symptoms. Evidence from a one-month test–retest study was found to bear out this hypoth- esis. In a later study using the HOQ (hysteroid–obsessoid question- naire) Foulds (1965) found a reasonably high correlation between self- assessments of hysteroid–obsessoid personality traits and external ratings of this personality dimension ($r = +0.68$) but a fairly low significant correlation with hysteric-dysthymic diagnosis ($r = +0.28$).

In conclusion, while clinical studies tend to show a close corre- spondence between obsessional illness and obsessoid personality, psychometric studies suggest that the relationship may be a somewhat weaker one and that it may depend largely on the way in which the obsessoid personality is defined. One possible reason for the discrepancy between clinical and psychometric studies may reside in the investi- gatory methods used. Clinical studies tend to rely on retrospective assessments of pre-morbid personality, whereas psychometric methods utilize concomitant investigation of illness and personality variables. The retrospective method may facilitate the discovery of similarities while the psychometric method may emphasize discrepancies.

THE NATURE OF OBSESSIONALITY AND ITS CORRELATES

In this section attention will be focused on three types of studies, namely:

1. studies employing special instruments designed to tap obsessionality,
2. studies aimed at relating obsessionality to more general parameters of personality such as extraversion/introversion and neuroticism, and
3. studies aimed at identifying more specific traits of obsessionality.

1. *Studies employing special obsessionality instruments*

Following Sandler and Hazari's factor-analytic study, some investigators have attempted to use their 40 items as a standard obsessionality instrument. Reed (1969) administered the Sandler–Hazari items to 20 patients with obsessional symptoms, to 20 patients with obsessional traits but without symptoms, and to 20 control patients matched for sex ratio. No significant differences were found between the three groups either with respect to the total 40 items or with respect to their 16 type 'A' items or their 17 type 'B' items. On the basis of this finding Reed criticizes the Sandler–Hazari study for both their selection of patients (i.e. they were unselected psychoneurotic patients) and their selection of obsessionality items. However, in fairness to the latter, it should be pointed out that they were not attempting to develop a standard obsessionality inventory, nor does Reed's result necessarily invalidate Sandler and Hazari's identification of two factors.

Orme (1965) administered 13 items of Sandler–Hazari's type 'B' (obsessional symptoms), together with Cattell's 13-item 'O' factor scale (emotional instability), to a variety of psychiatric groups and a normal group. The results indicated significant correlations between the two scales for both normals ($+0.518$) and obsessional and phobic patients ($+0.514$). On neither of the scales were the small groups of obsessional and phobic patients found to differ significantly. Orme concluded that 'the obsessional personality is, in fact, a personality that has general features of emotional instability'.

In a closely related study, Kline (1967) administered the MMPI, the Sandler–Hazari 16 type 'A' and 17 type 'B' items, and the Beloff (1957) test of anal obsessional traits to a group of 93 normal subjects. Six factors were extracted from a rotated factor analysis, three of which are relevant to the present discussion, namely:

Factor 1: general emotional instability
Factor 2: obsessional character traits, and
Factor 4: social introversion.

The Sandler–Hazari type 'A' items (traits) were found to load highly on the second factor, while their type 'B' items (symptoms) were found to load on the fourth factor. This finding was interpreted as supporting Foulds' sign-symptom/trait dichotomy. The fact that none of the obsessionality measures loaded substantially on the 'general emotional instability' factor was interpreted as being contrary to Orme's thesis, at least with respect to a normal population.

Another instrument which has been used to measure obsessionality is the HOQ (hysteroid–obsessoid questionnaire) of Foulds (Caine and Hawkins, 1963; Foulds, 1965). The HOQ consists of 48 self-assessment items which are scored in either a hysteroid or an obsessoid direction. Foulds (1965) quotes a test–retest reliability for the scale of +0·77 (over a six-week period), and an external validity correlation of +0·68. Barrett, Caldbeck-Meenan and White (1966) gave the HOQ, together with the MPI and a structured interview, to 98 territorial army personnel. They found that both the HOQ and the MPI 'E' scale correlated significantly with ratings by a TA psychiatrist along the hysteroid–obsessoid personality continuum. Furthermore, there was a highly significant correlation (+0·66) between the HOQ and the MPI 'E' scale. A similar result emerged from the study of Forbes (1969). He administered the HOQ together with Cattel's 16 PF questionnaire, to a mixed group of 58 neurotic and psychotic patients. On the basis of the HOQ scores the patients were then divided into a 'hysteroid' and an 'obsessoid' group and the two groups compared on the 16 PF scales. The 5 scales which discriminated the groups significantly all contribute to the second-order factor, extraversion, the obsessoid group obtaining lower mean scores on these scales. The overall correlation between the HOQ and the second-order PF factor of extraversion was found to be +0·79. Thus, there is evidence from these two studies of a very strong relationship between extraversion–introversion and the HOQ. This is in fact borne out by the data presented by Foulds and his co-workers (Foulds, 1965). They report correlations between the HOQ and the

MPI 'E' scale of $+0.84$ for 53 neurotics and of $+0.81$ for 35 normals. These correlations, it should be noted, are slightly higher than the test–retest reliability coefficient for the HOQ. From these data, therefore, it seems unlikely that the HOQ is tapping any specific variance which is not measured by tests of extraversion–introversion, such as the MPI 'E' scale.

A third special obsessionality inventory which has recently been developed is the Leyton Obsessional Inventory (Cooper and MacNeil, 1968; Cooper, 1970). This consists of 69 obsessional items, 46 symptom and 23 trait. As well as providing a wider coverage than previous inventories, it has the added advantage of two intensity scales ('resistance' and 'interference'), designed to tap the degree of resistance experienced by the subject to the symptoms and the extent of any resulting interference with other activities. It has been standardized on criterion groups of 17 obsessional patients, 25 house-proud housewives, and 60 normal women and 41 normal men, producing highly significant differences between the groups. The 'resistance' and 'interference' scales have been found particularly useful in discriminating between low-scoring obsessional patients and high-scoring normals. Preliminary test–retest reliability data are encouraging. One of the problems of the inventory noted by Cooper is its possible susceptibility to a non-specific 'complaint effect', similar to that noted by Orme (1965, 1968) for the Sandler–Hazari items. Cooper found high correlations between both 'symptom' and 'trait' scores and a shortened version of the Cornell Health Inventory, while Kendell and DiScipio (1970) found correlations of $+0.53$ and $+0.48$, respectively, between these two measures and the EPI 'N' scale, in a sample of 60 depressed patients after recovery from illness.

In conclusion, of the three special obsessionality inventories discussed, the Leyton Obsessional Inventory would seem to be the best because of both its wide coverage and its inclusion of intensity scales. One of the prominent features of all three is the high correlations with measures of introversion–extraversion and neuroticism. Let us then consider the relationship between obsessionality and these more general dimensions of personality more closely.

2. *The relation of obsessionality to neuroticism and extraversion–introversion*

The evidence relating obsessionality to these two general personality parameters comes from two sources, namely correlational and group-difference studies. The correlational data has been presented earlier and can be briefly summarized. A number of independent studies have produced significant positive correlations between obsessionality measures and a measure of neuroticism or emotional instability (i.e. Orme, 1965; Forbes, 1969; Cooper, 1970; Kendell and DiScipio, 1970) while a number of independent studies have found significant negative correlations between obsessionality measures and a measure of extraversion (i.e. Foulds, 1965; Barrett *et al.*, 1966; Kline, 1967; Forbes, 1969; Kendell and DiScipio, 1970; Rachman and Hodgson, 1971). In some cases the magnitude of the correlations is so great as to account almost entirely for the variance measured by the specific obsessionality inventories.

The second source of evidence comes from the group-difference studies of Eysenck and his co-workers and is an integral part of his personality theory. In the Eysenckian system two orthogonal dimensions are used to account for the psychoneuroses, namely neuroticism and extraversion–introversion. Hysterical and psychopathic disorders are classed as disorders of the neurotic extrovert while dysthymic disorders, including obsessional–compulsive disorder, are classed as disorders of the neurotic introvert. Despite the early controversy concerning the strength of the evidence (Sigal, Starr and Franks, 1958; Eysenck, 1958; Hamilton, 1959a; Eysenck, 1959a; Hamilton, 1959b) it would seem to be overwhelmingly in support of this descriptive system (Eysenck, 1957, 1959b, 1960; Eysenck and Claridge, 1962). This is particularly true in relation to the position of the obsessional neurotic within the two-dimensional framework. One glance at the manuals of the Maudsley Personality Inventory (Eysenck, 1959c) and the Eysenck Personality Inventory (Eysenck and Eysenck, 1964) reveals that the obsessional neurotic group is characterized by high N and low E scores relative to the normal group.

One study which appeared to be at variance with the system placing obsessional–compulsive and hysterical patients at opposite ends of a neurotic introversion–extraversion dimension was that of Hamilton (1957b). He administered a battery of 11 tests of perceptual ambiguity to 22 patients with anxiety states, 20 obsessionals, 20 conversion hysterics, and 40 normal control subjects. Of the 15 measures of perceptual conflict avoidance, the obsessionals and hysterics differed significantly on only 3 while the obsessionals and anxiety state patients differed significantly on 6. On the basis of these results, Hamilton attacks Eysenck's concept of dysthymia as a homogeneous entity and argues for a similar position of the hysterics and obsessionals on the introversion–extraversion dimension. The basic flaw in this interpretation seems to revolve around what is being measured by the tests of perceptual ambiguity. If they really do measure the extraversion–introversion dimension, then Hamilton's results must be considered a considerable embarrassment to Eysenck's system. However, it seems more likely that Hamilton's tests were measuring the neuroticism dimension, in which case Hamilton's results are quite consistent with other findings in this area.

In conclusion, there seems to be overwhelming evidence that a strong relationship exists between obsessionality and measures of neuroticism and extraversion–introversion; to put it another way, that the obsessional neurotic patient is a neurotic introvert.

3. Specific traits of obsessionality

Surprisingly few psychological studies seem to have focused on more specific traits of obsessionality. Asch (1958) found that the tendency to disagree (negative response set bias) is related to obsessive–compulsive traits; while Langer (1962) found that college students scoring high on a supposed index of compulsivity (the Dd factor in the Structured Objective Rorschach Test, O'Reilly, 1956) showed reduced flexibility in terms of a tendency to change their responses over time. Related to the Langer finding are the more recent studies of Reed (1969a, b). He found that patients with anancastic (obsessional) personality disorders, when compared with matched groups of psychiatric and normal controls, tended to over-define or over-specify both their verbal and nonverbal concepts, a tendency which Reed refers to as under-inclusion. However, this tendency might equally be conceptualized as one of reduced conceptual flexibility.

The psychoanalytic concept of the 'anal character' (the triad of obstinacy, parsimony and orderliness) has stimulated a number of psychometric studies. Barnes (1952) factor-analysed items thought to pertain to 'anal' characteristics and discovered no factor common to them. The Krout Personal Preference Scale (Krout and Tabin, 1954), which obtains a measure of the 'anal' character, suffered a similar fate. However, evidence of factorial validity for the 'anal' scales of the Dynamic Personality Inventory (Grygier, 1961) has been reported both by Barron (1955) and Kline (1968b), while Beloff (1957) developed an 'anal' scale, measuring a single general factor and having some degree of external validity as assessed by ratings by other people. While there is, therefore, some evidence for a syndrome of 'anal' traits, the evidence concerning psychoanalytic aetiology is sparse or contradictory. Kline (1968a) found positive correlations between the Beloff scale, the Sandler–Hazari symptom scale, his own 'anal' scale (A13), and a measure of 'anality' derived from the Blacky Pictures Test (Blum, 1949). However, it is not clear to what extent internal contamination may have contributed to this result.

In conclusion, there is some meagre evidence to suggest that obsessionality is associated with a tendency to disagree and to show decreased flexibility. In addition, there is some evidence for the coalescence of supposed anal character traits, although very little support for the psychoanalytic theory of its aetiology.

THE RELATIONSHIP OF OBSESSIONALITY TO CULTURAL, SOCIAL AND DEMOGRAPHIC VARIABLES

As far as the writer is aware only one cross-cultural study of psychometric differences in obsessionality has so far been undertaken; namely, the impressive and well-conducted study of Kelleher (1970). Kelleher administered the Leyton Obsessional Inventory to 72 English orthopaedic in-patients in London hospitals, to 73 Irish orthopaedic in-patients in hospitals in Cork, and to 12 Irish immigrant orthopaedic in-patients in London hospitals. The resulting data were analysed both in terms of quantitative and qualitative differences in obsessionality scores, which were then related to a fairly wide range of cultural, social and demographic variables.

1. *Quantitative differences*

The Irish obtained significantly higher scores than the English on both the symptom and trait items and also on the combined resistance and interference index. Thus, the evidence suggests that not only do the Irish have more obsessional symptoms and traits than the English, but that they are also more distressed by them. The Irish immigrants obtained similar scores to their kith at home. On closer inspection, it was found that the higher overall scores of the Irish were directly ascribable to a set of 23 symptom and trait items. Kelleher noted that these 23 highly discriminating items fall neatly into 4 categories; namely, a tendency to be preoccupied with personal cleanliness, a tendency to be house-proud, a tendency to have obsessional difficulty in decision-making and, lastly, a tendency to be disturbed by obsessional fears and phobias.

2. *Qualitative differences*

Separate principal component analyses were conducted on the English and Irish data. Of the first 5 components identified, 4 were common to both populations (i.e. 'methodical', 'checking', 'perfectionist' and 'regularity of function'). The fifth English factor, unnamed by Kelleher, seems to represent an amalgam of compulsive and hoarding items. While the fifth Irish factor, which had no obvious counterpart among the English group of factors, was named by Kelleher as 'obsessional doubt'. Thus, while there is evidence of similarity in the pattern of obsessionality in English and Irish populations, there is also some suggestion of at least one qualitative difference. These factors, however, must be regarded with caution in the light of the principal component analyses conducted by Cooper and Kelleher (1972) on much larger groups of subjects.

3. *Cultural, social and demographic differences*

A series of cross-cultural comparisons revealed that the significant differences between the English and Irish on the various obsessionality scores could *not* be accounted for by differences in:

    i) age (although within both groups age was negatively related to obsessionality scores)
    ii) type of injury
    iii) number of previous accidents
    iv) length of time in hospital
    v) previous physical or psychiatric illness
    vi) social class
    vii) type of religion
    viii) regularity of religious practice
    ix) number of siblings
    x) birth order
    xi) length of schooling
    xii) number of examinations passed
    xiii) occupational differences (in males)

However, within the Irish group three variables did seem to be related to obsessionality scores, namely:

i) Irish males who were unmarried obtained higher obsessionality scores than those who were married; and more Irish males were unmarried than English males.

ii) Irish females, who were rural dwellers, obtained higher obsessionality scores than those who lived in towns; once again there was a cultural difference with respect to this variable.

iii) Irish women who did not work outside the home scored higher than Irish women who did. A cultural difference was also observed with respect to this variable. As noted by Kelleher these three variables would all seem to have the effect of isolating the individual within the community. Whether such a tendency to isolation is a causative factor in determining obsessionality, or purely an effect, cannot of course be resolved from the simple observation of correlation.

In conclusion, Kelleher's study suggests that there are quantitative, and perhaps also qualitative differences in obsessionality between the English and Irish; and that the tendency for more obsessionality in the Irish may be related to cultural factors predisposing to greater isolation of the individual within the community.

GENERAL DISCUSSION AND CONCLUSIONS

A number of points seem worthy of discussion. Firstly, the evidence presented seems to support fairly strongly the distinction between obsessional personality traits and obsessional neurosis. The identification of separate trait and illness factors, in line with Foulds' 'ego-syntonic/distressful' criterion, would seem to have important implications for both classification and treatment. Let us consider the hypothetical case of two middle-aged housewives, who both report extreme concern with cleanliness and order. Female A spends a lot of time cleaning and tidying her home and is extremely proud of this; she is in no way distressed by her obsession with cleanliness and order, nor are her husband and children. Female B, on the other hand, equally spends a lot of time in cleaning and tidying her home; however, she is distressed by her obsession with dirt and order, is unable to resist it, and finds that it interferes with her everyday life. Her husband and children are equally distressed by her obsessional concern and behaviour. From the point of view of classification, it would seem absurd to apply the same label to both these women. Equally, it would be absurd to suggest that both are in need of treatment. The essential point would seem to be that neither the classification of obsessionality nor the indications for its treatment can be based solely on the observation of a person's behavioural repertoire (i.e. what he does). The effect of a person's behaviour on himself and on other people must be taken into account.

This point has largely been ignored in the development of specific tests of obsessionality, the notable exception being the inclusion of intensity scales in the Leyton Obsessional Inventory.

In the second place, the Cooper and Kelleher principal component analysis of the Leyton Obsessional Inventory suggested the possibility of a number of relatively independent clusters of obsessional symptoms as opposed to the single factor which has been identified by other workers. If this finding of multiple factors is replicated in further studies with obsessional patients, then it would seem to have an important implication for treatment. Namely, that not one but a number of different treatments may be necessary for dealing effectively with obsessional illness. Modification studies should therefore attempt to relate the treatment method to the type of obsessional symptoms with which it is effective.

Finally, the strong relationship between obsessional illness and neurotic introversion seems to be beyond doubt. In view of this, Kelleher's findings with regard to the cultural differences correlating with the higher obsessional scores of the Irish are of some interest. He found that the cultural factors which were related to increased obsessionality were those which would seem to lead to greater isolation of the individual within the community. And, by definition, one would expect the social introvert to be more isolated socially. The important question which is raised by these findings, of course, is the direction of the relationship between obsessionality and social isolation. Does social isolation predispose individuals towards obsessional illness, or does obsessional behaviour tend to isolate people socially? The answer to this question lies in the realms of future research.

PART TWO

Theory and Experiment

5

H. R. Beech and J. Perigault[1]

Toward a theory of obsessional disorder

Notional theorizing about the phenomena of obsessional disturbances has tended to dominate the description, explanation and treatment of afflicted patients. Such ideas have proved to be of little consequence, suffering, as they do, from all the defects of weak theories. Clearly what is required, and especially needed in the context of the disorder under consideration here, is a new and more adequate theoretical conception which is founded upon experimental study and directly related to the observed disabilities to be explained. Such conceptions are rare (Walker and Beech, 1969; Milner, Beech and Walker, 1971), but the recent revival of interest in obsessional behaviour has encouraged several authors to attempt the task. We would argue, however, that any new approach should not begin by stretching an existing theoretical framework to account for superficial impressions of the disorder. Behaviour therapists, for example, are especially prone to extend an over-simplified account of human functioning to new and inadequately researched topics (see for example, Wolpe and Lazarus, 1966) in an unhelpful way. While advocating objectivity and experimental analysis, both of which are strongly in the behaviourist tradition, we would stress the need for detailed application to the task of finding out more about what we wish our theory to explain, and this implies receptivity to all the available information, however puzzling and apparently contradictory, and often requires a lengthy period of uncontrolled observation. Out of these data the experimentalist will strive, by a process of induction, to introduce some system and order. The theory advanced by Beech and Perigault (1971) is an attempt to implement the

[1] Mr Perigault is supported in his research by the British Council and by Caja de Seguro Social, Republic of Panama.

principles to which reference has just been made. The basic data which were considered to be important came from an inquiry conducted by Walker (1967) and reported in part at a later date (Walker and Beech, 1969), and followed up by other experimental work by Milner, Walker and Beech (1971) and by Liddell and Beech (see Chap. 6). The findings and observations which seem to be of special interest might be briefly set out as follows:

First, paradoxes are evident in several aspects of the functioning of obsessional patients in which, for example, 'unavoidable' performance of rituals is sometimes completely suspended by the patient, or experiences which the obsessional might claim would lead inevitably to a ritualistic activity are sometimes disregarded. Furthermore, on occasions the patient might engage in a deliberate and purposeful act of contamination or, alternatively, show a degree of concern about some remotely possible contamination experience which is greatly exaggerated, even for patients of this kind. Such findings serve to erode any notion of the existence of a simple mechanical connection between some external event and a 'washing habit' (ritual).

It would not be unreasonable to argue (Beech, 1971) that such ordinary and typical misfortunes and vicissitudes as a slight or insult, a mild disappointment or criticism, and so on, seem to have a more profound effect (i.e. produce a more serious deterioration in mood state) in obsessional patients than in others. Furthermore, it seems that such changes, once induced, can show an unusual degree of perseverance in this group, and the question arises as to the mechanisms by which this enhanced intensity and endurance of emotional state comes about. The fluctuations and changes in mood are often well illustrated by patients' own descriptions of their problem. Mrs A., for example, reported that when her husband was about to make love to her ' . . . something quite trivial might happen . . . I might just bump my leg on something . . . and my mood changes completely to rage'. Or again ' . . . often things seem to take over my whole body . . . a tremendous intensity . . . even something ordinary like giving flowers to someone. . . .' Often it happens that the appearance of a pathological mood state seems not to be prompted by or related to any environmental event, although one cannot be certain of this. Such observations are of special interest and serve to emphasize two main conclusions which might be drawn. In the first place they suggest the primacy of mood in the causal chain which culminates in the performance of an obsessional ritual. Secondly, the cognitions which appear as part of the obsessional complex might be seen as *post hoc* accounts offered by the patients as a means of explaining the subjective experience of disturbance. In other words the individual who is subject to massive, unsolicited mood changes is prompted to explain these experiences and, in the absence of any 'real' external cause, will create a fiction or pathological idea (such as that concerning some source of contamination) and abnormalities of overt behaviour (e.g. rituals or avoidance behaviour) which are consistent with these ideas. Such a model certainly accords with the history of the disturbance which many patients provide, in which a deterioration of mood states has continued over a period of time until a certain critical level is reached. At this point in time some event, quite fortuitously it may seem, becomes linked with the intense arousal. Typical of such links is the description given by one patient in which, following a period of weeks characterized by feelings of increased disturbance, he had to swerve to avoid having an accident while on his motorcycle. From that moment the idea that he might unintentionally kill someone became insistent and 'irresistible' and, from that time, it became necessary first for him to check that such an accident had not occurred and, later, to check that the mere possibility of such an accident should not arise.

Such an account is not incompatible with the details of cases quoted by clinicians adopting a very different standpoint (Freud, 1948). However, the significance (symbolic value) attaching to the cue to pathological arousal (e.g. the 'rat' story told by Captain M.) has assumed an undeserved importance in analytical accounts and this has led to the tortuous, colourful, and insubstantial theoretical structures with which the reader is familiar.

In essence what we have in our own theory are two important elements; a predisposition to states of pathological arousal and some mechanism by which such a state leads to morbid thoughts and aberrant behaviour. Beech (1971) and Perigault have argued that the special conditions required for the development of obsessional ideas and behaviours might be described if we appeal to the evidence concerning habituation, the so-called Napalkov effect, and certain associative possibilities. The position adopted by us was that obsessionals are characterized by a tendency to exaggerated arousal and that such states may reach critical levels at which, instead of decrement being observed, additional stimulation may produce increased arousal. Such augmentation could arise if any stimulation is provided during the 'recovery' period from some previous stimulation, and any organism characterized by a slow recuperation would remain vulnerable for a longer period of time. Individuals who are susceptible to high arousal and slow recovery from stimulation might also be expected to show an increased number of spontaneous fluctuations of arousal state, thus creating more opportunities for special conditioning effects of the kind where the exceptional state of the organism becomes attached to discriminable environmental cues. These tendencies to pathology were seen by us as being relatively enduring so that, while attempts to disconnect ritualistic behaviour from certain specific cues might lead to temporary success, the basic vulnerability of the unstable arousal system is constantly providing further opportunities for pathological connection-forming. On the other hand, as we pointed out, there may be possibilities for useful therapy which aims at massive exposure to threatening stimuli (implosion) for obsessionals as their existing high state of arousal could take them closer to an emotional refractory phase, and the method outlined later in this book (see Meyer *et al.*) might derive its efficacy in this way. These theoretical conceptions depend, of course, upon the character and quality of the evidence which might be adduced in support of them. Much of this evidence comes from the study of Walker and Beech (1969), in which it is deduced from the data that in obsessional disorder the problem lies in the pathology of mood states or, translating this into preferred terminology, aberrations of the arousal system, which are basic to the development of those pathologies so characteristic of the condition. Such evidence is reviewed in some detail in Chapter 6 and will not be re-stated here.

However, other evidence concerning the elements involved in the theory, namely habituation, sensitization and the Napalkov effect, as well as those aspects of conditioning which seem to be relevant, require separate description and it is pertinent, therefore, briefly to recount the experimental status of these findings and phenomena which have led us to modify our earlier formulation.

HABITUATION

Habituation may be defined operationally in several different ways, and the criterion selected can be a product of technical convenience or personal preference. For example, among the criteria of habituation which have been used are the absence of response in 'n' consecutive trials, the slope of the regression line, the achievement of an asymptotic level of responsivity, the rank order correlation between response magnitude and the order of the tones, or decrements in certain variables such as the spontaneous fluctuations. Such plurality of criteria creates immense problems of comparability, which are further complicated by taking into consideration the fact that measurements are often taken at different behavioural or phylogenetic levels.

Habituation has been mainly studied in relation to the orienting reflex (Sokolov, 1963) and, in its simplest form, means a decrease of response to repeated stimulation. In relation to the factors affecting the habituation process, Thompson and Spencer (1966), working with spinal cats, identified nine stimuli and training parameters which had been verified by others. However, 'frequency' and 'intensity' are the stimulus variables which have been found to be most potent in influencing the final level of habituation (Groves and Thompson, 1970). Explanatory models of the mechanism of their habituation process have been put forward by Pavlov (1927 – 'Internal Inhibition'), Sharpless and Jasper (1956), Gastaut (1957), Roitbak (1960), Sokolov (1963) ('The Neuronal Model'), and by Groves and Thompson (1970 – 'The dual-process theory'). Of these theories, those of Sokolov and of Groves and Thompson, seem to be the most complete. The 'neuronal model' proposed by Sokolov states that the cortex develops an integral model of the parametric characteristic of the incoming stimulus and, when this model has been formed in the cortex, the CNS ceases to respond to the same stimulation.

Habituation of the orienting reflex, a complex reaction which appears to have the functions of preparing the organism for environmental change, has been studied in the context of clinical research in two ways. First, as an assessment procedure for the purpose of discriminating clinical groups, and mainly using measures of EEG and ANS. Commonly an habituation index has been employed to differentiate diagnostic categories, the effectiveness of drugs, and as a measure related to personality constructs, such as introversion/extroversion. In general these measurements have been employed as operational definitions of the 'arousal' or 'level of arousal' concept used to explain the nature of differences between personalities or behavioural disorders which are characterized by extreme levels of arousal.

Secondly, the habituation model is extrapolated to serve as an explanation of other processes. Thus, it is applied to treatment by desensitization considering both as decremental response processes with very straightforward parametric similarities, (Lader and Mathews, 1968). Empirical support for desensitization as an habituation process is found in the relationship between the level of arousal (defined as GSR rate of habituation and the number of spontaneous fluctuations in GSR level) and the outcome of treatment by desensitization (Lader, Gelder and Marks, 1967). In particular, the evidence is consistent with the possibility that patients showing more rapid GSR habituation tend to respond better to desensitization, while those showing a diminished rate, or absence, of habituation tend to respond poorly to that treatment.

Perhaps few writers feel that the picture is as clear cut as this, and certainly written statements urge only cautious acceptance of this simplistic relationship. There are, indeed, numerous difficulties and deficiencies in this area of study, some of which stem from the problems of an inadequate classificatory system, or a lack of comparability of subjects used in experimentation; others, perhaps, are attributed to faulty experimental design, inexplicit hypotheses, and an inability to assume an inductive approach in the face of discordant but interesting data. However, certain studies may be briefly reviewed as exemplifying the kind of findings which emerge from this area of research and as indicators of the kind of problems with which the researcher needs to contend.

In an early study Winokur *et al.* (1959) studied 67 psychiatric patients comprising 25 manic depressives, 17 schizophrenics, 7 chronic brain syndromes, and 18 psychoneurotics, using a conditioning paradigm, in which they compared the number of GSR responses to the CS during adaptation and extinction. While they reported a positive correlation (0·65) between the degree of reactivity (i.e. the number of responses to the CS during adaptation) and conditionability (i.e. the number of CRs to the CS during extinction), no relationship with diagnostic or other variables was found.

Stewart *et al.* (1959), using GSR measurements, studied a group of 70 psychiatric patients comprising 27 manic depressives (of whom all were in a depressed phase), 18 schizophrenics, 15 personality disorders (a very mixed group), and 10 anxiety neurotics (including 3 obsessive-compulsives). A classical conditioning paradigm was employed in which the CS was a 500 c.p.s. tone of 65 dB with a duration of 4 seconds, and the UCS was a shock of 46 volts of 1 second duration. It was found not only that the anxiety neurotics took significantly more trials to habituate to the CS during the adaptation phase than did others, but that there was a substantial correlation between the rate of CS habituation and the rate of extinction of the CR.

Berkson, Hermelin and O'Connor (1961), using EEG (alpha blocking time) and GSR (skin potential change), measured habituation to a frosted 60-watt bulb placed 5 feet from the subject's eyes and illuminated for one-fifth of a second. In their study 18 normals were compared with three groups of subnormals classified as 18 'feeble minded', 21 'imbeciles' and 20 'mongols'. They found, as expected, a decline of response to the signal but not a significant difference between the groups. It is interesting to note that they observed, in about a third of the subjects, that an initial decline could be followed by an increase in responsiveness. While the authors do not elaborate on this latter finding, it appears as an intriguing phenomenon with possible implications for the process by which sensitization might occur.

Reviewing Russian studies Vinogradova (1961)[1] pointed out three basic kinds of orienting reflex abnormalities, two of them apparently having a close relation to the habituation process. The first is an unusually powerful orienting reflex which is resistant to extinction. Such a pattern has been observed in early acute schizophrenia, 'infectious psychosis', and among neurotics. It has also been reported in other types of patients, for example those with cortical damage, in imbeciles and idiots, in senile patients, alcoholics and drug addicts. It is apparently rare in schizophrenia, Streltsova (1955) reporting that, in a population of 130 schizophrenics, 3 per cent had unusually large CR and 25 per cent needed many trials to habituate.

The second is a weakness of the orienting reflex, or even its complete absence, which is common among schizophrenics (65 per cent of the relevant population employed by Streltsova showed this tendency) and among subnormal patients. The third is a disruption of the relationship between the OR and the defensive reaction found in 'infectious psychosis', and among some schizophrenics, usually those with 'paranoid delusions'.

Lader and Wing (1964, 1966) compared a group of 20 patients with anxiety states and 20 normals, and examined 'habituation' to a random sequence of 20 tones of 1000 c.p.s., 100 dB and 1 second duration. 'Adaptation' was evaluated during a 'rest period' of ten minutes, and a 'stimulation period' of twenty minutes was employed. Four psychophysiological measures were taken, palmar skin resistance, finger pulse volume, pulse rate, and forearm extensor electromyogram. While the process of adaptation was assessed by using the four different measurements, habituation was evaluated only by GSR reactivity. It was found that the skin conductance was higher, and tended to rise, among the patient population, whereas the controls showed a lower level of skin conductance which tended to drop throughout the experiment. In relation to PGR habituation it was found that normals were characterized by large responses at the beginning, faster habituation, and smaller responses at the end of testing. In contrast, the patients had smaller,

---

[1] Cited by Lynn (1966), no details about the measurements or variables studied being reported.

earlier responses, failed to show habituation, and continued to give responses similar in magnitude to the earliest ones throughout the test period. Making use of the regression coefficient it was possible to classify the total population into 'habituators' and 'non-habituators', and this yielded the following picture:

	Habituators	*Non-habituators*
Normals	20	—
Patients	6	14

During the rest period it was also noted that spontaneous fluctuations declined while, during stimulation, a transient increase at the beginning followed by a decrease and a final slight rise was observed. The patients were characterized by showing a significantly greater number of spontaneous fluctuations.

In respect to pulse rate, highly significant differences were also found between the groups, with patients having a higher pulse rate than normals, but for other measures the results were not revealing of differences.

The next stage in the sequence of experiments carried out by Lader and Wing, was to compare the effect of amylobarbitone sodium and placebo on the same 20 patients. It was observed for patients on placebo, that the mean conductance rose throughout the experiment, whereas for patients on amylobarbitone sodium conductance tended to drop. Furthermore, it was observed that amylobarbitone sodium increased the rate of habituation so that patients who failed to habituate under placebo conditions succeeded in doing so when this drug was administered. Of interest too was the observation that spontaneous fluctuations were reduced by the drug.

The other measures (PV, PR and EMG) failed to reveal any significant differences between drug and placebo conditions, although it was noted that patients under placebo tended to show a greater pulse volume.

In the review published by Stern and McDonald (1965) on the physiological correlates of mental disease, several references are made to EEG and ANS habituation. In connection with schizophrenia, alpha desynchronization as an orienting response indicator is reported to be absent or inhibited among chronic patients, and in many catatonic patients defensive reactions are found to have habituated rapidly (Lynn, 1963; Kostandov, 1963). However, Hein *et al.* (1962) (chronic schizophrenics) and Fedio *et al.* (1961) (less chronic schizophrenics) have failed to find important differences between patients and normals in the habituation of the EEG desynchronization response. On the other hand, Titaeva (1962) has reported the discovery of two categories of catatonic schizophrenics. One of these is characterized by reduced EEG desynchronization responses, increased polyphasic skin potential responses, and a tendency to show an absence of skin potential responses.

With regard to depression, it was observed that alpha desynchronization persisted longer and there was 'a high level of muscle tension which was intensified by photic stimulation' in half of the group of 16 depressives (Wilson and Wilson, 1961). Longer and persistent orienting responses in the vasomotor system in depression have been reported by Vendeteva (1961) and by Traugott and Balonov (1961). In general the results suggest slower habituation in depressed patients than in controls, with the exception that Leibovitch (1959, 1961) reported rapid extinction of EEG orienting responses in depression.

In an investigation of 44 schizophrenics, Stern *et al.* (1965) studied electrodermal habituation to a sequence of 20 tones (500 c.p.s., 70 dB and 5 second duration) and to a word-association task (40 words, modified Rappaport list). Measurements were taken upon admission and again after five weeks of hospitalization, and were correlated with two prognostic categories, 'good' (needing hospitalization for less than seven weeks) and 'poor' (needing hospitalization for a lengthier period of time). The results indicated that patients with more rapid habituation on the second test occasion tended to have a more favourable prognosis than those who showed no such change.

Wolfensberger and O'Connor (1965), using EEG and GSR, studied the responsiveness, adaptation and habituation of 23 normals and 28 retardates. The stimuli used were lights of two intensities and three different durations (2, 3 and 15 seconds). The results of this study indicated that the retardates were more responsive in GSR but slower in alpha blocking. There was no evidence for an interaction between intensity or duration of stimulation on the one hand, and intelligence on the other, neither did the habituation measure differentiate normals from retardates.

Later, in 1967, these authors, using the previous data, tried to assess other aspects of GSR habituation. As measures of arousal and habituation, three different GSR variables were employed; latency, amplitude and duration. The experimental design took account of two intelligence groups, two stimulus intensities, three stimulus durations, with four block repetitions of six trials each. The purpose was to establish the discriminative power of the GSR variables and their relationship to the

E

experimental conditions. The results were inconclusive in relation to the main variables, which may be the outcome of using a design of too great a complexity. However, it was found that the 'duration score' was the most sensitive variable, followed by 'amplitude' and 'latency' scores.

Lader (1967) investigated 90 psychiatric patients comprising 18 anxiety-depressives, 16 anxiety states, 19 agoraphobics, 18 social phobics and 19 specific phobics. Five physiological variables related to skin resistance were studied, using a similar technique to the one employed in a previous experiment (1964). It was found that patients with specific phobias were similar to normals in having a rapid habituation and few spontaneous fluctuations (low arousal) and, in these respects, were differentiated from the other four groups. The predicted relationship was also established between habituation and levels of general and overt anxiety, and a significant correlation was found showing that 'high arousal subjects' respond better to sedative drug treatment.

Lader, Gelder and Marks (1967) also studied palmar skin conductance measures as a predictor of the degree of improvement in response to desensitization. The population studied comprised 11 agoraphobics, 8 social phobics, and 17 patients with specific phobias, the methodology being similar to that used previously. The results confirmed that specific phobics habituated more rapidly than did patients in the other two groups. Moreover, rapid habituation was associated with fewer spontaneous fluctuations, a lower level of overt anxiety reported by the patient, a lesser degree of social disability, and fewer reported panic attacks. Finally, rapid habituation was related to a better outcome in terms of the severity of the disorder and the degree of disability as assessed clinically. Unfortunately this study failed to provide a description of the basic parameters of the desensitization procedure applied, and the possibility exists, therefore, that the main source of variance in outcome measurements was a direct result of variations in the desensitization procedure itself.

Tizard (1968) studied a child population aged between 8 and 10 years, comprising 8 hospitalized overactive severe subnormals, 7 hospitalized severe subnormals who were *not* overactive, and 8 normal children. Habituation and responsiveness were assessed during waking and sleeping by EEG and skin potential measures and the results indicated that, during sleep, habituation did not occur in any group while, during wakefulness, only the normal group showed skin potential habituation. In relation to responsiveness no differences were found between groups or between states (awake–asleep).

Hare (1968), following previous investigations, explored the definitions of psychopathy in terms of an autonomic dysfunction. More precisely it was suggested that psychopaths were characterized by hyporeactivity or 'low arousal', with all the consequences that this basic assumption has for learning and conditioning. With 51 penitentiary inmates, comprising 21 primary psychopaths (P), 18 secondary psychopaths (S), and 12 non-psychopaths (NP), measures of skin resistance, heart rate, digital vasoconstriction and respiration rate were taken under conditions of 'rest' and 'stimulation'. The 'stimulation' period consisted of the random presentation of 15 tones (900 c.p.s., 2 second duration, 80 dB) followed by the presentation of a novel tone (250 c.p.s., and 10 dB) and, after five minutes' rest, a series of arithmetic problems.

At rest, 'primary psychopaths' showed a lower level of skin conductance than did 'non-psychopaths' and using a composite measure of autonomic variability, this group exhibited significantly less autonomic variability than did group NP. At a qualitative level it was observed that group P tended to show less spontaneous fluctuation than did group NP, and for groups P and S to have lower mean peak-trough differences in heart rate than NP. During the presentation of the tones groups P and S showed better skin conductance adaptation than did group NP. The three groups did not show any significant differences with respect to the magnitude of the responses, nor for the rate of habituation to the tones. Moreover, although not significant, it was observed that cardiac deceleration and digital vasoconstriction seemed to habituate more slowly for group P than for group NP. In spite of the fact that the empirical data gave only weak support to the basic hypothesis in terms of statistical significance, the consistency of direction of certain results appears to be promising.

Hutt (1968) set out to test the hypothesis that in brain-damaged children the 'exploration of new stimuli will show a slow rate of habituation'. The investigation was also concerned to show how this behaviour could be affected by two incentive conditions. Thus, habituation of the exploratory behaviour to an electric toy was measured under conditions of 'auditory plus visual' feedback produced by the manipulation of a lever. Under the 'auditory only' condition the 'manipulatory exploration' in normals showed a progressive increase until the fifth session, with a sudden drop in the sixth session, in contrast to the performance of brain-damaged children which followed a progressive decrease throughout the sessions. Under the dual incentive conditions (i.e. sound plus light) this same pattern was enhanced.

Manipulatory behaviour clearly suffers a qualitative change through-out the sessions, probably changing from exploration to play, which makes the variable for measuring habituation in this study a rather weak one. Furthermore, an analysis of variance revealed that the decrement in rate of investigatory responses was significantly slower in the brain-damage group than in the normal group, and that the recovery of exploratory responses after two weeks was greater among the brain-damage than among normal subjects. These results suggest that in brain-damaged children long-term habituation is impaired, although phasic or short-term habituation may not be affected. The dual incentive condition appears to increase the responsiveness of normals more than that of brain-damaged subjects, while in both groups this dual condition decreases the rate of habituation.

In another study Dykman *et al.* (1968) compared a group of 45 psychiatric patients with a normal control of 40 medical students. The psychiatric sample comprised a mixed group of schizophrenics, psycho-neurotics, personality disorders and organics. The experimental procedure lasted about half an hour and consisted of four stages. The first of these was a rest period of five minutes and the second was a random sequence of twelve tones. This was followed by a further rest period of five minutes and then, in the fourth period, by eleven questions to think about, but not to be answered aloud. During these four stages measurements of skin resistance, heart rate, respiratory rate and muscle potential (EMG) were taken.

As a whole the psychiatric patients were characterized by a faster rate of skin resistance habituation and lower magnitude of response than the students. Where heart rate and respiratory rate were concerned habituation to the tones used in this experiment occurred early, but this trend was reversed during the later presentation of tones. The shape of the skin resistance habituation curves was similar in the groups employed, although differences in level of function were observed. The heart rate habituation was similar in students, neurotics and schizophrenics, but it was very poor among those patients with person-ality disorders. In general, all the patient categories showed habituation in skin resistance, schizophrenics and neurotics showing some heart rate habituation, but respiratory rate habituation was not observed in any group.

Perhaps of most significance in this experiment is that habituation occurred at different rates in different systems. In the case of skin resistance for example organics showed the most rapid habituation but failed to remain in the habituated state, while schizophrenics tended to habituate more slowly than other patients. For heart rate schizophrenics showed the best habituation followed by the neurotics, while the personality disordered group responded with greater heart rate responses to the later tones than to the earlier ones, which suggests a reversal of the usual form of habituation, and which we might refer to as 'sensitization'. Furthermore, in no psychiatric group included in this experiment was there noted an orderly habituation of respiratory rate although it was noted that the organics and neurotics responded with greater variability than did other groups.

Finally, Brierly (1969) has reported on the forearm muscle blood flow in ten agoraphobics and ten normals, concluding that the habituation of forearm blood flow followed a similar pattern to that obtained by Lader on PGR.

Habituation is a phenomenon widely demonstrated at many different phylogenic, ontogenic and structural levels of the nervous system, and some of its basic parameters have also been identified, some of which are analogous to those of associative learning. However, there is still a need to integrate such a universally identified process into the general framework of biology and psychology. Thus, some authors (Razran, 1971) conceptualize it as 'learning what not to do', considering it as a more elementary or lower form of learning in the evolutionary scale, from which other forms of learning have subsequently evolved.

In our present context it is also necessary to consider the habituation process as a reflection of autonomic arousal. Such a conception, with its underlying notion of unidimensionality, poses important problems and some of the evidence which is available to us is in conflict with such a conception, added to which are the daunting technical problems of psychophysiological measurements. Yet, most studies, as a matter of fact, assume implicitly or explicitly that measures of habituation are measures along some unidimensional arousal continuum. Often we find that the conceptual framework is extended to embrace habituation, arousal, anxiety and emotions. Parsimony certainly has its value in scientific endeavour, but unwarranted over-simplification has many attendant dangers and offers no practical advantages to the researcher or the clinician. We would consider that one of the weaknesses of current approaches stems from employing a simple mechanistic model, in some ways comparable to the medical model appropriate in the context of physical disorders, where high arousal appears as a differentiating sign of psychiatric disorders, and a 'symptom' of which patients might be relieved.

The problem of what is in fact being measured in habituation remains unclear and there are various theoretical possibilities which are available to us. We would not deny the value of the concept of arousal, nor underestimate the importance of studies in this area, but it is pertinent to point to the peculiarities and discrepancies which emerge in the experimental study and which might best be dealt with by taking into consideration the characteristic temporal pattern of the arousal of each behavioural disorder. We feel it highly likely that arousal change follows a complex temporal pattern within the system, and between systems and, if we could but understand and describe these complexities well enough, we would find a pattern which might identify each behavioural disorder type.

A further important problem arises from the misuse of operational definitions. For example, 'arousal' has been defined both by the rate of habituation and the number of GSR spontaneous fluctuations, presumably on the assumption that a direct correspondence exists between habituation rate and the frequency of spontaneous fluctuations.

In practice, however, divergencies from such an association are common and make it difficult for us to make meaningful statements about 'arousal level' from a variety of measures. Nevertheless, dismaying though such discrepancies may appear, we may hopefully see in them the basis for a more complex and sophisticated descriptive framework.

As an illustration of the kind of problem we may be facing in relation to the temporal dimension, we might consider the following. The behavioural disorder can be characterized by having 'N' (A, B, C, D, E) different discriminable stages of arousal through a given time period. These stages may represent specific patterns of arousal between systems. If we take measures at two different times 'X' and 'Y' (see Fig. 5.1), for a number of subjects, we may see two important possibilities. First we must note that the different subjects were at the time of the measurements at different qualitative stages, and secondly that the central tendency measures and the possible estimated correlations from these measurements, will be misleading, because we are amalgamating things which are qualitatively different.

Clearly a great deal of experimental work and sophisticated theorizing will be required before we can make use of the concepts of arousal and habituation with any degree of confidence. However, even in our present state of knowledge it is apparent that the kind of experimental findings which have been provided, and which have been presented briefly here, are of sufficient interest to stimulate our thinking about abnormalities of process and the way in which use may be made of these findings in our own model concerning obsessional disorder.

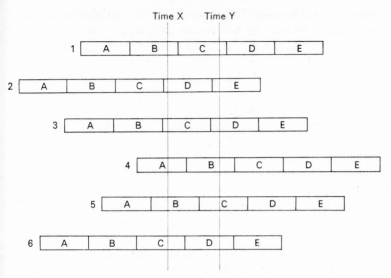

Fig. 5.1 The Methodological problem of characterizing patients under specific categories as having 'high arousal' without considering the temporal dimension of the behavioural disorder.

Note: The numbers (1, 2, 3, 4, 5, 6) represent different S's with the same behavioural disorder.
The letters (A, B, C, D, E) represent different qualitative states, not different degrees of the same state.
Time X and Y are similar observations (measurements) at different times.

PSEUDO-CONDITIONING

This term has been used to refer to 'the formation of a set to respond to a formerly inadequate stimulus following a series of presentations of some strong unconditioned stimulus' (Grant and Dittmer, 1940), and it must be stressed here that the CS and the UCS are never paired as is ordinarily the case in conditioning. Thus, pseudo-conditioning procedures differ from those in classical conditioning in that the former do not involve associative factors. On the other hand, sensitization is held to differ from pseudo-conditioning in that any increment in reactivity attributable to the former is obtained with repeated presentations of a CS without any involvement of UCS manipulation.

Pseudo-conditioning has been mainly studied with the purpose of evaluating the effect of associative and non-associative factors on increases in responsivity, but at this point in time the factual evidence is scarce and it is difficult to establish clear cut differences between associative and non-associative procedures. In explaining the response increments obtained under pseudo-conditioning some theoretical interpretations have been put forward. An early example was that of 'cortical dominance' as employed by Sears (1934), and Harlow (1939), and is, in fact, the principle of dominance as originally applied to neural activity by Ukhtomsky,[1] although it was used at first in philosophy by Avenarious (1890).[1]

According to Ukhtomsky, 'Sufficiently stable excitations, cumulated in any neural centre, acquire a dominant position with respect to excitations in other centres so that stimulations directed to the other centres increase the excitation of the dominant centre and decrease the excitation in their own subordinate centres' (Razran, 1971). This same principle has also been extended to cover the so-called 'state of readiness' of the effectors or much better named effector dominance (Wickens and Wickens, 1940).

Some, such as Grether (1938), and Harlow and Toltzien (1940), have tried to explain pseudo-conditioning in terms of 'expectancy', while others (Wickens and Wickens, 1940) have considered that pseudo-conditioning could be a case of 'true conditioning with associative or contiguity factors present'. Finally, the possibility has been considered that the state of 'drive' of the organism is transformed by the non-paired UCS presentations creating a functional state which permits increments of response from previously habituated or innocuous stimulations. Although crude and speculative it seems to us useful to explore the possibilities of a redefinition in terms of arousal. So that we may have a better understanding of the contemporary state of the evidence some of the most important literature available in pseudo-conditioning of humans may now be presented.

In an early and very brief communication, Grant and Hilgard (1940) reported on an experimental group which, during the acquisition trials, received forty UCS's, while a control group spent the same period of time under conditions of visual fixation. The results showed an increase in frequency of eyelid responses in both groups and no extinction during a retention test. They concluded that 'non-associative increases supplement associative increases'. It must be observed also that the fixation condition produced increases in eyelid responses which might possibly be explained as a consequence of a state of disinhibition following a period of activity (fixation).

Grant and Dittmer (1940), in another relevant study, examined the tactile generalization gradient resulting from pseudo-conditioning.

[1] See Razran, 1971.

They applied four differently located vibro-tactile stimulators as CS's, and a shock as the UCS, to a sample of fifteen male students. The conditioning consisted of nine alternated sequences of CS and UCS. They were able to demonstrate a clear-cut generalization gradient of response amplitude following non-paired UCS's, and it was suggested that this finding required an alternative or complementary explanation of conditioning which might be in terms of 'spatial contiguity'.

In another experiment Wickens and Wickens (1940) studied conditioning in full-term neonates who were less than ten days old. They used a classical conditioning paradigm group, a pseudo-conditioning group and a control group with a time lapse of two days between tests as a control for maturational factors. They found that the classical conditioning group and the pseudo-conditioning group were practically identical in extinction and spontaneous recovery. In the control group 'only one out of 12 S's used gave any response to the CS on the second test'. In accounting for these findings, ideas about the 'state of readiness' of the effectors and the possibility of non-controlled associative factors embedded in the procedure, or in the environment, were offered by the authors.

A study published by Grant and Meyer (1941) studied the formation of generalized response sets under a pseudo-conditioning paradigm. Samples of the group were exposed to either a warning or no-warning condition and multiple recording of responses was made. It was found that after a series of UCS's the formerly neutral stimuli elicited a significantly high frequency of hand withdrawal and that this responsivity had also generalized to different CS's and to different sensory modalities.

Harris (1941) also studied forward, backward and pseudo-conditioning, and adaptation of the finger withdrawal response in a sample of 41 students using a loud tone as the CS, and an electric shock as the UCS. Pre-training included 3 CS's and 3 UCS's, the training being specific to each of the four groups and, during extinction, 10 CS's were presented. It was observed that in the pseudo-conditioning group an initial very high level of response was followed by a sharp falling off. In general the results again suggest the existence of non-associative factors in conditioning.

Grant (1943a), using a population of students comprising an experimental group and a control group, assessed the pseudo-conditioning of the eyelid response. The CS's consisted of a light and three different intensities of sound, while the UCS was a puff of air. This experiment revealed a clear-cut response to the pseudo-conditioning of eyelid responses to light consisting of 'a highly reliable frequency increase' in the 170–450 m.s. latency range. Good retention was observed over a period of one week and there was resistance to extinction (no evidence of extinction after 24 CS trials) with broad sensory generalization.

In yet another study Grant (1943b) compared the effect of pseudo-conditioning, classical conditioning, a visual fixation condition and a control condition respecting eyelid responses. In this experiment the pseudo-conditioning procedure consisted on day 1 of 4 CS's followed by 40 UC's followed by 4 CS's once again with this procedure being repeated again on day 2. Clear-cut increases in frequency were found in the pseudo-conditioning, fixation and control procedures, and good overnight retention was observed in all groups, although the conditioning group showed the best results. It was also observed that there was no tendency to extinction in any of the groups. Qualitatively, orthodox CR's differed from those responses resulting from sensitization in that they tended to be of greater duration and had a lower modal latency with greater overnight retention.

Grant (1945) explored some factors relating to the sensitization of Beta responses (those having latencies from 120 to 240 m.s.). A sample of 60 students was employed, grouped under three different pre-stimulus illumination conditions. The procedure consisted of alternated series of different random intensity light presentations, secondly, fixation periods of eight minutes and, thirdly, rest periods of two minutes. It was shown in this experiment that beta response increments occurred without UCS presentations at all. However, there is a conceptual confusion in this paper since the procedures basically involved sensitization under rest and fixation, rather than pseudo-conditioning considered as non-paired presentations of CS and UCS.

Kimble, Mann and Dufort (1955) carried out a series of four experiments in an endeavour to explore some critical factors in eyelid conditioning under classical and instrument procedures although, for our purposes, the relevant experiment is the fourth in this series in which they examined the effects of associative factors and the 'acquired drive'. One group which served as a control and had 60 classical conditioning trials, while two other control groups, in addition to having CS–UCS trials, were given a proportion of trials (between 10 and 20 of the total of 60 trials) with only the UCS being administered. It was reported that the omission of the CS had no detrimental effect on learning, and that the two experimental groups had a significant superiority during extinction. The authors commented upon the existence of two factors in eyelid conditioning, one being the associative and the other a 'per-

formance factor, probably a drive which is acquired with the presentation of the UCS' (Kimble and Dufort, 1956). Thus, the CS omission
did not interfere with the progress of conditioning.

Champion and Jones (1961) have also explored and reported upon
forward, backward and pseudo-conditioning of the GSR. Using a tone
as the CS and a shock as the UCS an increase in performance was
observed in both forward and backward groups, while in the pseudo-
conditioning group there was a small, although non-significant decrement which resembles in some way an habituation curve.

In another study of 112 adolescents, Martin (1962), using a light as
a CS and a tone as a UCS, studied the effect of a different number
of trials on the classical and pseudo-conditioning of the GSR. Also
examined in this experiment was the relationship of the procedures
with the level of skin resistance (BSR) and GSR responses to the tones.
Highly significant increases of response were observed from the first
to the final light with higher efficiency being shown for the paired trials.
Furthermore, the number of trials was positively related to responses
during the final presentation of lights, although this relation was clearer
with the pseudo-conditioning group. The BRS became lower after the
tones, but did not differentiate the groups.

Prokasy, Hall and Fawcett (1962) studied a population of students
using different conditioning paradigms of the GSR. In this experiment
forward and backward conditioning was studied, two forms of sensitization and adaptation conditions and a pseudo-conditioning procedure.
Observation showed that the response magnitude to the shocks remained constant and did not differentiate between the two sensitization
groups and the pseudo-conditioning group. Furthermore the response
levels of backward and pseudo-conditioning decreased drastically after
the first test trial, and forward conditioning differed significantly only
from adaptation on the first extinction test trial. Finally the test trials
did not differentiate between the performance of the two sensitization
groups on the one hand and the pseudo-conditioning group on the
other.

Prokasy and Ebel (1964) studied conditioning and sensitization of
the GSR in relation to two different inter-trial stimuli, the measures
of GSR being magnitude of response, amplitude, latency and recruitment. During acquisition trials they found that classical conditioning
produced greater magnitude and recruitment than did sensitization.
Also, spaced practice was associated with greater magnitude and
recruitment in responses, and sensitization was characterized by a
decrease in magnitude. During extinction, longer latency of sensitized

responses and greater magnitude occurred in connection with spaced practice.

Stolz (1965) studied the conditioning and pseudo-conditioning of the vasomotor response in humans using a photocrystal plethysmograph. The subjects were exposed to one of the following conditions: classical conditioning, pseudo-conditioning, and pseudo-conditioning plus extinction. Using a light as the CS and a 50 dB buzzer as the UCS, no differences could be found between classical conditioning and the pseudo-conditioning procedure.

From this review it is only possible to conclude that the empirical evidence, while scarce, indicates that increments of response can occur under non-associative procedures. The principal aim of most of the studies has been centred upon disentangling the importance of associative factors from non-associative and, since these studies were designed for this special purpose, the basic parameters of pseudo-conditioning and other possible extraneous factors have not been properly scrutinized. It is also evident that, apart from some interesting theoretical speculations emerging from earlier studies, most researchers have been concerned only with empirical outcome without any undue concern for theoretical sophistication.

The possibility of obtaining response increments under pseudo-conditioning procedures has very interesting implications indeed for clinical psychology. While classical conditioning seems to us to be a probably rare event in the real world, pseudo-conditioning would seem to be a distinctly more frequent possibility and, consequently, offers an interesting paradigm for the acquisition of neuroses. Furthermore the pseudo-conditioning paradigm offers other decided advantages. In the first place, it makes the more or less rigorous temporal relations required by classical and operant conditioning irrelevant and, secondly, there is considerably greater freedom to manipulate those CS's or UCS's that are either seldom or never under the control of the experimenter.

ONE-TRIAL LEARNING

The impressive empirical support now available for the existence of one-trial learning has given to the clinical psychologist a potentially useful model for the acquisition of neurotic behaviours. Moreover, an important element always embedded in conditioning experiments, and from our point of view crucial to the one-trial paradigm, is the problem of 'paradoxical enhancement' (Rohrbaugh and Riccio, 1970).

The process of '*paradoxical enhancement*' is different from *incubation* which implies an increase in responsivity over a particular time interval (Eysenck, 1968). The incubation procedure consists initially of a conditioning procedure in which there are CS and UCS paired presentations, then an interval with no further presentations of either stimuli until the association is reassessed. To account for increments in responsivity following the 'rest' period, Eysenck (1965) put forward an explanation in terms of reminiscence or consolidation of the memory trace. In contrast with this procedure 'paradoxical enhancement' refers to increments in response which are attributable to exposure to non-reinforced CS's ($\overline{CS}$) following an initial period of CS–UCS association. Eysenck has pointed out that the notation $\overline{CS}$ has certain important advantages.

Lichtenstein (1950) studied 'feeding inhibition' in 14 dogs using an instrumental avoidance paradigm involving shock (85 volts, a.c., 2 second duration) contingent upon eating. There were two experimental groups, the first of which received 20 shocks during food presentation in the first session, and shocks during eating in subsequent sessions, while the second was consistently shocked during eating.

All the dogs developed an inhibitory response to food, but a big difference was observed in speed of acquisition in favour of the second group.

In general the outcome of the procedure was characterized by the fast acquisition, only one to four shocks trials during eating being necessary in the majority of the cases. The inhibition was also very stable, lasting for weeks or even months. Other behaviour changes were also observed, such as passivity or immobility in the experimental situation, active avoidance resistance to the shock, tremors, disturbed respiration, and tic-like movements during the experimental sessions. Furthermore, the animals refused to eat in their living cage, showed increased aggression against cage-mates, and a lowering of the general activity level.

Maatsch (1959) was concerned with the theoretical problem of extinction either as interference or as a reactive-inhibition process. The procedure involved developing a learning situation in which on the one hand, 'interference' would be minimized while, on the other, the effort and rate of response maximized. Thus, if 'interference' is the main mechanism involved, extinction would be minimal, while, if reactive-inhibition ('. . . work-inhibition interpretation of extinction . . .') is the crucial process, rapid extinction of the CR would be expected.

The experimental environment was an open box (24 × 12 × 10 ins) surrounded externally on the top by a ledge and the floor covered with a grid. The procedure was extremely simple. The rats were tamed, adapted to the experimental manipulation and tested in the box for absence of 'jump habit'. Each of the rats received one trial in which it was placed on the charged grid which remained charged until the animal jumped. During extinction two different treatment groups were arranged. The 'massed' group received an extinction trial every 20 seconds for the 15 initial trials and, after that, every 5 seconds until two successive 2-minute no-jump trials. The spaced group, on the other hand, received a maximum of 15 extinction trials delivered every 5 minutes. Latency of the 'jumpout' response decreased markedly during extinction, the extinction curves of the 'massed' and 'spaced' groups being similar. The number of trials necessary to obtain extinction criterion in 6 individuals of the 'massed' group were 641, 911, 848, 134, 260, 177, 18 and 28, the responses appearing 'extremely stereotyped, relaxed and ballistic; . . . the behaviour commonly associated with "abnormal fixation" . . .'. It was also observed that the latency changes suddenly, the medians in the last ten trials changing from 0·5 seconds to 120 seconds. The author interpreted the results as confirming the interference theory of extinction.

Napalkov (1963, *see also* Eysenck, 1967b) in his experiment involving 5 dogs, employed only one classical CS–UCS presentation. During extinction the CS was presented using an inter-stimuli interval of 3 to 5 minutes. The initial CS presentations produced an increase of 30 to 40 mm rise in blood pressure in all the animals, and during the sixth and seventh CS presentation the blood pressure reached a level of 50 to 60 mm, while in the following days, a level of 190 to 230 mm was reached. This hypertensive state persisted for a lengthy period (with observations being made over 16 months) without decrement even though the dogs were excluded from the experimental conditions in which the response had been acquired.

Napalkov explains this extraordinary outcome in terms of cybernetics, although Eysenck has commented that this account is not very enlightening. Eysenck's own explanation, in terms of autonomic feedback, is more coherent than Napalkov's, but again falls short of being complete.

Campbell, Sanderson and Laverty (1964), using 5 male alcoholics, studied the CR's during extinction following a single traumatic conditioned trial. The UCS was a temporary interruption of respiration induced by succinylcholine chloride dehydrate ('Scoline'), while the CS was a tone (600 c.p.s., 70 dB, 5 second duration, 30 ISI – 90 second). Thus, as the 'Scoline' was administered through a saline drip flow, the conditioning procedure appears to be a case of extero–interoceptive conditioning (CS is exteroceptive and the UCS is interoceptive).

The experimental procedures consisted of: a) an adaptation period of CS presentations until no GSR response appeared for 5 consecutive trials; b) one paired trial, followed by a rest period of 5 minutes, and c) three different extinction sessions, the first, 30 CS presentations following 5 minutes of rest, the second 30 CS after a period of 3 weeks. As control 3 subjects received CS only and 3 others only UCS. For the control S's no data is available for the last extinction series (40 CS after 3 weeks).

For the experimental group significant shifts were observed between periods of the experiment in relation to GSR spontaneous fluctuations. Following conditioning the rate of spontaneous fluctuations increased very sharply and in the last two extinction series 'it rose even further'. The absolute level of skin resistance did not show substantial change between periods. The CR to the tone did not diminish in amplitude or frequency. In relation to latency measurements it was observed that, throughout the conditioning procedure, the GSR and cardiac components developed shorter latencies and the respiratory and muscular components of the CR developed longer latencies. Thus, taking into consideration latency and amplitude as indices of strength of the GSR conditioned response, it may be concluded that the CR's showed increase in strength throughout the time (enhancement) following the single traumatic trial.

Finally, although few details are given, two additional extinction procedures of GSR CR were tried in some subjects. The first was 10 or 20 CS presentations with no inter-stimulus interval (ISI), and the second, CS presentation during sodium amytal slow administration. Under the first procedure although the amplitude became smaller the latency did not change, and following a rest period of 30 to 60 seconds, the response was elicited again at full strength.

The second procedure shows that the CS responses diminished and disappeared while the subject passed through the sedation threshold and reappeared again when the subject was almost asleep.

Rohrbaugh and Riccio (1970) carried out two experiments which combined the use of one-trial learning and the effect of different subsequent CS exposure.

In the first experiment a group of albino rats deprived of food and water for 48 hours was used. During conditioning they received 10 inescapable shocks of 2 second duration during $5\frac{1}{2}$ minutes of confinement in a box. Afterwards, during the next hour, groups of S's (N = 12) were exposed to the box environment (CS) for 0, $\frac{1}{2}$, 5, 15 or 50 minutes. The measures taken were of latency and the amount of food and water (now available in the same box) intake during 15 minutes. It was found that the 5-minute CS exposure group showed greater fear than did the 15- and 50-minute groups.

In the second experiment 32 young male rats were employed. For conditioning each rat was put in the black wall side of a double compartment box and during a 5-minute period it received 5 shocks of 2 second duration. Following this the gate was opened and the rats were permitted to stay on the white (safe) side for 5 minutes. During the next two weeks the rats were re-exposed to the discriminative stimuli (black and white sides) for 0, 30, 60 or 300 seconds on three different occasions.

Finally a test was carried out two days after the last exposure in which the animals were assessed for spatial avoidance to the black side (normally preferred by rats). Now, with the gate lifted, the time spent on the white side during 20 minutes was recorded. The results indicated that 30- and 60-second exposures were more effective in producing the avoidance reaction.

Although the results are inconclusive with respect to enhancement, it seems reasonable to argue that certain forms of short CS exposure led to subsequent stronger responsivity to the learned CS cues. On the other hand it is clear that one-trial conditioning schedules can be a very powerful source of learned fear.

EVIDENCE BEARING UPON THE BEECH–PERIGAULT THEORY

Essentially our theory, as indicated earlier in this chapter, has two important elements. First, it postulates an unusual state of arousal, experienced by patients and interpreted by them as powerful emotional states. Secondly, it postulates some means by which these emotional states, which in the theory have primary importance, became attached to certain cognitive events. It is not envisaged that the abnormality of arousal is fixed or unchanging, indeed such would not be in accord with clinical observation. More likely is that the condition is a fluctuating one, reflecting both spontaneous interval changes as well as a special *vulnerability* to environmental events, rather than a steady state of abnormality.

We also feel it necessary to argue for some means by which environmental cues of a wide variety can become attached to the feelings of disturbance experienced by the patient, the latter, at least during the early stages of the disorder, probably intensifying until some critical level is reached. This need arises again from clinical and empirical considerations which argue the necessity to account for the vagaries of behaviour and ideas which are encountered in these conditions. Such ideas and behaviour, however, tend to incorporate an important common element, namely that they are those which are *ordinarily* capable of elevating emotional states. In this way, the theory argues, existing high arousal levels are given additional impetus to raise them to the critical levels at which special connections can be formed of a kind which are *resistant to extinction*.

It must be emphasized that such a formulation can only be regarded as tentative, although we feel that it has the merit of being in accord with empirical observation. Furthermore, we feel bound to indicate that our own evidence is of an extremely preliminary kind, being based substantially on GSR assessment, with its own very particular proneness to interpretative problems, and on relatively few patients.

Finally, we are obliged to point out that, at this stage, our preference has been for a more qualitative rather than quantitative analysis, in which we emphasize an exploratory study of individuals, rather than large-scale studies in which the results of examining substantial numbers are combined. Recognizing, of course, that our theory is couched in general terms and argues a common pathological mechanism for all patients exhibiting certain abnormalities, we feel – and are persuaded by the evidence – that wide individual differences may be found even among patients bearing the same diagnostic label.

A number of different studies have been conducted in our laboratory, mainly employing obsessionals, patients with social phobias and agoraphobias of a severe kind, and normal subjects. Of these we feel that three experiments have special relevance for our theoretical position, and the outcome may be briefly summarized as follows:

1. *Evidence for pathological states of arousal*

While for various reasons, we have not been anxious to gather our data in a way which permits quantitative analysis, our impression is that there is evidence for abnormal levels of arousal as being characteristic of the obsessional patient. In this respect they are differentiated from normal individuals, although perhaps not significantly so from severely disturbed agoraphobics and social phobics.

We would not feel that the failure to differentiate obsessionals from the other abnormal groups affects our theory; indeed, we would feel it likely that the mechanisms we postulate in respect of obsessionals may well apply to the two other groups mentioned. We would argue, for example, that in all three abnormal groups under consideration here, the evidence for causation in terms of specific conditioning is lacking and, in this respect, such patients tend to be differentiated from other kinds of phobias in which particular events in the patient's history might be seen as having a direct causal influence upon the behavioural abnormality.

Further evidence for the pathology of arousal level comes from an

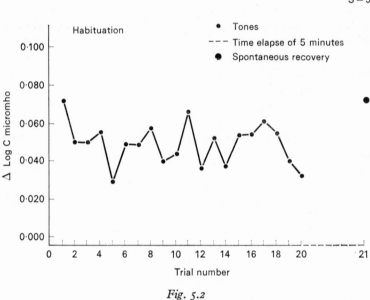

Fig. 5.2

inquiry into the habituation of our patients. Our impression, at this stage, is that obsessionals, more than any other group, experience difficulty in habituation and, instead, show a continued tendency to GSR responsivity to repeated stimulation. An example of this tendency in an obsessional patient is shown in Figure 5.2.

2. *Evidence for one-trial conditioning, and the 'Napalkov Effect'*
Clinical evidence strongly argues for a single important environmental event which serves to provide a cognitive framework around which the obsessional organizes his behavioural abnormalities, and which becomes, thereafter, an enduring connection. While we have argued elsewhere

that abnormal mood state (pathological arousal) has greater importance as a determinant of obsessional behaviour, it is also clear that certain cues, under appropriate 'mood' conditions, have acquired some capacity to affect the individual.

We have found tentative evidence for obsessionals to be especially susceptible to one-trial conditioning and, while other patients may

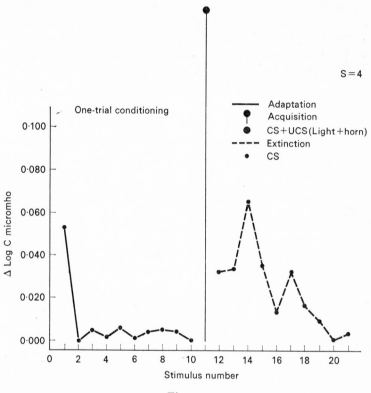

Fig. 5.3

show this they have done so, in our experiments, to a lesser extent. On the other hand, normals have not reflected this tendency in our study. An example of a positive response in an obsessional patient is shown in Figure 5.3.

We have argued elsewhere (Beech, 1971) that the special status of the obsessional patient will render him particularly vulnerable to incrementation of his already abnormal arousal level (Napalkov Effect). So far, we have not found evidence in any of our patients, obsessional or

otherwise, for such incrementation to occur under conditions of repeated presentation of the CS. This failure is of some interest to us and
further experiments are planned to examine the problem in greater
detail.

3. *Evidence for pseudo-conditioning*

While it is not an essential part of our theoretical conception that
obsessionals should show susceptibility to pseudo-conditioning, it
seems to us that the world outside the conditioning laboratory would
be more likely to provide for acquisition in this way. Indeed, our model
would appear to lend itself particularly well to this effect and, accordingly, we include reference to the evidence so far obtained.

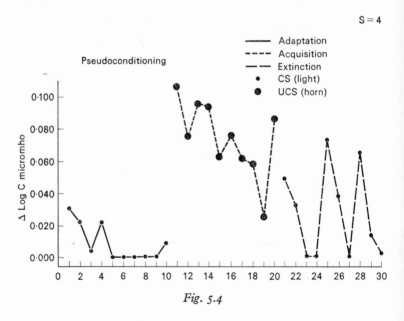

Fig. 5.4

In fact, as Figure 5.4 illustrates, we have found it relatively easy to
demonstrate pseudo-conditioning in our obsessional patients, although
it is pertinent to observe that our other severely disturbed neurotic
patients showed equal susceptibility while normals did not. As will be
seen from Figure 5.4, incrementation of responses occurs in accordance
with prediction, but perhaps an even more important, and unantici-
pated, phenomenon was also apparent, namely the absence of a 'normal'
extinction curve. While we can only repeat our emphasis upon the
speculative nature of our reasoning and the tentative character of our

preliminary results, we may here have the beginning of an explanation of the extraordinary preservation or fixation of abnormal behaviours among obsessionals. It may be that acquisition by the process described above is, for some reason, relatively unamenable to the decremental process ordinarily expected.

Clearly the data we have provided is extremely limited, both in terms of number of patients and important controls. Only further intensive effort in collecting evidence will inform us of the value of the theoretical formulation outlined above.

6

H. R. Beech and Andrée Liddell

Decision-making, mood states and ritualistic behaviour among obsessional patients

Many references have been made to doubting and indecision as salient characteristics of the obsessional neurotic patient. Schachtel (1969), for example, associates this feature with a kind of vigilance maintained by the obsessional who tends to be hyperalert, watchful, and ready for battle against other people, the environment, and against mistakes which he himself might make. He attributes the source of the uncertainty, the feeling of precariousness and the doubting to a pervasive confusion about whether the other person and the world in general are friendly or hostile, accepting and approving, rejecting and blaming. Schachtel points out that this preparedness for battle, which has also been described by Freud, and the extreme vigilance maintained by the obsessional, are characterized by intense affective experience. In short the readiness to fight and the search for 'the right rules' are matters of exaggerated emotional importance to the patient.

Reed too (1968), in drawing up a list of nine categories of difficulties, sees one of these as concerned with decision-making. Much of the distress experienced by his patients appeared to be related to their inability to categorize, terminate, organize and structure their experiences, which they themselves referred to as a 'lack of decision'. Or, looking at another aspect of this indecisiveness, Reed described all the patients as explaining that they were quite capable of 'making decisions' through deductive reasoning but that they were harassed by a lack of conviction about the *conclusions* which they had drawn. Again, such patients tended to claim that the indecisiveness did not apply to the use of old-established skills of the kind involved in riding a bicycle, putting on make-up, or playing table tennis but to matters where choice or novelty were concerned such as for example, deciding whether to ride a bicycle fast or slow, or learning some new activity. But, as

Reed indicates, often the difficulties in decision-making do not seem to bear any obvious relationship to the importance or emotional significance of the situation. Indeed often the greatest agonies of mind are experienced when handling quite trivial issues.

Two other points made by Reed are of interest. The first is that all patients claimed that the emotional reactions which they experienced in decision-making situations were the result, rather than the cause, of their obsessional doubting. This stands in some sharp contrast to the viewpoint which we will argue in this chapter, although there is little doubt that obsessional patients are prone to see emotional responsivity as an effect rather than a cause of their vacillation. The second point is that, contrary to the assumption which is often made by the learning theorist, the patient's attempts to enforce structure by compulsive behaviour or by engaging in ritualistic activities, do not serve to reduce their anxiety. In this last particular we would agree with Reed and argue that no simple 'connectionist' theory can explain the phenomena to be observed. Certainly, where ritualistic hand-washing is concerned, the anxiety-reduction model is limited, as several authors have pointed out.

The literature on obsessional neurosis is also replete with references to the presence of adverse mood states, especially to depression, as an accompaniment of an obsessional condition. Lewis (1934), for example, reported that 23 per cent of his sample of depressed patients showed obsessive–compulsive features, while Kendell and DiScipio (1970) have also noted the correspondence between these two features in 414 of their 4,793 cases.

Stengel (1945) remarks that many psychiatrists tend to think of this duality of symptomatology as evidence that obsessional symptoms occur as a *reaction* to the depressive disorder. However, Stengel disagrees firstly because depression often occurs in the *absence* of obsessions and compulsions and, secondly, because a depression can both precede and also outlive any obsessional characteristic. In his view depression has '. . . an unmasking and aggravating effect . . .' upon obsessionality.

A further complication is introduced by Sargant and Slater's (1950) observation that, *obsessional symptoms* are common among patients who do not have *obsessional personalities*, and Gittleson (1966) has reported that one-third of depressed patients without obsessional features as part of their illness *did* have obsessional pre-morbid personalities.

In his four papers (1966) Gittleson remarks upon the relationship between obsessional symptoms and depression, noting both types of symptom in one-third of his 398 cases. He found that obsessions were common in the course of depressive psychoses and that they appeared to be based upon the activation of existing pre-morbid traits. Furthermore, they seemed to have a marked protective effect where suicide attempts were concerned. Further illustration of the interplay between these two types of symptoms came from his comparison between 39 obsessional neurotics who retained their obsessions during their depression, and 85 depressives who gained obsessions during their depression – not having exhibited these symptoms previously. Gittleson concluded that a pre-existing obsessional neurosis *per se* tended to produce earlier onset of a depression and accounted for a greater incidence of obsessional phenomena in depressive attacks.

In another study, by Rosenberg (1968a), the case notes of 144 obsessional neurotics were compared with those of a similar number of anxiety neurotics treated at Netherne Hospital. The findings of this inquiry suggested that depression is indeed a common complication of obsessional neurosis although, interestingly, other hazards such as alcoholism, drug addiction or suicide appeared to be reduced risks for this group.

Further evidence concerning the frequency with which depressive symptoms are encountered among obsessional patients is provided by Solyom (1971), and in a very striking way by Mellett (see Chap. 3).

There is no doubt, therefore, that depression and obsessionality often appear in association but what is the particular nature of this relationship? In her own inquiry, Vaughan (1971) has approached this problem by arguing that certain apparent contradictions in the evidence might be reconciled by assuming that a *particular form* of depression may be implicated and which occurs with greater frequency in both depressives with pre-morbid obsessional personality and among patients showing obsessions and compulsions as part of their depressive illness. In fact her carefully contrived retrospective study of 168 sets of case notes failed to provide any evidence for a significant association between obsessional personality and the symptoms of depression. On the other hand, where obsessional symptoms occurred in depressive illness, there did appear to be a particular depressive pattern which was characterized by increased agitation, anxiety, over-activity, rapid mood changes, and less retardation. In such cases, as Vaughan points out, if we assume that obsessions are the consequences of depression, then therapy would first be directed to the modification of the abnormal mood state.

The problems arising out of the relation between mood state and obsessional–compulsive symptoms were the primary concern of Walker (1967), who began by noting that no existing theoretical framework could satisfactorily account for the range of abnormalities which are encountered in the obsessional states. Psychoanalytic theory, for example, may postulate a conflict between sexual or aggressive impulses on the one hand and guilt and anxiety on the other, but there is little evidence to support such an explanation. Similarly, Walker felt there was little support to be found for the over-simplified view of the orthodox behaviourist. Indeed, in certain respects the psychoanalytic and behaviourist frameworks share the common misconception that rituals serve to reduce anxiety and are preserved on this account. This displacement theory has some indirect evidence to support it and still finds favour among contemporary writers. For example, Worsley (1970) assumed that rituals are a learned habit because of their anxiety-reducing function, and argued that we need not expect them to be effective on every occasion because partial reinforcement would be enough to ensure preservation of the habit. Where *deterioration* in mood state occurs following the performance of a ritual, Worsley argues this could be seen as the patient's unfavourable reaction to the failure of the ritual to provide the expected relief. However, the most compelling evidence is that rituals often fail to secure the reduction in anxiety postulated. Certainly Solyom *et al.* (1971) have reported that almost 40 per cent of abnormalities of behaviour exhibited by obsessional patients are found to increase the amount of experienced anxiety rather than to reduce it.

In search of a cogent explanation for the ritualistic behaviour of obsessional patients, Walker decided upon an experiment comprising the intensive investigation of several individual patients who were marked by clear-cut ritualistic behaviour. Patients with marked hand-washing rituals were chosen. Among the measurements which Walker made were the time at which the ritual occurred, the time taken to perform it, the number of repetitions involved, the event which was alleged by the patient to have provoked it, the degree of disturbance which this event produced for the patient, and the time at which he judged himself to have recovered from the disturbance. A drive-reduction model was tentatively adopted in which it was supposed that certain 'contaminating' experiences produced an enhanced state of arousal which only dissipated slowly. Furthermore, it was assumed that rituals would occur only when the drive reached a certain peak elevation, this level being at its highest immediately before a wash and decreasing thereafter. In addition, numerous observations had led

Walker to assume that washing itself aroused an unpleasant feeling state which could not be reduced by washing, but which would dissipate with the passing of time.

This detailed experiment failed to confirm many of the propositions included in the model, but certain important conclusions could be drawn from the kind of inquiry carried out. In the first place it became apparent that *mood state* was of paramount importance as a determinant of ritualistic behaviour and that depression and hostility, rather than anxiety, were the adverse mood states which most affected our patients. Secondly, it became clear that the performance of a ritual does not necessarily lead to a termination of the state of experienced abnormality. Indeed, on numerous occasions the performance of a ritual appeared to produce an exacerbation of the adverse mood state. Such a finding is obviously at variance with a simple displacement hypothesis. It was also discovered that deliberately curtailing ritualistic behaviours, such as hand-washing, tended to produce favourable rather than unfavourable consequences for the patient. It has generally been assumed that any attempt to interfere with a performance of a ritual in this way would inevitably lead to a greater disruption and disorganization of the patient's behaviour, with a consequent increase of unfavourable affect. Such, however, was not the case and the experimental work clearly advised that any attempt to reduce the extent of the ritual by offering instructions and advice to the patient, or in some other way preventing him from carrying out his full ritualistic experience, would tend to produce a more favourable outcome and a more rapid return to stability than if no such attempt were made.

These experiments on a few single cases have established for us a quite different picture of the nature of obsessional disorder than that which is generally found in a psychiatric textbook. The emphasis which had been placed upon contaminating events in the environment of the afflicted individual, was now shifted to the variability and intensity of mood state as the most important determinant of ritualistic performances. Secondly, it was discovered that we must disabuse ourselves of any simple-minded notion that the ritual serves the function of reducing anxiety as it certainly does not do so on many occasions and, indeed, as often as not leads to incrementation of the adverse mood state. Furthermore, rather than anxiety being the most prominent of the pathological states found among obsessional patients, as is commonly assumed by behavioural psychologists, hostility and depression would appear to be the most important abnormalities. Finally, these simple experiments served the important purpose of rejecting the psychiatric adage that interfering with the ritualistic performances of obsessional patients inevitably produces a worsening of state, for among our patients, curtailment of the ritual had led to an improvement over and above that which we would have expected had the patient been allowed to complete his ritual. Several other observations of a more clinical-anecdotal kind were made and, of themselves, had an important bearing upon the validity of the generalizations set out above. Two of these may be mentioned here as they serve to point up the emphasis given to adverse mood states as a major determinant of the ritualistic behaviour. The first concerns our observation that the obsessional patient can choose to suspend the performance of ritualistic behaviour despite having encountered many environmental contaminating experiences. In other words, what may appear to be a rigid and inflexible system in which the performance of a ritual inevitably follows an experience of contamination is not that, for contaminating experiences may be set aside by the patient under certain prescribed conditions which appear to have most to do with the prevailing mood state. Secondly, we could observe that patients might, under certain conditions which we would describe as those in which the patient felt himself in a highly abnormal state, engage upon 'deliberate' self-contamination for which he would then have to wash. In this latter case, from the patient's viewpoint and, indeed, from casual observation, it might well be erroneously concluded that contamination leads to a ritual, and such an account would leave out of the causal chain the important prerequisite of adverse mood state.

At this stage Walker chose to concentrate attention upon the problem of why some rituals last a good deal longer than others, and why the performance of a ritual often leads to deterioration rather than improvement in mood state. In the first place, it was argued that rituals are instances of situations where change from one activity to another is abnormally postponed. Such an assumption would appear to be very reasonable in terms of what may be easily observed from the behaviour of obsessional patients. When such individuals are confronted with a choice, for example, as to whether to terminate a ritual or to continue, there are two alternatives, each of which may have unpleasant consequences: continuing the ritual causes additional delay, discomfort, lateness for appointment, and perhaps even some physical strain; terminating a ritual before one can be sure that it is complete leaves the obsessional patient vulnerable to the pervasive uncertainty he experiences. However, the unpleasantness of the consequences and the probabilities involved are different for the two alternatives. One might say that in the one case there is a high cost for error but a low probability of a mistake being made, so that stopping the ritual would be seen as having very dire consequences if one is wrong, but the chances of being so would be low; on the other hand a decision to continue the ritual would have a relatively low cost but a high probability of unpleasant consequence. In other words, to continue the ritual would be less unpleasant but that limited unpleasantness would be fairly certain to come about.

Walker then set out to examine this proposition by arranging choice situations where the costs and probabilities could be manipulated, predicting that obsessionals would tend to choose the low cost/high probability alternative (LC/HP) in preference to high cost/low probability (HC/LP) more frequently than will other persons. In short, obsessionals would show less willingness to take risks.

Walker considered that the deterioration in mood states which often accompanied the performance of rituals, might be explained in terms of the above model. It was argued that, after each repetition of the ritual, the obsessional patient is faced with a choice as to whether or not to terminate the ritual and is thus placed in a conflict between two avoidance tendencies. The result of this is a state of unpleasant high arousal which is reflected in the measures of mood states of hostility, depression and anxiety. As every exposure to this conflict situation increases the arousal level, the result is that a longer ritual, which involves more repetition and, therefore, more choice points (where a decision to terminate might be considered), must lead inevitably to a still greater deterioration in mood.

The task chosen was an expanded judgement test involving the discrimination of shapes where the patient could elect to make additional observations before reaching a decision. Comparing obsessionals with other neurotic patients and with depressives having obsessional features, confirmed the main prediction that obsessional symptoms would be associated with the need to make more observations on the expanded judgement task, and the related prediction that they would show longer response latencies on the unlimited time task. However, the prediction that the mood of the obsessional subject would show deterioration during the performance of an expanded judgement task, which involved the manipulation of cost and probabilities, was not confirmed. In fact the mood state showed a tendency towards improvement rather than deterioration.

Nevertheless, the initial mood state of the patient before taking part in the expanded judgement task showed a tendency to correlate with the number of additional observations which the patient required during the performance of that task. Walker goes on to comment that although the obsessional's abnormality is not confined to the ritualistic behaviour situation, it is obvious that not *all* everyday activities which are performed by him are characterized by hesitancy and postponement and, similarly, extra postulates are needed to deal with these exceptions.

It was argued that two additional assumptions are needed, the first being that the patient's estimate of the unpleasantness of the mistake or the probability of committing some error, deviates more from the normal as the perceived cost of making the mistake increases. In other words, for any given mistake the obsessional patient will tend to view this with greater seriousness, will be more disturbed by it, and will rate it as being a more unpleasant event, than will other types of patient. Secondly, the obsessional patient's estimate of the probability of making a mistake will deviate from the normal as a function of the abnormality of mood state. In her main experiment, in which she used twenty obsessionals, twenty anxiety neurotics, and the same number of normal controls, matched for age, sex and intelligence, Walker examined several propositions deriving from her model, using a specially constructed questionnaire to examine the extent to which obsessionals would view everyday mistakes with greater seriousness and with greater feelings of unpleasantness than would other groups. She found that some obsessionals did in fact offer abnormally high estimates of the unpleasantness. Paradoxically, however, other obsessionals offered abnormally low estimates of this characteristic and it was suggested that the explanation for this disparity was that the obsessional may react abnormally strongly only to those mistakes which applied to certain areas of his life, and that he might react relatively weakly to mistakes which occurred in certain other areas. These areas could be different from patient to patient. On the other hand, no abnormality specific to the obsessional group was observed in estimates of the probability of everyday mistakes occurring, and this finding failed to confirm the hypothesis put forward.

Respecting a second part of her thesis, and contrary to expectation, no tendency was found in the expanded judgement task for obsessionals to ask for more information before reaching a decision. However, for both the risk preference task and the expanded judgement task, the obsessionals tended to show some deterioration in their mood state as the task progressed. While we may say that the results of this experiment did not offer unqualified support for the theory, and that the interpretation of many of the findings was open to doubt, while yet others were inconsistent with the theory, there was some general support for the propositions involved which might be summarized as follows. In the first place, obsessionals offered abnormal estimates of the unpleasantness of a mistake. Secondly, the changes in the mood state of obsessionals had an important effect on the perceived unpleasantness of the mistake and, thirdly, that in certain circumstances, obsessionals show abnormal postponement of a final decision in an expanded judgement task. Finally, while bearing in mind that the findings were based upon a limited number of cases, it is of interest that the measures of hostility, depression and anxiety, were all strongly related to each other. Furthermore, the evidence was consistent in showing that a deterioration in mood state as measured by the three variables, is associated with an increased severity of obsessional symptoms.

In a later follow-up study (Milner, Beech and Walker, 1971) the propositions that ritualistic and checking behaviour could be regarded as the result of an overpowering need for certainty in decisions to terminate activities was re-examined. Here a group of six patients with obsessional symptoms and a control group of eight patients without such symptoms, comprised the research sample. The task involved detection of eight auditory tone signals under two conditions. In condition A the subject was required to indicate the presence or absence of the tone with a 'Yes' or 'No' response on every trial, while, in condition B, trials could be repeated until the subject felt ready to respond 'Yes' or 'No'. Under both conditions tones were in fact delivered on only half the trials, on a random schedule. The results of this experiment showed that requests for repeats of trials among the obsessionals were significantly greater than for the control group, and a comparison with the results under condition A showed clearly that this tendency could not be attributed to lower signal detectability.

A study directly related to Walker's work was conducted by Carr (1970) who began by using psychophysiological measures in assessing the patient's status as a function of the ritualistic behaviour which that patient performed. One of the most important hypotheses initially tested in this research was that compulsive rituals would be accompanied by decreases in activation, which Carr related to reaching a decision to perform a ritual. The results were found to be consistent with expectation in that performance of a compulsive ritual *was* associated with decreases in levels of physiological activity, while non-performance was accompanied by high activation levels.

While faults in the experimental design and the lack of important controls make it difficult to draw firm conclusions from these results, they appear to be somewhat at variance with Walker's findings. It could be that the apparent discrepancy is largely attributable to the artificiality of the special conditions in Carr's experiment, but it is not inconceivable that the two sets of findings can be reconciled by assuming, as Walker reported, that only certain rituals produce incrementation of arousal, while others do not. Alternatively, it is quite possible that while the initial effect of the ritual is to reduce activation, a persistence of those behaviours allows for increases in pathological status.

In his next experiment Carr set out to test the proposition deriving from Walker's study that the compulsive neurotic had an abnormally high estimate of the probability of an unfavourable outcome in decision-making. In particular it was predicted that the normal group, when responding under low cost conditions, would show significantly smaller stress or responses than would the compulsive group, but that these inter-group differences would not be evident under conditions of high cost.

The results appeared to indicate that, when operating under conditions of high cost for errors, normals appeared to behave like compulsive subjects, and that this similarity was not evident when the conditions were those of low cost. Generally speaking, under high cost conditions the pattern of responses was one of apparent increased activity where decisions of greater difficulty were concerned. In short, normal subjects made the same appraisal of threat as compulsives did under objectively low cost conditions. It was concluded that the patterns of motor response latency and anticipatory EMG indicated that the behaviour of compulsive patients was characterized by a relatively high level of uncertainty and the data supported the basic contention that in all situations the compulsive neurotic entertained an abnormally high subjective estimate of the probability of an unfavourable outcome. This finding is entirely consistent with Walker's results.

Hodgson and Rachman (1972) are well aware of the limitations of the anxiety-reduction model as a complete explanation of obsessional behaviour. Furthermore, recognizing the problems of an account which deals solely with anxiety, they label their measure of the distress experienced by obsessional patients as anxiety/discomfort.

Their study involved an attempt to test three specific predictions: that a 'contamination' experience deliberately contrived in a laboratory setting would produce increases in 'anxiety/discomfort' (that is, in the feeling which would indicate an abnormal reaction to the experimental condition), secondly, that when the patient was allowed to complete a ritualistic performance such as hand-washing, the state of 'anxiety/discomfort' would be diminished, finally that the interruption of a ritualistic behaviour would be accompanied by the enhancement of the experienced state of 'anxiety/discomfort'. Using as their measure a simple rating scale to indicate the degree of subjective experience of discomfort occasioned by the experimental condition, and a measure of pulse rate variability as an objective indication of emotional activity, the authors investigated the reactions of twelve obsessional patients all characterized by marked and easily quantifiable rituals.

The results indicated that touching a 'contaminated' object produced increases in both pulse variability and an enhancement of feelings of 'anxiety/discomfort', while the completion of a washing ritual had the opposite effect. On the other hand, there was no evidence at all for changes in state which could be attributed to a condition in which the ritual was interrupted by the experiment. Hodgson and Rachman interpret their results as being consistent with the anxiety-reduction hypothesis and at variance with the findings of Walker and Beech. The suggestion is made that the discrepancy in outcome in the two studies might be attributable to sampling difficulties, with the obsessional patients employed by Walker and Beech being possibly characterized by more marked checking and doubt than their own patients. It was considered that the former type of patient might be more likely to find difficulty in deciding whether or not to terminate a ritual and, as a result of this dilemma, suffer a deterioration in mood state. However, Hodgson and Rachman point out that the natural decline in experienced discomfort among their own patients as a result of conducting their washing ritual, was not particularly large and there were some patients who did not show this tendency at all. Furthermore, this natural decline may have been influenced by the patients' knowledge that they would be permitted to carry out their washing ritual.

It may be, as Hodgson and Rachman suggest, that differences in sampling could account for the discrepancies between their own findings and those of Beech and Walker, although other differences between the two studies could well have played an important role. It seems likely, for example, that the patients in the latter study were more severely disturbed but, in our view, other difficulties could assume even greater importance. In particular it would seem to us that the laboratory situations employed in the Hodgson and Rachman study with a specially contrived contaminating event is quite unlike the naturalistic setting with which the obsessional patient usually deals,

F

and as Beech (1971) has reported, the assumption of a systematic relation between contaminating event and ritualistic performance is probably erroneous, although patients themselves tend to subscribe, on
interrogation, to this view. Indeed, Hodgson and Rachman point out
that 'cognitive appraisal' of a situation could have influenced the
outcome. Patients understood, for example, that washing was going to
be permitted at some time, and that there was no risk of the contamination being spread from their hands to other objects in their
environment. Such a situation, in our experience, should produce
minimal disturbance, and is quite unlike the conditions which the
patient experiences outside the laboratory setting.

Again, the situation described by Hodgson and Rachman, does not
take account of what Walker and Beech found to be a crucial factor
determining ritualistic performance, namely that of existing mood
state, nor is their measure as sophisticated as those employed by
Walker and Beech in which depression, hostility and anxiety were
assessed separately and found to be relevant to predicting the duration
of ritualistic behaviour. Hodgson and Rachman confined themselves
to asking the patient 'How bothered are you now?' and indicating this
on a scale of o to 100. As Walker and Beech (1969) and Beech (1971)
have emphasized, discrepancies between a patient's self-report and his
mood state are sometimes at variance with the mood state as assessed
by others, and it may well have been that a fuller and more detailed
inquiry into existing mood state of the patients would have revealed
the tendencies which Walker and Beech had noted.

Nevertheless, the function which the ritual serves for the obsessional
patient remains unclarified and further experimentation is needed to
resolve the apparent discrepancies between findings.

A number of interesting and relevant hypotheses concerning this
topic area have recently been examined by Liddell (1974). In her study
Liddell was concerned with differences between a group of obsessionals,
a group of mixed neurotics, and a group of normals, who had been
carefully matched on a variety of important variables. Using the
Sandler and Hazari questionnaire (1960) she was able to show that
there was a predictable and highly significant difference between the
three groups in terms of the self-report of obsessional symptoms.
Furthermore, by selecting from this test the four items which were
directly concerned with decision-making, she was able to demonstrate
that the obsessional group complained significantly more frequently of
decision-making problems than either of the other two groups concerned.

Again, using the Kogan and Wallach questionnaire (1964) it was possible to demonstrate a highly significant difference in 'riskiness' between the three groups, with the obsessionals appearing as the most conservative of the three.

In another part of her experimental work Liddell was able to compare the performance of her three groups of obsessionals, mixed neurotics and normals on four discrimination tasks which required decisions in

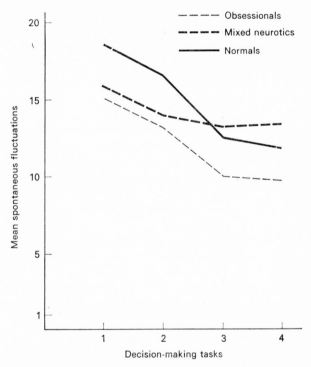

Fig. 6.1 Overall spontaneous fluctuations in GSR under 'punishment' condition.

respect of differences in tone, weight, quality of design, and judgements concerning the characteristics of people depicted in photographs. While on the last two tests of decision-making the obsessional group showed a tendency to ask for more repeats of each item before reaching a decision, no differences on this measure were found on the other tasks. This differentiation on the decision-making tasks was also reflected in the speed at which the task was completed by the three groups concerned, with the slowest performance coming from the obsessionals, and being largely attributable to the number of repeat trials requested by that group. Slowness of functioning *per se* could not explain this trend for it was possible to show that a simple test of speed of functioning (the Digit Symbol Test of the WAIS) failed to differentiate the three groups, and this suggests that it is particularly under conditions of decision-making that obsessionals appear to be slow.

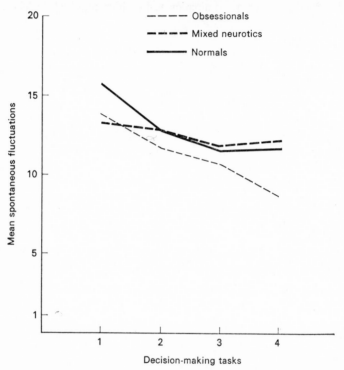

Fig. 6.2 Overall spontaneous fluctuations in GSR under 'neutral' condition.

One of the most interesting aspects of Liddell's research was concerned with the assessment of GSR responsivity in decision-making tasks. Using the same three groups of subjects, and concerning herself with the four decision-making tasks referred to earlier, Liddell examined the spontaneous fluctuations in GSR responsivity exhibited by the subjects under conditions which she described as 'neutral' and 'punishment'. 'Punishment' here refers to the use of a loud and unpleasant tone which subjects were told indicated an incorrect decision. The 'neutral' condition refers simply to the omission of this aversive stimulus.

In fact, as will be seen from Figures 6.1 and 6.2, the general level of spontaneous fluctuations among obsessionals is lower than that found in the other two groups in both 'punishment' and 'neutral' conditions and over the four kinds of decision-making tasks employed. Such an outcome was directly contrary to the expectations set out by Liddell who had predicted a significantly higher general level of spontaneous fluctuation among the obsessionals. On the other hand, the immediate

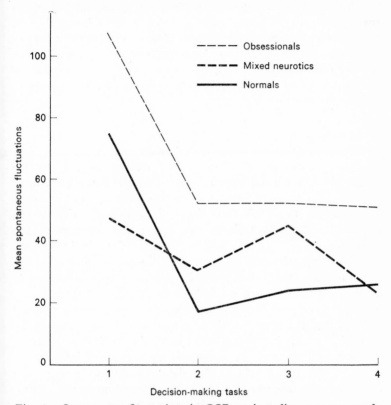

Fig. 6.3 Spontaneous fluctuations in GSR as immediate response to the aversive stimulus on four decision-making tasks.

response to punishment in terms of level of GSR reactivity showed very significant differences between the obsessional patients and the other two groups, with obsessionals showing markedly heightened increase in this measure as the immediate consequence of the buzzer presentation, as is shown in Figure 6.3.

We have, therefore, what is, at least at face value, a discrepancy between the general level of GSR activity, in terms of spontaneous fluctuations, and the specific reactivity to particular circumstances, with obsessionals showing a lower level of spontaneous fluctuation in the former conditions, but a very much higher level on the latter. These findings tend to suggest the existence of some important mechanism which not only produces some degree of regulation of fluctuations in arousal but which also offers the capacity for heightened or exaggerated responsivity to salient stimulation. That the general level of spontaneous fluctuation should be lower than that for normals over the task conditions might suggest the existence of some suppressor mechanism which may perhaps have some important protective properties, and that the true nature of the hyper-responsivity of the arousal system of obsessional patients can be detected only under special stimulating circumstances.

While we would be disinclined to emphasize an exclusively environmentalist viewpoint to account for the observed differences in reactivity to punishment between obsessionals and others, we would hold out the possibility that there are special environmental circumstances in the history of obsessional patients which have rendered them more susceptible to this form of reaction. Indeed, questioning of obsessionals in an interview situation tends to leave one with the impression that they view their history as being pitted with many more traumas, and more keenly experienced effects of traumatic episodes, than is the case with most patients. While Walker had to some extent concerned herself with this particular problem, Liddell directed her inquiry specifically to asking whether there was in fact any evidence that obsessionals had suffered more unpleasant events in their history and had attached greater significance to them. Accordingly, patients were asked to recall those unpleasant happenings which had occurred in four age periods (from 0 to 5 years, from 5 to 10 years, from 10 to 15 years and after the age of 15). The total number of events recalled in these categories failed to differentiate the three groups, with all three samples remembering fewer unpleasant events for the younger age period, but rather more episodes of this kind more recently. While the total number of such events recorded by patients was not different for the three groups, differences did emerge when the events categorized into four types. The outcome of this more detailed analysis revealed, as Liddell points out, that obsessionals tend to remember worrying a great deal more about events that *had not happened but could possibly happen*, while they appeared to recall fewer events of an unpleasant character that had actually happened to them when compared with the other two groups.

It would seem from this finding that a simple conditioning explanation in terms of environmental circumstances producing a predisposition to avoid painful consequences or punishment does not fit the data. Much more likely appears to be the possibility that obsessionals, perhaps throughout their lives, have been specially alert to the possible harmful consequences of interacting with their environment, and have shown an exaggerated sensitivity to aversive circumstances.

In addition, the subjects of this experiment were asked to categorize the intensity with which they experienced the unpleasant events which they had noted. But, while as expected, the obsessionals tended to use the category of extreme unpleasantness to describe their feelings rather more than did the control group, they were not differentiated from either the mixed neurotics or the normals in terms of this variable.

Another interesting facet of this part of her inquiry was concerned with the special attention given to punishment which had occurred at home or at school, and with special disagreements or quarrels with friends, the subjects being asked whether such incidents had occurred often in their history, seldom, or not at all. Here, while normal controls made the same use of the 'often' category as did obsessionals and mixed neurotics, there was a substantial difference between the normal control and the other two groups in that far more frequently no evidence of punishment or disagreement was cited by the obsessionals and mixed neurotics. It would appear to be rather unusual that anyone should fail to recall evidence of punishments or serious disagreements with friends, and a possible explanation of this is that the two neurotic groups feared the possibility of punishment so much that they went to extreme lengths to avoid this kind of occurrence. A similarity between the obsessionals and mixed neurotics has a bearing upon this explanation for, when subjects were asked to rate the degree to which they were disturbed by punishment or disagreements, it was found that both these groups attached far more concern to such noxious events than did the normal controls.

There is a large measure of agreement in the reports detailed above and our knowledge of the special problems of the obsessional patient is enhanced to some extent by these findings. It is now abundantly evident, for example, that decision-making difficulties are characteristic of this group and are easily demonstrated, although it seems unlikely that this abnormality is to be found under all circumstances. While it may be said that this is simply a confirmation of long-established clinical observation, we are now in a position to elaborate the decision-making difficulty and doubting into a costs and probability model, and thus relate the whole problem to a new set of parameters and theoretical propositions.

Liddell has added the idea that the emphasis may be placed upon *anticipated* unpleasantness of decision-making consequences and, furthermore, that there is no good evidence that this attitude emerges from special environmental circumstances in which the obsessional has been placed. This does not exclude the possibility that the reaction of obsessionals to actual stress *per se* is abnormal and, indeed, Liddell's findings suggest that such reactions are distinguishable as being greatly exaggerated compared with those of other groups in the context of decision-making.

There seems, also, little room for disagreement concerning the importance of mood state among this group of patients, and Walker's elaboration of adverse feeling states into depression, hostility, and anxiety, must be regarded as a useful contribution.

Perhaps too little work has been concerned with mood as a predictor of rituals, and this important pointer deserves our closest attention. Inquiry into this aspect would, among other things, throw light upon the significance of the relationship between 'contaminating' experiences and ritualistic behaviours. On this point there appears to be some room for differences in opinion and, in particular, the position adopted by Walker and others can be contrasted with the anxiety-reduction hypothesis. It may well be that these viewpoints are reconcilable in that both may turn out to have validity; existing mood state having a pronounced effect upon rituals, but the latter having some degree of effect upon the former.

The precise nature of the relationship between mood, rituals, and decision-making, remains unclear, although there is sufficient evidence for a connection of some kind to make further inquiry worthwhile. The effects of interruption of rituals have also to be fully investigated.

It seems likely that continued experimental work in these areas will lead to a better understanding of the abnormalities of functioning among this little-understood group of patients.

7

H. C. Holland

Displacement activity as a form of abnormal behaviour in animals

INTRODUCTION

Some readers may think it odd to find a contribution concerned with the behavioural abnormalities of animals in a volume designed to illustrate the parameters of a specific disorder which, at first sight, seems to be a disorder only of humans (Eysenck, 1962; Lewis, 1965). The conception of restriction to the human species may have arisen because of the pervasive 'cognitive' contribution which frequenly attends obsessional disorders in the context of clinical experience. It is freely admitted that, in the present state of knowledge, it would be unwise to draw inferences about cognitive activity from animal behaviour. Nevertheless, it is felt that observation of the latter may help to elucidate some of the problems surrounding the overt behavioural manifestations of the disorder, in particular the ritualistic acts so commonly performed by obsessionals. Indeed, it should be made clear that the purpose of this contribution is to present the evidence and discuss the case for the assertion that obsessional behaviour, with its victim's apparent preoccupation with repetitive acts (Taylor, 1963), is an example of abnormality stemming from displacement activity. Further, it is suggested that, as this activity has been most systematically studied in the total behaviour of infra-human species, it is in this area that a useful beginning may be made towards understanding the human condition.

Our starting point, therefore, is the assumption that important advantages may derive from the systematic observation and investigation of animals. These advantages have been clearly stated by Munn (1950) and Broadhurst (1958), and need not be laboured further here. However, it should be stressed that not the least of these advantages is the insight that such endeavours may provide into the causes, mechanisms and cures of human pathologies for which species or regime might have direct or analogue relevance (Levy, 1952; Bates, 1970). This statement appears undeniable to the author, nevertheless it has been challenged by many. Much opposition to the idea of extrapolation from animal to human being arises when abnormal behaviour is to be the subject of study. Some seem to go so far as to assert that abnormalities cannot exist in the behaviour of animals. Such claims are based upon the argument that it is virtually self-evident that the particular responses of the infra-human organism in the *natural* state cannot be abnormal, as such would be, by definition, unadaptive and consequently lack survival value. Hence, either the whole organism or its particular response would have disappeared within the unrelenting process of a natural selection based upon survival of the fittest (Fingerman, 1969). However, the shortcoming of this argument seems to lie in the fact that it is applicable only to organisms living in their *natural* state, i.e. their optimal environment. For animals *never* to become victims of ab-normalities in their physical or functional capacities would require that they lived in a fixed, unchanging world, which provided for them an environment of which they were an equally fixed, unchanging com-ponent, unaffected by age, disease, or any other developmental change brought about by accident or 'design'. Such a static conceptualization is unlikely and unacceptable. Some degree of variability is inescapable in the environment and, therefore, essential in the animal, as is implied in the concept of 'adaptation'. Indeed, it is firmly asserted here that, under quite a narrow range of deviation from optimal conditions, animals can, and do, develop abnormalities and that these may be indicative of the sorts of behaviour that are likewise to be developed by humans under similar conditions.

ANIMAL ANALOGUES OF OBSESSIONS

The most distinctive feature of obsessional acts are their stereotyped, repetitive nature and their apparent lack of appropriateness to the situation in which they are employed. Thus, the minimum requirement for any acceptable analogue of obsession must be that it possesses these characteristics. Hopefully, it will also resemble the human disorder in some finer details, such as the nature of the repetitive response.

Careful surveillance of the relevant literature suggests that two clear examples of stereotyped, repetitive, inappropriate acts may be extracted from the vast spectrum of animal behaviour. The first is experimentally induced fixated behaviour, where the animal persists in a well-learnt response, despite a change in the stimulus situation. The second, and more exciting, is displacement behaviour. As intimated in the introduction, the author's main concern is with the latter. However, the former will be reviewed briefly so that the extent of its similarity to displacement activity may be appreciated.

Fixated behaviour

The resemblance of fixated behaviour to obsessions has been noted and discussed by Metzner (1963). As he ably reviews the animal experimental work on fixation, no attempt will be made to do so here, and the reader is referred to this authoritative paper. However, it is of interest to cite briefly the three types of experimental situation in which Metzner considers that a response may become fixated:

1. 'A positive approach response may get fixated when it also becomes an avoidance response, so that the response which satisfies the approach response also reduces a learned anxiety (double reinforcement). . . .'
2. 'An instrumental avoidance response may get fixated by being punished, i.e. by becoming an unsuccessful avoidance response. . . .'
3. 'Avoidance behaviour may also be fixated by the delivery of free 'shock', i.e. shocks not contingent upon any behaviour that the animal shows. . . .'

On Metzner's own admission, the analogy drawn between fixated behaviour and obsessions is far from perfect. Such fixated responses are repetitive in the sense that the same response is repeated each time the animal is placed in that particular situation, and stereotyped in that the gross form of the response is always the same, e.g. the rat always turns right at the choice point. Fixated responses are inappropriate to the extent that they are not adaptive in the experimental situation. It is not sensible for the rat to continue in its approach-response-with-avoidance-value (1. above) when neither positive nor negative reinforcement is being administered.

In fact, the mere recognition that fixated behaviour resembles an obsessional act does little to clarify the nature of the latter. As Metzner points out, it seems probable that the acquisition and extinction of avoidance responses represent far more complex processes in humans than in other animal species. However, there is one aspect of fixated responding which, the author feels, may be applicable to the human case: Metzner's three situations outlined above all seem to be geared to produce a state of high arousal in the organism; and high arousal, as will be indicated below, may well prove to be a crucial determinant of obsessional behaviour.

Displacement activity

Tinbergen's (1949) sticklebacks provide a now famous example of displacement activity. When two male sticklebacks meet at the boundaries of their adjacent territories, each might be expected either to attack the other or to flee from him, as both responses would be elicited to equal degree by the boundary stimuli. But in fact they do neither, but instead begin to dig nests with incredible enthusiasm! This nest-digging appears not only to be inappropriate, but also downright maladaptive. It is this 'out of context' behaviour (Zeigler, 1964) that has been termed 'displacement activity'. Such behaviour is not merely a property of fish but has been observed in a wide variety of species, ranging from invertebrates to apes and encompassing a considerable proportion of the phylogenetic scale.

Despite interspecies differences, there appear to be three constant characteristics of such behaviour which have become the recognized hallmarks of displacement activity:

1. The 'out of context' behaviour is usually an identifiable component of one of the following activities: feeding, grooming or cleaning and, in birds and fish at least, nest-building. Other behaviours do occur (see below) but these are rare.

2. The response appears to be inappropriate, i.e. to the casual observer, the stimuli which *usually* elicit the behaviour are not salient in the situation in which it takes place.

3. Displacement activity occurs under a very restricted range of circumstances. All the stimulus situations giving rise to these responses are such as to induce one of three (or possibly four) motivational states in the animal. As Delius (1970) has observed, these are 'motivational conflict, or competition between drives for control over behaviour; frustration, when the animal fails to obtain the terminal or consummatory stimulation appropriate to its drive state; or thwarting, where the animal is prevented from executing behaviour for which it is motivated'. Delius (following Bindra, 1959) also states that the effects of exposure to novelty could be added to this list, but suggests that such may often be reducible to one of the other three conditions.

If obsessional behaviour is to be regarded as a form of displacement activity, it too should show these three characteristics. Indeed, the first of them has immediate, although perhaps anthropomorphic, appeal; the animals' preoccupation with grooming (and nesting?) seems to bear some resemblance to the obsessional's indulgence in washing and tidying rituals. Moreover, the motivational conditions cited in 3, may tempt the more psychodynamically minded to extrapolate to the intrapsychic conflicts assumed to underlie neuroses. (It might be noted in passing, that a more general interpretation of the organism's state will be considered below.)

Unfortunately, the characteristic inappropriateness of displacement activity seems to be as dissonant with the accepted conceptualization of obsessional disorder as the other two features are consonant. To be sure, the obsessional's washing is inappropriate in the sense that it may be executed more frequently or continued far longer and with far greater vigour than is warranted by the situation. *But*, there is (nearly) always a clearly definable eliciting stimulus. The obsessional appears to know exactly which contaminated object he has touched, and where it has touched him. How can this be reconciled with the fact that the appropriate eliciting stimulus is not salient in the displacement situation? The answer to this question must lie in the interpretation of the term 'salient'. Early theorists have assumed that displacement activity was not under stimulus control, but occurred as a result of an overflow of energy or frustrated drive (see Zeigler, 1964, for an historical review). With this conceptualization there was no need to seek eliciting stimuli and so, *ipso facto*, none was found. However, more recently the movement away from 'reservoir' theories has led to a comprehensive search for appropriate 'causes' of displacement behaviour. Indeed, much evidence has now been accumulated which conclusively demonstrates that displacement activity is not merely a random event. The form and intensity of the response are largely determined by the stimuli impinging on the animal. Responses other than those involved in grooming, feeding and nesting may occur as displacement activity if stimuli appropriate to them are present in the environment. For example, a bird in a conflict situation will go through the motions of settling down to incubate if there is an egg available. In the absence of an egg, displacement preening takes place (Zeigler, 1964).

This observed stimulus control over displacement activity not only suggests that obsessional checking may be explicable in terms of displacement, but also provides some possible reason why washing rituals constitute such a common feature of obsessional disorder. Indeed, how easy it is to say that the obsessional washes *because* he has touched an offending object in his contaminated world. (If confronted with gas taps, he would be expected to check, not wash.) Unfortunately, such a glib description does not explain why he should believe that so many innocuous objects are contaminated, and perceived as a potential source of danger. This is a question which carries the discussion deep into the realm of cognition, an area which, as has already been mentioned, lies outside the scope of animal research. However, animal studies may be of help in clarifying the issue, if the emphasis is shifted from 'contamination fears' to the fact of 'having touched', or 'being dirty'.

Rowell (1961) has shown that the form of displacement response executed by chaffinches depended upon the peripheral stimulation which they were receiving at the time. By means of carefully controlled experiments he found that, in a conflict situation, the resulting displacement activity consisted of *body grooming* if the birds had previously been sprayed with water, but *bill wiping* if their beaks were messy from eating sticky seed. In fact it could be said that the birds' displacement cleaning was directed toward the parts where they felt 'dirty'. It appears that the input from peripheral receptors signalling 'dirt present' acted as the eliciting stimulus for the displacement activity. Could it be that similar input triggers off washing in obsessionals? At first sight the answer appears to be no, since it is characteristic of obsessionals that they wash in the absence of any obvious trace of dirt. If there is no dirt, there can be no source of input signalling dirt, *unless* 'messages' indistinguishable from those produced by the presence of dirt were emanating from the periphery. Morris (1956) and Andrew (1956) have pointed out that many autonomic changes occur in mammals and birds in a conflict situation. These include respiratory, circulatory and thermo-regulatory changes which would be reflected in altered and increased input from the blood vessels and the skin. The same authors also state that such internally produced stimulation from the periphery would be expected to elicit a variety of grooming responses. It is suggested that obsessionals may undergo similar changes in internal state which likewise evoke stimuli from the skin which serve to elicit washing behaviour. When faced with sensations arising from his skin and the feeling that he wants to wash, the obsessional concludes that he must be dirty. In an attempt to be rational he assumes that as the 'dirt' is invisible it must, therefore, be germs (i.e. contamination) and that such must have an identifiable source. The most likely candidate is the object that he last touched. Hence there may arise a complex system of beliefs which have obvious implications for future action.

THE AROUSAL HYPOTHESIS

It may have been observed that the foregoing discussion relied heavily on the assumption that obsessionals experience an internal state which is equivalent to that found in animals in displacement situations. So far, the only reference to the nature of this state has been the observation that it involves considerable autonomic changes. We must now consider this matter in more detail.

Bindra (1959) was the first to recognize that the situations giving rise to displacement activity (i.e. conflict, frustration and thwarting) were those which produce a high degree of arousal in animals. This observation led him to postulate that displacement activity occurs as the result of high arousal; or, stated more generally, that high arousal elicits behaviour with high habit strength. Such a reformulation could well assume some explanatory value were it not for the fact that there appears to be no universally accepted definition (operational or other) of 'arousal'.

The term 'arousal' has been applied either to the state of behavioural alertness of the animal, or to the degree of cortical activity present (as measured by electroencephalographic techniques). More commonly it has been applied to both, the assumption being that the two co-vary and, moreover, are causally related. In fact the nature and extent of the relationship between these two variables is as yet unknown. However, there is some well-documented evidence from ablation studies in animals which suggests that the two variables are indeed intimately related. For example, the early work of Moruzzi and Magoun (1949) demonstrated that lesions in the reticular formation of cats produced behaviourally comatose animals with EEG recording indicative of sleep. It was this work which first suggested that the reticular formation and other medial brain-stem structures formed a single system concerned with the regulation of behavioural and cortical alertness.

Unfortunately this picture did not remain simple for long. More recent work has demonstrated that a lack of correspondence between cortical and behavioural state may be produced by lesions at slightly different sites. Feldman and Waller (1962) found that cats with lesions in the midbrain reticular formation showed EEG synchronization, but were not behaviourally asleep. Some anomalies have led Routtenberg (1968) to postulate that there are, in fact, two arousal systems, rather than one. Arousal System I is the 'Reticular Activating System' delineated by Moruzzi and Magoun (1949), and extends through the medial core of the brain stem. It is thought to be concerned with drive, or organization of response. Arousal System II is the limbic midbrain system suggested by Nauta (1958), and is thought to be concerned with incentive or reward. The interested reader is referred to the original paper by Routtenberg. Mention of this theory is made here only as a means of highlighting the complexities which surround the construct of arousal and hence of the dangers inherent in adopting the customary simplistic conceptualization of arousal. Such caution is necessary for, in spite of the complexity suggested in the ablation and stimulation studies, many psychologists have persisted in regarding arousal as a general facilitator or energizer of all forms of action. This situation appears to have arisen because, despite the difficulty in defining arousal, it is undeniable that the general alertness and responsiveness of the animal varies as a function of its circumstances.

Delius (1970) circumvents many of the problems of description by providing an operational definition of arousal couched in terms of the information processing rather than energizing function of the brain-stem systems outlined above (i.e. Routtenberg's Arousal System I and possibly also II). He argues that, before a stimulus can elicit a response, the afferent stimulation it produces must be processed by the animal. The rate of processing depends, to a large extent, upon the amount of information 'contained' in the stimulus. The more information that is present in the situation, the faster will have to be the rate, if it is to be processed efficiently. As it happens, those stimuli which contain a great deal of information (i.e. are complex, novel or of particular significance) generally also elicit high degrees of arousal as conventionally described. In fact Delius contends 'that arousal is equivalent, or at least related to the overall rate of processing in the nervous system (Welford, 1962). He suggests that the organism anticipates its energy requirements from its rate of information processing as well as from more specific in-formation. Situations necessitating rapid processing usually promote extensive action, and considerable autonomic changes are a prerequisite of such action. Thus rapid processing is indicative of the need for great autonomic activity, and in Delius' opinion, is usually sufficient to produce the required changes.

It is clear that Delius considers that the rate of effective information processing is greatly influenced by the amount of information present in the environment. He does not suppose, however, that this rate of processing can increase indefinitely but rather that there is a definite limit to the organizer's processing ability. He uses the conventional (if somewhat misleading) term 'limited channel capacity' to refer to the fact that there is an upper limit to the amount of information which the organism is able to process efficiently. This channel capacity is not considered to be constant but changes over time as a function of the metabolic state of the animal. Moruzzi (1966) has demonstrated that information processing and metabolic recovery are at least partially incompatible. Thus, if the animal's nervous system is engaged in metabolic recovery, its channel capacity (information processing rate) will be reduced. Moreover, in addition to these intra-individual fluctuations, it would be expected that there would be inter-individual differences in channel capacity.

Delius postulates that if the environmental input is so taxing as to cause this unit to be exceeded, processing becomes inefficient and prone to error. It would be deleterious to the animal to remain in a situation where it was not processing effectively, but physical escape may not always be possible. Thus it would be consonant with the concepts of adaptation and homeostasis for the animal to possess some arousal-inhibiting 'mechanism' which would serve to reduce the information processing rate, and which could be switched into action automatically when the input exceeded the channel capacity. Delius suggests that such a mechanism may exist in the activation of the sleep system. Evidence that the sleep system may be set into action as a direct consequence of high arousal is to be found in the work of Dell, Bonvallet and Hugelin (1961). They discovered that strong activation of the reticular formation led to spontaneous activation of the sleep system which, in turn, inhibited the reticular formation. Koella (1966) demonstrated that activation of the sleep system affects the afference of the sensory information. Delius postulates that this leads to an overall reduction of information input and thus of processing rate (i.e. arousal) through efferent inhibition of the primary sensory systems, i.e. those concerned with vision and audition.

HYPER AROUSAL AND DISPLACEMENT ACTIVITY

This postulated autonomic de-arousal function of the sleep system allows Delius to resolve an as yet unmentioned paradox concerning displacement activity. As has already been noted, grooming behaviour constitutes a very common form of displacement activity. In the atypical displacement situation, it occurs when the animal is highly aroused. Yet, in marked contrast, under normal circumstances grooming is accompanied by a state of very low arousal; indeed it characteristically occurs just prior to sleep, or when the animal is still drowsy upon waking. Bolles (1960) has confirmed this observation experimentally. By analysing the behaviour patterns of normal rats in terms of transition probabilities, he showed that grooming regularly precedes and follows sleep. Delius, himself, has demonstrated a further link between grooming and sleep. Electrical stimulation of certain areas of gulls' brains elicited a series of actions terminating in preening accompanied by drowsiness and sometimes followed by sleep. From the results of many studies of this kind, as well as from casual observation, Delius concludes that grooming and sleep are intimately related. Indeed, he tentatively suggests that they may be causally related. Grooming, by virtue of its repetitive nature, may well promote sleep, for Roitbak (1960) has shown that repetitive stimulation of cutaneous afferents is extremely efficient in producing sleep in the cat.

Of course, the above relationship does not indicate why grooming normally occurs in a state of low arousal. Delius feels that the reason for this association is fairly obvious. Behaviour such as grooming has low priority in the animal's response repertoire. It can easily be postponed in order to allow other more important activities, such as feeding and fighting, to take place. Further, the rather stereotyped mechanistic actions involved in grooming seem to be minimally under the control of external stimuli. These features of grooming make its operation during a state of low arousal both feasible and adaptive. Hence, Delius thinks it reasonable to assume that a built-in 'organizational pattern', facilitating the occurrence of grooming in the presence of reduced arousal, has been selected for in evolution.

Having acknowledged that grooming behaviour is associated not only with low arousal, but more significantly with sleep, it is not difficult for Delius to 'explain' the paradoxical occurrence of displacement activity in a state of high arousal. If it is assumed that the environmental stimulation has great informational value and consequently overloads the processing system, then the hypothesized de-arousal mechanism would be automatically switched into play; i.e. the sleep system would be activated. Such activation would serve to switch the animal's attention away from the input from its primary sensory receptors. As a consequence of this switch, there would be a relative facilitation of the secondary systems, including that concerned with cutaneous sensation and the behaviour associated with them. Thus the animal would become more 'aware' (though not necessarily at a conscious level) of the stimuli issuing from its skin and would be likely to respond to these with grooming behaviour. The persisting autonomic response resulting from the previously high state of arousal would be sufficient to ensure that fairly strong cutaneous stimulation is always present in displacement situations (Morris, 1956, Andrew, 1956).

IMPLICATIONS FOR A MODEL OF OBSESSIONAL RITUALS

If obsessional rituals are to be considered as a form of displacement activity, their occurrence must be viewed as being a consequence of the activation of the sleep system. As it has been suggested that this system is automatically activated when the organism's processing channel is overloaded, it must follow that obsessionals must experience such an overload just prior to the execution of their rituals. But what causes their channel capacity to be exceeded? It has already been argued quite strenuously that, at least initially, the obsessional's sighting of 'contaminated' objects is a consequence and not a cause of his ritualistic washing. Thus the presence of environmental input of extremely high informational value cannot be put forward as the cause of the overload as it is in animal displacement activities. Fortunately, the notion of overload does not necessitate that the incoming information is excessive. It merely requires that the amount of incoming information is too great for the particular processing system to handle effectively. This essential relativity between input and channel capacity implies that the latter may be as influential in determining the occurrence of overload as is the former. A system with a low maximum rate of processing (i.e. very limited capacity) would be expected to be thrown into chaos by relatively smaller amounts of channel capacity than other people, there is no need to search for avoidance of information-laden external (or internal) stimuli in order to account for the overload. The obsessional is not being bombarded with input, but is simply unable to deal effectively with amounts of information which other people process with ease. By virtue of his rather limited capacity the obsessional is more susceptible to overload and hence to the automatic activation of the sleep system. He, therefore, exhibits ritualistic displacement activity in situations in which most other people are functioning efficiently.

Having suggested that the obsessional possesses an abnormally limited channel capacity, it seems desirable to attempt to explain why this should be the case. Of course, the all-pervasive law of individual differences instantly springs to mind. It is only necessary to postulate that there exists a normal distribution of channel capacity within the human population and obsessionals immediately become identifiable as those who are lodged in the left-hand asymptote. Unfortunately, this statistical 'explanation' lacks substance and there would be greater satisfaction if we were able to locate a definite abnormality in obsessionals which not only differentiated them from 'normals' but also accounted for the postulated limited channel capacity.

Again, the animal studies may provide a clue as to where such a search might begin. It may be recalled that Moruzzi (1966) found that information processing and metabolic recovery were at least partially incompatible. The more the nervous system is involved with metabolic activity, the more limited its information channel capacity must become. Thus an animal which is suffering from an abnormality of metabolic recovery may well also exhibit an impairment of its information processing capacity. The reduced channel capacity automatically increases the likelihood that incoming information will overload the system and thereby give rise to displacement activity in the animal. Thus indirectly metabolic malfunctioning may lower the threshold for displacement activity.

Stated in this way, the relationship between displacement activity and metabolic abnormality bears some resemblance to that observed between obsessions and depression. Stengel (1945), Gittleson (1966b) and many others have noted both that obsessions may arise with the onset of depression and disappear when it is alleviated, and that already existing obsessions may become worse during depression. Indeed, as the presence of metabolic abnormality is heavily implicated in depression, it is tempting to argue that the nature of depression is such as to produce a reduction in the information processing capacity of the organism. However, such a conclusion would seem to be unwarranted in view of the fact that the exact role of metabolic disorder is unclear, and has not yet been established as a *sine qua non* of depression. Nevertheless, it is tentatively suggested that in some cases the emergence of rituals may be precipitated by a reduction in processing capacity occurring as a function of depression.

The hypothesized relationship with depression cannot be used to explain the characteristic intractability of obsessional rituals. Once they are established the obsessional may continue to exercise his obsession for the rest of his life, often without exhibiting any pronounced depression. There are at least two possible factors which could account for the resilience of the rituals in such cases. It could be postulated either that the obsessional's information processing capacity must have become permanently reduced (perhaps through some functional or structural change in the Reticular Activating System), or that his capacity has returned to normal but that his environment has changed and now frequently overloads him with information. Although admittedly the former is plausible, the latter occurrence appears to be the more likely.

If, as was suggested earlier, the obsessional begins to label things around him as being 'contaminated', he is in effect altering his environment. What heretofore were familiar objects requiring little consideration, now become potential threats demanding considerable vigilance. In fact the belief that they are 'contaminated' drastically increases their information value. It is possible that after such labelling the information input from these stimuli is great enough to overload the now normal channel capacity. The ensuing activation of the sleep system would thus precipitate washing as before.

8

Fay Fransella

Thinking and the obsessional

There has been a quite exceptional dearth of experimental work on the thought processes that could underlie the behaviour of obsessional neurotics. Perhaps one reason for this is the compelling nature of the behaviour itself. This behaviour is so obviously distressing to the patient that it seems almost irrelevant to ask what manner of thinking could lead a person to act in this seemingly self-defeating way.

Explanations do not have to be sought to account for why man behaves at all, but only why he behaves as he does. If one rejects the idea that man responds blindly, at the whim of a stimulus, or that he is goaded on by some psychical force in the nether regions of his mind, then one can look at the man himself and seek there reasons for his acts. The explanation must be such that it tells why one man becomes incapacitated by, say, obsessional rituals, while another is content to be precise, punctilious and true.

No attempt will be made to tease out the relationship between personality type and neurotic disorder, as this has been done in full by Slade in Chapter 4. Comparison of studies of obsessional thought processes has been made considerably more difficult by the fact that investigators have not all studied the same type of person. Thus, in the following discussion, note will simply be made of whether it is those with obsessional personality or obsessional neurosis who are the subject of investigation.

PATTERNS OF INTELLIGENCE

One of the early studies of the cognitive structure of obsessionals was that by Rapaport *et al.* (1946). This attempted:

to demonstrate that the different types of maladjustment tend to have different distinguishable and recognisable impairments of test performance. It will be shown, however, that certain deficiencies due to the educational environment, or assets due to cultural predilections, may cloud or exaggerate some of these diagnostically distinguishing features of impairment. (p. 39).

Indeed, in spite of testing 271 people (sub-divided into several diagnostic categories and including 54 normal subjects) on the Wechsler–Bellevue intelligence test, Rapaport failed to demonstrate convincingly any clear scatter on the scales that could be related to diagnostic categories. Wechsler (1965) discusses this problem in relation to his own work and comes to the following conclusion:

> Considering the many possible sources of error, the over-all agreement in the findings on most subtests is rather substantial. This is not equally true for all the syndromes. The consensus is much better for organic brain disease than for schizophrenia, better for schizophrenia than psychopathic personality, and generally poor for the category neuroses, whether treated as a broad category or broken down to sub-groups, like conversion hysteria, obsessions, etc.
>
> In view of the limited agreement as regards the neurotic signs as originally described in the earlier editions of the *Measurement of Adult Intelligence*, and also their limited usefulness in practice, this category has been dropped from our present summaries. (p. 173)

As to the broader category of Verbal as opposed to Performance scores on the Wechsler test, nothing need be added to the summary given by Gurvitz more than twenty years ago.

> In obsessive–compulsives there appears to be real preponderance of Verbal over Performance scores with a higher average Verbal IQ and with 2 out of 3 cases having a higher Verbal IQ. If we use the concept of a significant difference of 11 points, however, we will not regularly find more than 25 per cent showing differences of this magnitude. Unfortunately, many other groups, notably early schizophrenics, have a similar relationship between verbal and performance abilities. (Gurvitz, 1951, p. 19)

No convincing evidence has been produced since these studies to make one alter his opinion that the obsessional does not differ significantly from any other group in the ways he performs on standard intelligence tests.

TOLERANCE OF AMBIGUITY AND RIGIDITY

No attempt is going to be made to give a critical review of the vast literature on rigidity and tolerance of ambiguity as this has been ably done elsewhere (e.g. Chown, 1959; Leach, 1967). But mention will be made of the few studies that have used these concepts in an attempt to differentiate obsessionals from other types of neurotic and non-psychiatric populations.

In 1949, Frenkel-Brunswick suggested that a person's ability to tolerate ambiguity in his environment may be specifically related to his method of dealing with conflicts and anxieties. Following this line of thought, Hamilton (1957a) gave a variety of groups (including obsessional neurotics) eleven tasks to perform. These included weight, brightness and length discriminations, block sorting and that used by Luchins in his investigation of 'Einstellung' rigidity. In this latter task, ambiguous drawings gradually change from, say, a car to a dog, and a measure is based on how long the person 'hangs on' to the original concept. Amongst other things, Hamilton found that the obsessional group had the lowest number of 'can't decide' responses and that, in general, they tended to avoid ambiguity more than others. He comments that while obsessional doubt may be present while reaching a decision, a decision is nearly always made in an attempt to achieve psychological stability. He concluded that avoidance of ambiguity indeed serves to minimize anxiety and conflict.

The notion that relative inability to tolerate ambiguity was a personality characteristic of obsessional people was supported by Rosenberg (1953). He studied students attending a psychiatric clinic who had obsessional–compulsive profiles on the MMPI. He found that they made greater systematic errors in the direction of 'symmetry' on a visual task than did a group of non-psychiatrically disturbed students. No mention was made, however, as to whether this was a characteristic of 'neurotic' students generally.

In an earlier study, Balkan and Masserman (1940) analysed verbal responses to TAT cards. They found that obsessional neurotics differed in some respects from groups of normal controls, patients with anxiety states and those with conversion hysteria. They scored *highest* on 'compulsions' e.g. I have to . . ., I must . . ., and on a qualification/certainty ratio (expressions of qualification/expressions of certainty). They scored *lowest* on a pro/con ratio (expressions of possibility and probability/expressions of impossibility and improbability) and on a certainty/uncertainty ratio. These linguistic tendencies, coupled with an extensive use of 'special expressions' (such as 'sort of', 'this is how'), generally increased the average length of production. Foulds (1951) also found that obsessionals were slower than all groups except depressives on a Porteus Maze Test – a performance as opposed to a verbal task. It is a possibility, therefore, that the verbal vacillation that occurs before an obsessional makes a decision is reflected also in his nonverbal behaviour.

Recently, Milner, Beech and Walker (1971) carried out a further investigation relating to tolerance of ambiguity in the obsessional. They state that the rituals and ruminations of the obsessional neurotic are 'the result of an overpowering need for certainty in decisions to terminate quite ordinary activities'. Under conditions in which the subjects were allowed to ask for repetitions of a sound occurring amidst 'white noise', the obsessionals asked for significantly more repeats than did a control group. The authors also reported a high correlation (0·79), across obsessionals *and* controls, between age and the response 'no' when a definite decision was required on each occasion. The obsessional is thus seen as deferring decisions to an abnormal extent. But also, with increase in age there is a growing reluctance in all subjects to risk being wrong in identifying the *presence* of a stimulus; it is better to be wrong for saying 'no' than for saying 'yes'.

RIGIDITY AND AGE

If the results of Milner and his co-workers cannot be attributed to differences in auditory acuity, then the finding that there is an increasing reluctance to report the presence of a signal with increasing age, is in accord with observations that there is increasing 'rigidity' with age. There is resistance to anything that may lead to the necessity of dealing with new information which will have to be incorporated into the existing conceptual system.

Propositional construing (Kelly, 1955) becomes less common and rigidity of thought more the order of the day. This type of thinking is of the 'any roundish mass may be considered, among other things, as a ball' type. One is quite prepared to admit that balls can be all sorts of things other than roundish masses. The opposite type of construing, in construct theory terms, is 'constellatory'. This is of the 'since this is a ball, it must be round, resilient, and small enough to hold in the hand' type. It is the sort of thinking that leads people to say 'the young are a lot of layabouts and drug takers', without taking into account the possibility that they may also be kind, poor or parents. The elderly can be seen as increasingly using constellatory type of thinking – they constrict their thinking so as to be more able to deal with events that occur. They tend to increase the predictability of life events by ensuring that their room is always the same from day to day, that clothes are taken off in the same order and that the daily constitutional is taken at the same time and along circumscribed routes. By doing this they are reducing the chances of being caught unawares by an event which may present difficulties of interpretation.

The narrowing of horizons, whether seen in information or construct theory terms, also has hazards for people. It leaves them vulnerable to being overwhelmed by anxiety. They may be made to realize that *the events with which they are confronted lie outside the range of convenience of their construct system* (Kelly, 1955). If the world ceases to be orderly, if prized possessions are moved, then chaos throughout their whole environment is a possibility.

CONCLUSIONS

Studies using several measures of tolerance of ambiguity or rigidity have been fairly consistent in reporting very low correlations between the measures (e.g. Kenny and Ginsburg, 1958; Pervin, 1960). As concluding remarks to his section on this topic, Mischel (1968, p. 29) says:

> ... investigators frequently measure and describe a purportedly general dimension of behaviour only to discover later that it has dubious consistency. As a result the popular dimensions of personality research often wax and wane almost like fashions. Research on the generality of the behavioural indices of personality dimensions has generated its own truisms. Over and over again the conclusions of these investigations, regardless of the specific content area, are virtually identical and predictable. The following paragraph, from Applezweig's (1954) own summary, is essentially interchangeable with those from a plethora of later researches on the generality of many different traits:

> *The following conclusions appear to be justified: (a) There is no general factor of rigidity among a number of so-called measures of rigidity; the interrelationships of these measures appear to vary with the nature of the tests employed and the conditions of test administration as well as behavioural determinants within S's. (b) Scores obtained by an individual on any so-called measure of rigidity appear to be a function not*

*only of the individual, but also of the nature of the test and the con-
ditions of test administration.* (Applezweig, p. 228)

CREATIVITY

Snyder (1967) linked the notion of tolerance of ambiguity with that of
creativity when discussing the relative intellectual needs of science and
engineering students. He was suggesting that perhaps creative thinking
for the engineer involves intolerance rather than tolerance of ambiguity.
However, it is more commonly held that creative thinking is linked to
'a willingness to accept some uncertainty in conclusions and decisions
and a tendency to avoid thinking in terms of rigid categories' (Guildford, 1959). This ability to think up as many novel answers as possible
to a question (the usual test of creative thought) has been discussed also
as a personality trait – there are said to be convergent and divergent
thinkers.

> An individual described as 'convergent' is, by implication, good at
> walking, blinkered and unquestioningly, along a prescribed groove;
> it is understood that the groove is narrow, arbitrary and leads, if
> anywhere, to somewhere dull. On the other hand, the person des-
> cribed as 'divergent', it is suggested, is lively, enterprising and free-
> ranging in exciting, unexplored territory. (Heim, 1970, p. 43)

However, yet again there is evidence accruing to show that creativity
as a personality trait is too simplistic a notion. For instance, Hudson
(1970) found that, when given specific instructions, the 'convergent'
child can obtain scores which fall well within the range of those of the
'divergent' child. It seems much more likely that these are thinking
strategies, encouraged or discouraged during childhood, rather than
opposite poles of a personality trait dimension.

Kelly (1955) sees creative thinking as being part of a cycle, which
'starts with loosened construction and terminates with tightened
validated construction'. Discussing the two extremes of the tight–loose
dimension he says:

> A person who always uses tight constructions may be productive –
> that is, he may turn out a lot of things – but he cannot be creative;
> he cannot produce anything which has not already been blueprinted.
> . . . A person who uses loose constructions exclusively cannot be
> creative either. He would never get out of the stage of mumbling
> to himself. He would never get around to setting up a hypothesis for

crucial testing. The creative person must have that important capacity to move from loosening to tightening. (p. 529)

Bannister (1960) has argued that the schizophrenic who thinks in a characteristically disordered way, could be viewed as having such a loose connection between the concepts he uses that he has mostly lost the capacity to make predictions about his world and to put his predictions to the test. Those describing the obsessional as a characteristically 'rigid' thinker, are placing him at the tight end of this same dimension. But, just as Bannister demonstrated that there are varying degrees of thought disorder within the thinking of each schizophrenic, so it is suggested here that there are varying degrees of 'rigidity', creativity or tightness–looseness, within the construing systems of each obsessional. It is not an all-pervasive personality trait. The degree of tight construing for any particular individual will depend upon how he construes the type of task he is being asked to do.

EXTREMITY RATINGS

Just as some have related creativity to notions of rigidity or inability to tolerate ambiguity, so others have seen a relationship between rigidity and the tendency to use the extreme positions on rating scales rather than the more intermediary ones. Hamilton (1968) takes the view that 'to respond in the extreme is here seen as an effort to achieve a greater degree of structure in the environment, thus reducing ambiguity', and cites several experiments that support this notion. One of the very few studies reporting specifically on the response styles of obsessionals is that of Marks (1966). The obsessionals used the *central* position of the scales significantly more often and the intermediary, more discriminatory, positions significantly *less* often than did the non-psychiatric control subjects. It presumably could be argued that the central position on a scale is at least as unambiguous for the obsessional neurotic as are the scale extremes.

Bonarius (1970) categorized the experiments mentioned by Hamilton under three headings: i) rigidity or intolerance of ambiguity, ii) drive or anxiety, and iii) cognitive development (an inverse relationship between age and extremity ratings) and subsumed these under the general heading *maladjustment*. The various authors cited argue that the data state that the more maladjusted a person is the more extreme his ratings will be. In a series of experiments, Bonarius proceeded to make the case for an Interaction Model, involving the three variables of rater, object being rated and scale contrast. In these experiments he tested the *maladjustment* hypothesis and a *meaningfulness* hypothesis. This latter suggests that the more meaningful the task is, the more extreme will be the ratings (e.g. O'Donovan, 1965; Landfield, 1968). He concluded that there was no evidence to support the *maladjustment* hypothesis, since he failed to find a relationship between neuroticism (as measured on a questionnaire) and extremity of rating. However, it needs to be borne in mind that his subjects were non-psychiatrically disturbed students.

On the other hand, he showed quite clearly the importance of personal relevance or *meaningfulness* of the task for the individual. The

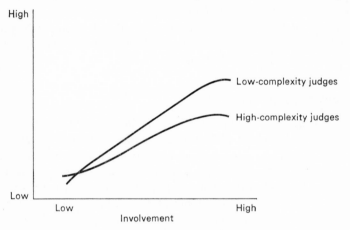

Fig. 8.1 Interaction between cognitive complexity, involvement and extremity ratings. (Redrawn from Warr and Coffman, 1970)

more the scales and object being rated were personally meaningful to the judge, the more extreme was the rating. He states that 'extremity rating is not the characteristic of certain people as compared to others, but rather the kind of relations between components of the rating'.

Warr and Coffman (1970) also discuss the interaction effects between judge, scale dimensions and stimulus being rated. They invoke the term 'involvement' to help explain the consistent failure to find relationships between rating extremity and personality variables. They differ from Bonarius in that they report a general tendency for subjects to be consistent across tasks in the extremity of their ratings. They also failed to find a difference between meaningfulness of *scale* and extremity of rating. However, they attribute this latter result to lack of range of meaningfulness in the scales used. The data left the authors in no doubt about the importance of the meaningfulness of the *concept* in determining extremity of rating – they correlated 0·83. Warr and Coffman conclude by suggesting that extremity ratings are only related to personality factors on tasks in which subjects are highly involved. They produce slight evidence that cognitive complexity is implicated – the more extreme scorers being those having both low complexity of thought structure and high involvement in the task (see Fig. 8.1). Bieri (1966) defines cognitive complexity as the tendency to construe social behaviour in a multidimensional way 'such that a more cognitively complex individual has available a more versatile system for perceiving the behaviour of others than does a less cognitively complex person'.

Once again it would appear that a seemingly straightforward form of behaviour is complex. One not only has to look at the situation in relation to the person involved, but also at *how he interprets that situation*.

INDUCTIVE VERSUS DEDUCTIVE REASONING

Instead of examining types of people, Reed (1969b, c) looked at types of thinking. He put forward the notion that the thinking of obsessional neurotics is related to a relative inability to organize and integrate experience. He goes on to say that 'this failure is expressed in the overstructuring of input and in maladaptive over-defining of categories and boundaries'. To test this idea, he gave a 'deductive' task (the Essentials Test) to three groups consisting of twenty-five people with either a) a variety of psychiatric disorders, or b) no demonstrable psychiatric disturbance or c) obsessional personality disorder. The people in the three groups were matched for sex, age, occupation and education. They were required to underline words considered essential in the description of a word. For example, the word DOG would be followed by *Head, Collar, Legs, Kennel, Tail* and *None*. The person would be expected to consider that *Head, Legs* and *Tail* would be underlined as essential elements to make up a DOG.

By conventional scoring, that is by a simple totting of items in which *all* words were correctly underlined, there was absolutely no difference between the three groups. However, Reed argued that a study of differences in *types* of error rather than global counts would differentiate the groups. He predicted that the obsessional would be overspecific in his interpretation of a given category and therefore select very few of the possible alternatives as being members of that category or class. The difference was indeed demonstrated (p < 0·001), eighteen obsessionals, two non-obsessional psychiatric patients and only one normal subject giving too few alternatives.

Reed suggests that one of the reasons Rapaport (1946) and Wechsler (1965) failed to find specific patterns of thought structure, was that they used the conventional scoring methods rather than analysing the errors into types.

The obsessional's style of thinking is likened by Reed to that described in normal psychology as 'category width' (Pettigrew, 1958). In abnormal psychology he makes a comparison with the notion of over-inclusiveness, although the obsessional thinks in the opposite or under-inclusive manner. One problem with this concept is that there is no theoretical basis from which one can deduce how people come to be 'inclusive' in the first place and how some 'over' or 'under' do it. Another point to be taken into account before irrevocably linking Reed's work to the concept of over-inclusion is that the various measures of the concept fail to correlate in an acceptable way (Hawks, 1964).

Reed followed up this first experiment with another (1969b) in which he predicted that 'when required to produce his own categorical system his (the obsessional's) over-specifying tendency will result in his allotting fewer items to each class than would the non-anakast. Thus, to classify all the items in any given array the anakast will require more classes.' He used three matched groups, this time ten people in each. The task was the standard Vigotsky test of concept formation, consisting of twenty-two blocks in five different colours, six surface shapes, two heights and two sizes of horizontal surface. The anakasts did produce significantly more categories than the normal controls as predicted, but not more than the psychiatric controls. In a second part of the experiment, the subjects were asked to use as *few* categories as possible. Under these conditions, the anakasts produced significantly *more* categories than both the normal controls ($p < 0.02$) and psychiatric controls ($p < 0.03$). Reed comments on the indecision and doubt that characterized the obsessionals during the task and considers that 'this identification of remote or unlikely complicating features may be taken as colourful evidence for anakastic over-structuring'.

One of the most interesting features of these studies is the suggestion they make that the thought processes of obsessionals and some schizophrenics could be investigated by thinking of them along the same continuum. Not only might this lead to a greater understanding of disordered thought but would help describe more clearly the observed clinical relationship between the psychiatric categories of schizophrenic and obsessional neurosis (e.g. Rosenberg, 1968a).

COGNITIVE STRUCTURE

A recent study of the thought processes of obsessional neurotics adopted a construct theory approach and used repertory grid methodology (Makhlouf Norris, 1968). In the first instance, she sought to determine the degree of cognitive complexity (Bieri, 1966) shown by eleven people diagnosed as obsessional–compulsive neurotics and eleven people with no demonstrable psychiatric disorder.

Measures of cognitive complexity and others were derived from Kelly's Role Construct Repertory Grid using the Self Identification Method of administration. The subject was asked to name twenty people he knew (each name being written on a card) who fit certain role titles, such as friends, authority figures, family figures or those disliked and including actual, ideal and social selves. The subject was then presented with three of these cards at a time, one always being the actual self, and asked to state an important way in which two of the three people were alike and thereby different from the third. Makhlouf elicited sixteen constructs from each of her subjects in this way.

Most forms of grid involve the sorting of *elements* in terms of certain *constructs*. These elements may be people known to the person (as in Makhlouf's study) or strangers, or cars or noses, depending on the sub-system of constructs being investigated. In Makhlouf's case, the subjects rated each person known to them, in terms of each of the bipolar constructs that had been elicited from them, along a seven-point scale. Product moment correlations were calculated between all possible pairs of constructs. These correlation matrices were then analysed into their principal components for each individual.

Not only did Makhlouf find no difference in the degree of complexity between the two groups – the obsessionals were no 'simpler' in their construing of people than the group of normals, but there was also no difference in the degree to which the concepts were intercorrelated (Bannister's Intensity score, 1960). The consistency of the scores was measured by giving a re-test over a ten-minute interval. The range of consistency scores for the normal subjects was 0·73 to 0·97 while, among the obsessionals, nine scored over 0·90, one had a correlation of 0·86 and one of 0·42.

Finding no difference on these measures, Makhlouf proceeded to look at other aspects of structure. For instance, she examined the clustering of constructs having significant relationships ($p < 0.05$) with each other. She considered clusters in which all constructs were significantly related to one another as 'primary'. The remainder she divided

G

into i) 'secondary' constructs (those significantly related to one or more constructs in a primary cluster); ii) 'linkage' constructs (those significantly related to one or more constructs in two or more clusters); and iii) 'isolates' (constructs not significantly correlated with any other constructs). Figures 8.2, 8.3 and 8.4 show the three main types of conceptual organization found (Makhlouf Norris, Jones and Norris 1970).

Figure 8.2 represents a structure described as monolithic and was

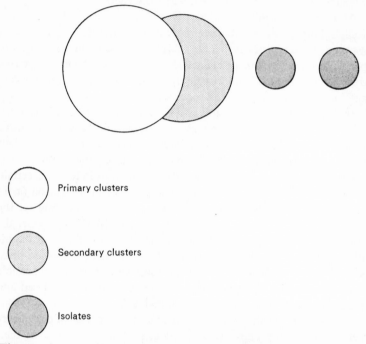

Primary clusters

Secondary clusters

Isolates

Fig. 8.2 A monolithic structure of constructs consisting of one primary, one secondary clusters and two isolates. (Redrawn from Makhlouf Norris, Jones and Norris, 1970)

found in an obsessional patient. This monolithic structure combined with the segmented structure shown in Figure 8.3 were categorized as non-articulated systems. These can be compared with an articulated system found in most normal control subjects shown in Figure 8.4.

Makhlouf points out how restricting monolithic or segmented systems must be. The segmented structure permits only 'discrete cataloguing of the separate aspects of a person, but cannot bring these together into a single identity'. With a monolithic structure 'independent judgements with opposing implications cannot be made. Therefore the tendency is to make judgements which mean the same thing.' Makhlouf argues that monolithic or segmented systems are not able to be adequately modified in the face of repeated invalidation. This would lead the obsessional to avoid those situations likely to require the need for making predictions or decisions and 'in uncertainty he creates islands of certainty in which he can control events, he tries to create a condition

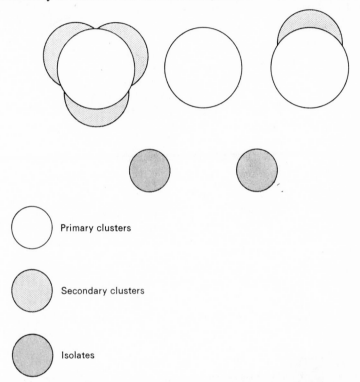

Primary clusters

Secondary clusters

Isolates

Fig. 8.3 A segmented structure of constructs consisting of three primary and four secondary clusters and two isolates. (Redrawn from Makhlouf Norris, Jones and Norris, 1970)

in which his objective probabilities are invariably 1·00 – an obsessional idea or compulsive act. It is a symbolic miniature act, with a dual function; that of bridging the gap between self and ideal self, and also of confirming the inferiority of the self . . .' (1968).

Apart from discussing the theoretical implications of the features of cognitive structure she found in the obsessionals, Makhlouf places considerable emphasis on the fact that obsessionals were found to have significantly greater distances between their construing of their *actual*

self and *ideal self* and that the *actual self* was usually seen in an unfavourable light. She argues that, because of the degree of separation
of *actual* from *ideal self*, the construct system of the obsessional has the
task of construing itself, rather than construing external reality. Because
of this internal preoccupation, it is not an efficient system for construing events and thereby making valid predictions.

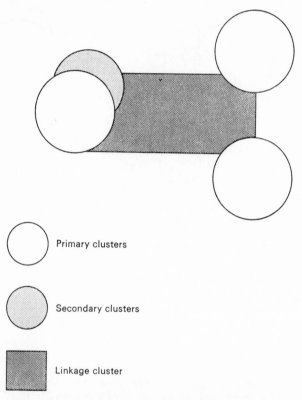

Primary clusters

Secondary clusters

Linkage cluster

*Fig. 8.4 An articulated structure of constructs consisting of three primary
and one secondary cluster and one linkage cluster. (Redrawn from Makhlouf
Norris, Jones and Norris, 1970)*

Both the Reed and Makhlouf studies show how global methods of
measurement can hide important differences which are found to exist
when results are looked at in more detail. At different levels, they
suggest that those with obsessional personalities as well as those with
obsessional symptoms tend to use relatively discrete conceptual
categories, both in operational and in construing terms.

It may be that Makhlouf would have found such non-articulated systems in a group of neurotics had she included them in her investigation, as monolithic systems have been found to occur in people other than obsessionals. The existing evidence is, however, only suggestive at the present time. First, there is the finding that those suffering from some form of clear-cut brain damage show a bi-modal distribution in terms of Intensity and Consistency of construing as measured on the Grid Test of Thought Disorder (Bannister and Fransella, 1966, 1967). Also, part of an investigation of the construing of patients with dysphasia involved a single case investigation of a man diagnosed as having severe receptive and expressive dysphasia (Fransella, 1970a). He was found to have near maximum scores on the Grid Test. That is, he could organize and relate certain constructs and maintain the relationships as others do, even though he related them more rigidly. Further investigation revealed that what he could not do was fix the correct verbal label to the elements. He could meaningfully rank elements such as cloth, sandpaper, ashtray in terms of weight, softness, colour and so forth, but he could not point to them when they were identified by name. It was suggested that the tightness or rigidity of construing he showed was an attempt to impose as much structure as possible on the events of which he could make some sense, because so many things were confusing to him.

A second source of evidence concerning the greater generality of non-articulated systems is the finding that some obese patients have unidimensional systems (Fransella, 1970b; Fransella and Crisp, 1970), as well as some patients being treated for anorexia nervosa (Fransella, 1971a).

While Makhlouf found no simple relationship between tightness or the measure of Intensity and cognitive structure, the possibility that there is such a relationship cannot be ruled out. Differences between two groups of eleven people have to be considerable to be significant and one of her eleven patients had the segmented system which would tend to reduce the overall Intensity of the group. To support the idea that people with 'problems' may tighten their construing systems is the evidence that neurotics score more highly on Intensity than normals or other diagnostic groups (Bannister and Fransella, 1967; Bannister, Fransella and Agnew, 1971).

So far we have been discussing construct sub-system structure almost in trait terms. But there is no reason to suppose that a person cannot have parts of his system on a monolithic pattern, other parts segmented and the remainder articulated. Each may even change style during the

act of living. In the instances mentioned, the dyphasic man was construing objects or people in photographs unknown to him and no self
constructs or elicited constructs were used. It can be argued that a man
who over-structures his construing of strangers and objects, all unrelated to self, may have this as a feature of virtually the whole of his
construct system, as outside these rigid boundaries is total chaos – no
structure whatever. For the obese and anorexic patients, as well as for
Makhlouf's obsessionals, various self constructs were used and elements
and other constructs mainly obtained from the individual concerned.
In this situation the grid would be expected to have near maximal
meaningfulness for the person. However, there is no reason to suppose
that other construct sub-systems of these patients are equally as
monolithic or segmented.

The relative importance of the *self* in the construct systems of the
obsessionals was shown by the fact that they rated them significantly
more highly on constellatory constructs than did the normals. A constellatory construct 'permits its elements to belong to other realms
concurrently but fixes their realm membership'. Stereotypes belong to
this category – they are of the 'anything which is a ball must also be
something which will bounce' type. Makhlouf operationally defined
constellatory constructs as the first five constructs with the highest
loadings on the first component of a principal component analysis.
These notions of *self* 'anchored' the whole conceptual system (as
measured) for the obsessionals, while the controls 'anchored theirs on
other people'. Perhaps it is that within the general context of tightening
of construing, there is a decrease in relative tightening as the *self*
becomes less immediately relevant. In general it could be said that the
more meaningful or personally relevant the grid content and the more
construing centres around the *self*, the tighter and the more monolithic
will be the conceptual structure.

A THEORY OF OBSESSIONAL THINKING

Construct theory (Kelly, 1955) has the advantage of being a theory
concerned with both normal and so-called abnormal people. Thus its
fundamental postulate and eleven corollaries can be applied with equal
validity to the construing systems of all people (and animals for that
matter) who make discriminations and so predict and hope to control
to some extent events in their environment. The only well-thought-out
application of construct theory to abnormal thought processes at the
present time is that of Bannister (1960, 1962, 1963). He described the

disordered thinking typically found in schizophrenics in terms of a general loosening between constructs, operationally defined as low correlations between constructs on a repertory grid.

It was in the course of testing groups of psychiatric patients to establish normative data for the Grid Test of Thought Disorder, which stemmed from Bannister's work, that an uncontrolled observation provided the basis of a tentative theory of obsessional thought processes. It was observed that some scores of obsessional neurotics overlapped with those of thought-disordered schizophrenics, whereas there was little overlap of scores for other neurotics. This was unexpected since, implicitly using notions of the rigidity/intolerance of ambiguity sort, and data from other forms of grid used with obsessionals, it had been expected that they would have strong relationships between the constructs in the test. In view of this observation it was hypothesized that the obsessional must have a very tight construing system within the range of constructs relating to himself and his symptoms but that, outside this range, his system was very loose.

The fact that this observation of obsessionals obtaining very low scores differs from Makhlouf's, who found they did not differ in Intensity or Consistency from normals, probably results from the different grid contents. Makhlouf used as elements people known to each person personally, whereas in the Grid Test, the elements are photographs of strangers. Also, in Makhlouf's study, the constructs were elicited (and therefore presumably meaningful) for each person, whereas on the Grid Test the constructs are supplied and standard.

It is argued that the more symptom/self related the grid of an obsessional is, the tighter will be the correlations between the constructs. Where the obsessional is expected to differ from other neurotics is in the great *reduction* in the size of interconstruct correlations with *decrease* in meaningfulness or personal relevance of areas outside the direct construing of *self* and *symptoms*. This reduction in Intensity is also seen as being directly related to length of illness and severity of symptoms. The more entrenched in his symptom world the obsessional becomes, the looser and looser becomes the remainder of his construct system until he can be seen as 'living in the only world that was meaningful to him – outside the area of his obsessions all was vagueness and confusion' (Bannister and Fransella, 1971, p. 172).

In conjunction with this notion of differential loosening between construct sub-systems, account needs to be taken of Makhlouf's findings concerning the non-articulation of the structure of the obsessional's construing system. Kelly's Fragmentation Corollary states that *a person may successively employ a variety of construction sub-systems which are inferentially incompatible with each other.* Talking of the implications of this corollary he states that

> There is no clearer example of the limitation of one's ability to adjust to the vicissitudes of life, due to the impermeability of his super-ordinate constructs, than the case of a compulsion-neurosis client who is undergoing a marked decompensation process. The construct system of such a client is characteristically impermeable; he needs a separate pigeonhole for each new experience and he calculates his anticipations of events with minute pseudomathematical schemes. He has long been accustomed to subsume his principles. The variety of construction subsystems which are inferentially incompatible with each other may, in the train of rapidly moving events, become so vast that he is hard put to it to find ready-made superordinate constructs which are sufficiently permeable or open-ended to maintain over-all consistency. He starts making new ones. While he has very little successful experience with concept formation at the permeable level, these are the kinds of concepts he tries to develop. They may turn out to be generalized suspicions of the motives of other people. They may have to do with reevaluations of life and death. They may lead him to anticipate reality in very bizarre ways. (Kelly, 1955, p. 89)

Makhlouf's demonstration of the articulated and non-articulated systems of obsessionals and normals is related to this discussion of Kelly on the implications of the Fragmentation Corollary. The obsessional can be seen as having insufficient 'linkage' constructs to pull his remaining meaningful sub-systems together. Even if he were able to do so, the possibility of loosening or increasing the range of applicability of the construing of himself and his symptoms so as to increase the predictability of the whole system would be too threatening. Threat is seen as the *awareness of imminent comprehensive change in one's core structures.* It would indeed be threatening for the person with only a very limited part of his system functioning as an integrated whole, to be confronted with the prospect of letting even a limited part of it go momentarily out of his control – he must hang on at all costs. Thus, he over-defines, under-includes, he misreads the evidence, he does anything to help him hang on to meaning when he perceives threat to his system. He insists on validation, willingly making type 2 errors, that is, missing many opportunities for validating his predictions so as to avoid invalidation. Invalidation is a threat to the total system. Outside this non-articulated self/symptom sub-system, there is no threat. Construing is so loose that it enables few predictions to be made about events that cannot readily be fitted into the self/sympton complex. When the obsessional is brought face to face with an event that is not self/symptom related, he would be expected to experience anxiety, defined by Kelly as *the recognition that the events with which one is confronted lie outside the range of convenience of one's construct system.*

If, in the Kellian sense, the person goes on and on fragmenting his system, this should theoretically lead to thought disorder characteristically found in some schizophrenics. Bannister found it necessary to invoke the notion of consistency to differentiate the thought-disordered schizophrenic from the 'super' cognitively complex person. What Bannister showed was that the normal loose construer or cognitively complex person was consistent in his construing, whereas the thought-disordered schizophrenic was not.

Bannister talks of unusual or delusional thinking as being a bus-stop on the way to thought disorder.

> This leaves open the question of why, if paranoia is a bus-stop on the way to schizophrenic thought disorder, some patients get off the bus there, while others carry on to thought disorder. The answer may lie in the original state of development of the construct system at 'point of impact'. Thought disorder may be the fate of the person whose construct system had never developed beyond a relatively embryonic level and paranoia may be the result of pressures on a construct system which was largely workable until particular interpersonal difficulties were met. (Bannister and Fransella, 1971, p. 170)

The segmentation of thought structure found in the obsessional could be a different route to disintegration of thought. He can be seen as someone who had a previously tightly knit system. He continues along this path until such time as events in his environment start to produce unacceptable, invalidating evidence. At first he may try and tamper with the evidence or cook the books (show hostility in the Kellian sense), or he may repeat the experiment to see if he read the results wrongly the first time. But if people and events continue refusing to comply with his rigid predictions, he constricts his system further. *When one minimizes the apparent incompatibility of his construction system by drawing in the outer boundaries of his perceptual field, the relatively repetitive mental process that ensues is designated as 'constriction'.* Kelly goes on to say:

> When a person moves in the direction of constriction he tends to limit his interests, he deals with one issue at a time, he does not

accept potential relationships between widely varying events, he beats out the path of his daily routine in smaller and smaller circles, and he insists that his therapist stick to a sharply limited version of his problem. (1955, p. 477)

The focusing becomes more and more confined and more and more desperate until all the obsessional is doing is searching for certainty. He must maintain control at all costs, until all he has left are small nuggets of behaviour on which his whole life depends. If something undermines this one remaining area of workable construing, he has nothing to fall back on – he faces disintegration of his whole system.

THERAPY

Any proposed theory of some psychological phenomenon should have implications for the changing of that phenomenon. If one takes the point of view that obsessional thinking is concerned more and more with less and less, then the aim of therapy would be to start to reverse this process. It would enlarge the range of events with which the patient is prepared to concern himself. In the same way that the stutterer is helped to reduce his stutter by experiencing (and thus construing) what it is like to be a fluent speaker (Fransella, 1971b), so the obsessional hand-washer might reduce his rituals by being helped to experience (and thus construe) what it would be like to be someone *not* concerned with hand-washing. Psychotherapy would be directed towards enabling him to construe himself along lines other than those to do with his ritualistic behaviour. Of course, 'experience' does not simply mean going mechanically through an act. Kelly (1955) comments that one can have ten years' experience of, say, being a teacher, if one reconstrues along the line, or one can have one year's experience repeated ten times if one fails to reconstrue. The construct theory approach to therapy is aimed at facilitating such reconstruction.

A central issue in the approach is that behaviour is related to how one construes the world of events with which he is confronted. If something is construed as dangerous or contaminating, the person will take what, to him, is the appropriate action. Thus, changing construing is expected to lead to change in behaviour. The behaviour therapy literature is currently much concerned with this issue (e.g. Marcia, Rubin and Efran, 1969; Rimm, 1970), although this is not our present concern. However, there are a few studies which clearly relate improvement in the obsessional patient with change in attitude.

Frankl (1960, 1969) describes a technique he calls 'paradoxical intention'. This procedure involves the person, perhaps a phobic patient, in thinking or doing precisely that thing which he fears. Frankl sees the patient as strengthening his symptom by trying to fight to suppress ideas about it. By getting him to perform the act or think the thought that he constantly avoids, he comes to be detached from it and to laugh at it. Frankl states that '. . . the logotherapist, when applying paradoxical intention, is concerned not so much with the symptom in itself but, rather, the patient's *attitude* toward his neurosis and its symptomatic manifestations. It is the very act of changing this attitude that is involved whenever an improvement is obtained' (Frankl, 1969, p. 245). Gertz (1966) used this procedure with phobic and obsessional patients. With the latter, he recommends logotherapy together with intensive phenothiazine therapy. The sort of instructions given to a patient include, for example, telling him to say 'I love to make my hands as dirty as possible. I'm crazy about germs. Who wants to be clean anyway?'

With this technique, the patient is being encouraged to produce massive polarization in his construing of himself in relation to, say, contamination. He is not someone who fears contamination, he is someone who just does not care about it, or even loves it. It can be argued that such a polarization in construing can only be lasting if the patient can be made to mark, learn and inwardly digest all the implications that are involved in being a person who does not care about contamination. Gertz comments on this point:

> . . . we do not merely use the technique of PI, but intensive efforts are made to understand the patient and his symptoms in his uniqueness as a human being, in terms of his life history, his present life situation, his conflicts, and finally, in the light of his future, that is to say, the meaning of his existence. Paradoxical intention is to supplement dynamic therapy, not to replace it. (Gertz, 1966)

Meyer (1966) treated two long-standing severe obsessional patients with a similar technique, but speaks of modification of expectations instead of paradoxical intention. Both his patients improved by being made to perform acts that were most difficult for them and so having 'their expectations invalidated'. They found they were not struck dumb, or flattened by a thunderbolt or made impotent.

Whether the patient is rather gently introduced to the notion of a symptom-free self or more positively by the paradoxical intention method, both have the effect of getting the patient to reconstrue himself along new dimensions of action. Once he has seen that the alternative ways of seeing himself are viable, he can elaborate them and so invalidate notions of himself as a symptom-bound person.

A construct theory approach to obsessional disorders offers a way of incorporating existing evidence and therapeutic techniques within one framework. It allows detailed predictions to be made about the factors underlying change, provides a technique of measurement so that aspects of cognitive change can be monitored, and suggests ways of comparing psychological processes across psychiatric diagnostic categories.

9

John D. Teasdale

Learning models of obsessional–compulsive disorder

INTRODUCTION

An essential element in the scientific approach to a problem is the formulation of hypotheses which can be tested by experiment. Such hypotheses might be derived from any source; the most important thing is not where they come from, but whether they are useful in generating predictions which withstand experimental test, and, in the case of clinical problems, in suggesting viable treatment approaches.

This chapter is concerned with hypotheses of the nature of obsessional–compulsive disorder which have been derived from experimental studies of animal and human learning.

In deriving such hypotheses one could adopt one of two, broadly distinguishable, strategies. One of these would be to base one's hypotheses simply on experimentally observed general rules of behaviour such as 'if a neutral stimulus is repeatedly paired with an aversive event the stimulus itself acquires aversive properties'. The hypotheses derived to account for obsessional–compulsive disorder using this strategy would be of the simple form 'phenomenon X in obsessional–compulsive behaviour is simply another example of the general class of phenomena Y'. This is at a low level of 'explanation', but it enables predictions to be made about phenomenon X by virtue of what has been experimentally established to be true of behaviours which conform to the general class of phenomena Y. In other words, by classifying behaviour into a number of categories we can, hopefully, make predictions about one member of a category from what we know about other members of that category. I shall refer to hypotheses at this low level as Type A hypotheses.

The other type of hypothesis (Type B) would be derived, not directly from empirical generalizations about animal or human learning, but from hypothetical models advanced to explain these empirical generalizations. An example of this would be to use elements of the two-factor model of avoidance learning (Mowrer, 1960) to account for aspects of obsessional–compulsive behaviour.

Although broadly distinguishable, there will probably exist some overlap between the two types of hypotheses.

THE BEHAVIOUR TO BE EXPLAINED

Before examining hypotheses constructed to explain obsessional–compulsive behaviour, it would be as well to get a description of the behaviour that is to be explained.

The definition offered in a standard textbook of psychiatry (Mayer-Gross, Slater and Roth, 1955) is as follows: 'The essential nature of the obsessional or compulsive symptom lies in its appearance as a mental content, an idea, image, affect, impulse or movement, with a *subjective sense of compulsion overriding an internal resistance.* This resistance from the healthy part of the personality, in which the symptom is recognized as strange or morbid, is the essential characteristic by which truly compulsive phenomena can be distinguished from other phenomena of a related or similar kind. . . . Compulsive symptoms tend to take on a *precisely determined form*, and to be repetitive, especially if they consist in a movement or have a motor component, as with a gesture.'

This definition can be illustrated, and the ensuing discussion made more concrete, by the descriptions of three cases of obsessional–compulsive disorder that follow.

Case 1 (Meyer, 1966)
'A 33-year-old intelligent school-mistress, married with one child and with a 3-year history of severely disabling washing and cleaning rituals, was admitted under the care of Professor D. Hill.

Some compulsive checking (doors, lights and marking of school papers) occurred 3 years prior to the main complaint. A few months after the birth of her baby she began to over-wash the nappies so that no diaper rash would occur. After the birth of the child she started to worry about anything which might be "dirty". A wide range of objects and situations e.g. door knobs, blankets, clothes, dustbins, meat, animals, men, sexual intercourse, were considered as "contaminated by dirt" and led to almost continuous washing and cleaning. It appeared that the reason for this behaviour was due to a fear of "dirt" which was grounded in the belief that any contact with it would result in her baby and/or her being "eventually afflicted by some disease due to contamination".

Prior to the first hospitalization the main symptoms of her illness were: she would only touch foreign objects with tissue paper; would not allow her daughter or her husband to touch any of the "contaminated objects"; unless the husband and the daughter were "clean" she would not permit them to touch her; stopped having sexual intercourse; became housebound because of the fear of "contamination"; touching any of the "contaminated objects" evoked excessive washing of hands; spent most of her time washing and rewashing clothes and scrubbing her house (used £3.10.0 a week worth of soap, detergents and disinfectants and developed a severe dermatitis on her hands).'

Case 2 (Meyer, 1966)
'A 47-year-old school-mistress of superior intelligence, married with one daughter and with a history of 36 years duration of compulsive thoughts and rituals, was admitted under the care of Professor D. Hill.

Recalls that at the age of 10, after hearing a passage from the Bible – "to blaspheme against the Holy Ghost is unforgivable" – became preoccupied with this thought. Shortly afterwards, words like "damn", "blast", "bloody" came to her mind despite all her attempts to resist them. These "blasphemous thoughts" elicited guilt and anxiety which she found could be alleviated by repeating any activity on hand a certain number of times. By the age of 13, these intrusive thoughts became of a direct sexual nature, centred on the sexual words and the idea of having sexual intercourse with the Holy Ghost. The associated anxiety continued to be allayed by performing repetitive acts e.g. dressing and undressing, writing and rewriting, walking up and down staircases, retracing her steps.

At 29, attended a psychiatrist for 9 months with little improvement. At 31, deteriorated and was admitted for 3 months; had ECT and drugs and left unimproved. Soon after developed a compulsive urge to kill her husband and daughter and was leucotomized at the age of 32. Two years later embarked on psycho-analysis and continued with it for 11 years. At the end of the analysis was much worse. Now not only the intruding sex words and thoughts about the Holy Ghost evoked ritualistic behaviour, but also any activity with sexual meaning e.g. shutting drawers, putting in plugs, cleaning a pipe, wiping tall receptacles, putting on stockings, eating oblong objects, doing things four times (association with four letter Anglo-Saxon words), stepping on patterns in the shape of sex organs, entering underground trains etc. Whenever possible avoided these activities e.g. stopped eating bananas and sausages, and her life became a "misery". For instance, it took her hours to dress or to travel short distances. Attributes this change to the psycho-analysis since in it she learned about the extent of sexual symbolization. After 2 years of supportive psychotherapy and drugs with another psychiatrist, was referred to the National Hospital to be considered for another leucotomy. This was decided against and was referred to this Department for behaviour therapy in March 1964.

On the ward appeared mildly depressed, constantly agitated and frequently engaged in avoidance and ritualistic behaviour. These were more pronounced when on her own. Said she felt constantly afraid waiting for the thought to "strike her". Symptoms appeared to subside when occupied with interesting and important tasks e.g. writing children's stories. The illness did not prevent her from working as a part-time supply teacher of children. While teaching, to which she was dedicated, the symptoms did not trouble her. It was interesting that marital sexual intercourse was completely satisfactory and did not give rise to her ritualistic behaviour.

Regarded her rituals as "acts of repentance for being a sinner". Felt that her non-performance of rituals would result in her family being eventually "afflicted by some disorder" and was convinced that she herself would face an "eternal damnation". Did not regard herself as religious but had high moral standards.'

Case 3

This is a case described by Wolpe (1958), which he presented as an example of an anxiety-elevating obsession.

'When a motor mechanic of 45 had neurotic anxiety exceeding a fairly low level, he would have a terrifying though always controllable impulse to strike people. From the first moment of awareness of the impulse he would feel increased anxiety, and if at the time he was with an associate or even among strangers – for example, in a bus – he would thrust his hands firmly into his pockets "to keep them out of trouble". ... In 1942 this motor mechanic, on military service, had been sentenced to 30 days' imprisonment in circumstances which he had with some justice felt to be grossly unfair. Then, as he had resisted the military police rather violently in protest, he was taken to a psychiatrist who said there was nothing wrong with him and that the sentence should be carried out. At this his feeling of helpless rage had further increased and he was taken out by force. Then for the first time he had "this queer feeling" in his abdomen and had struck a military policemen who tried to compel him to work. Horror at the implications of this act intensified his disturbed state. The obsession to strike people made its first appearance in 1953, eleven years later. He had been imprisoned over-night (for the first time since 1942) because, arriving home one night to find his house crowded with his wife's relatives he had shouted and been violent until his wife had called the police. After emerging from jail, burning with a sense of injustice much like that experienced during his imprisonment in the army, he had felt the impulse to strike a stranger who was giving him a lift in an automobile, and then again, much more strongly, a few days later toward his wife at their first meeting since his night in jail. This time he had gone into a state of panic, and since then, for a period of five months, the obsession had recurred very frequently and in an increasing range of conditions e.g. at work he would often have a fear-laden desire to hit fellow workmen with any tool he happened to be holding.'

The discussion here can be usefully divided into consideration of acquisition, maintenance, and treatment of obsessional–compulsive disorder. While, chronologically, discussion of acquisition should precede discussion of maintenance, this order will be reversed here as it is easier to gain information on the current variables affecting perform-ance of a behaviour than historical information on the conditions rele-vant to its acquisition. Thus, acquisition will be discussed in relation to the conclusions drawn about maintenance, rather than vice versa.

THE MAINTENANCE OF OBSESSIONAL–COMPULSIVE BEHAVIOUR

Ritualistic behaviour

As will be apparent from the case histories presented, not all patients display overt motor obsessional behaviour, or rituals. Where these are present, the paradigm of animal and human learning which has been most often considered relevant is that of avoidance learning (e.g. Metzner, 1963; Bandura, 1969; Meyer, 1966; Walton and Mather, 1963). Avoidance learning is defined as 'a training procedure in which the learned movement circumvents or prevents the appearance of a noxious stimulus' (Kimble, 1964, p. 477). The utility of this paradigm in describing the maintenance of ritualistic obsessional–compulsive behaviour will be considered in terms of both types of hypotheses described in the introduction.

i) *Type A hypotheses*

Two main types of situation have been used experimentally to study the avoidance conditioning paradigm. The first, discriminated avoidance, is exemplified by the shuttle-box training procedure (e.g. Mowrer and Lamoreaux, 1942). A rat is placed in a small box with an electrifiable floor, a light or sound stimulus is presented, and is followed after a short interval by a shock, from which the rat can escape by running to the opposite side of the box. If the rat makes this response after the light or sound stimulus is presented and before the time when the shock is due, then shock is not presented and the animal is said to have made an avoidance response. Rats do learn to make such avoidance responses, and thus avoid the receipt of shock. The second, free-operant avoidance, is exemplified by the procedure used by Sidman (1953). In this situation, the rat is placed in a chamber, with an electrifiable floor, through one wall of which protrudes a lever. Shock is delivered at a fixed frequency, say every ten seconds, as long as the animal fails to respond by depressing the lever. In this situation, the avoidance response, depression of the lever, has the effect of postponing the next shock for a certain period, say twelve seconds, so that if the animal continues to press the lever at intervals of less than twelve seconds it can indefinitely avoid receipt of shock. Rats can learn to make such avoidance responses.

Cases 1 and 2 demonstrate obvious motor rituals. In terms of the type A hypothesis under consideration, the continuous washing and cleaning in Case 1 and the performance of repetitive acts such as dressing and undressing in Case 2 would be classified as 'active' avoidance responses, in that the patients avoid noxious stimulation by making an active response. The abstention from touching 'contaminated' objects in Case 1, and from eating bananas and sausages in Case 2, would be classified as 'passive' avoidance responses in that the patients avoid noxious stimulation by refraining from certain responses. In each case, the immediate noxious stimulus that is avoided by such responses is the increase in discomfort contingent upon the non-performance of the avoidance response. In both cases, there are also delayed consequences perceived as resulting from the non-performance of the avoidance response (in Case 1, disease of the patient or her baby, in Case 2, disaster for the patient's family and eternal damnation for the patient).

Whilst it is an interesting exercise, this equation of aspects of obsessional–compulsive disorder with aspects of the behaviour of animals in a contrived experimental situation is not particularly useful unless it can help us understand some of the oddities of obsessional–

compulsive disorder. Differences which it has been suggested differentiate obsessional–compulsive rituals from other 'normal' forms of human avoidance behaviour (such as putting on a raincoat before going out into the rain to avoid getting wet) include:

1. The high frequency of occurrence, persistence and repetitiveness of the behaviour.
2. The stereotyped form of the behaviour.
3. The subjective sense of compulsion to perform the behaviour overriding an internal resistance against the performance of the behaviour.
4. The behaviour appears senseless to others and embarrassing to the patient.

Can the results of experiments on avoidance learning help clarify these differences between obsessional–compulsive rituals and 'normal' human avoidance behaviour?

1. *The high frequency of occurrence, persistence and repetitiveness of the behaviour.* The most commonly used measure of persistence of behaviour in experimental studies is resistance to extinction, by which is usually meant the number of times the experimental subject performs the behaviour in the absence of the reinforcement used to train the behaviour in the acquisition phase of the experiment. As a number of writers (e.g. Morgan, 1968) have pointed out, the concept of extinction poses problems when applied to avoidance learning; extinction is defined by the experimenter disconnecting his shock supply, but, as far as the subject is concerned, his avoidance responses are still 'successful' in that they prevent the occurrence of shock. This stands in contrast to the situation in studies of positive reinforcement, where extinction is defined, for example, by the experimenter disconnecting the machinery that dispenses food pellets when the animal presses a bar, and results in the animal's bar press responses no longer being successful in obtaining food.

There follows a list of empirical generalizations, derived from experimental studies of avoidance learning, about the frequency of occurrence and persistence of avoidance responses, which may be relevant to an understanding of obsessional–compulsive rituals.

a) *Once trained, the frequency and persistence of avoidance responses is greater in the condition where shock is contingent on the non-performance of the avoidance response than in the condition where shock is no longer contingent on the non-performance of the avoidance response (extinction).* This very obvious generalization simply says that, in situations where introduction of the extinction procedure by the experimenter eventually leads to cessation of responding, the frequency and persistence of avoidance responses is greater in the phase where the experimenter arranges conditions to maintain avoidance responding than in the phase where the experimenter arranges conditions to extinguish avoidance responding.

b) *Where the shock contingent on non-performance of the avoidance response is of high intensity, responding is more consistent in the maintenance phase and more resistant to extinction, than where the shock contingent on non-performance of the avoidance response is of low intensity.* One of the attractions of the avoidance paradigm to psychologists speculating about the nature of maladaptive behaviour, which appears to persist in spite of the absence of any apparent external reinforcement, has been the alleged resistance to extinction shown by responses trained on an avoidance schedule. However, while avoidance responses may take some time to extinguish, the majority of studies have, in fact, found that the responses do sooner or later extinguish (e.g. Sidman, 1966; Kimble, 1955). The best-known study in which there appeared to be little, if any, tendency for the avoidance response to extinguish is that of Solomon and Wynne (1953). The shock used to generate avoidance responses in this study was described as 'traumatic' (it was, in fact, the most intense shock that could be given the experimental animals without tetanizing their muscles). The most obvious difference between this study and those which have failed to generate avoidance responses highly resistant to extinction is the intensity of the shock used, suggesting that this may be an important variable in determining the resistance to extinction. Boren, Sidman and Herrnstein (1959), in a study of free operant avoidance, did in fact obtain a positive relationship between intensity of shock and degree of resistance to extinction. However, Kimble (1955) and Brush (1957) failed to obtain this relationship when studying discriminated avoidance learning. These results were against the experimenter's expectation, and Solomon and Brush (1956) have suggested that the failure to obtain the expected relationship was a result of the complicating factor that avoidance responding terminated the warning signal in these two experiments.

In their study, Boren *et al.* (1959) also found that the rate of responding during the phase when the shock contingency was operating was positively related to the intensity of shock used.

c) *Rate of avoidance responding is higher in the absence of a stimulus which can be used to discriminate occasions when shock will be delivered from those when it will not.* In the discriminated avoidance situation, the experimental animal typically learns to make the avoidance response at a high probability in the period immediately after the onset of the warning stimulus, and at a low frequency in the absence of the warning stimulus. In this sense, it can be said that the avoidance response has been brought under the stimulus control of the warning signal, and that the animal can successfully discriminate between the stimulus situation where the avoidance response is required and that where it is unnecessary. The importance of providing a warning signal to the animal to allow it to discriminate situations where avoidance responding is required from those where it is unnecessary, and thereby make avoidance responding most effective, is illustrated by an experiment of Sidman (1955). He found that the effect of introducing a warning signal into a free-operant avoidance procedure was to make avoidance behaviour more effective in terms of the animal receiving fewer shocks, while emitting fewer responses.

Another demonstration of stimulus control is reported by Sidman (1966). In this experiment, a monkey learned to discriminate the situation in which failure to make the avoidance response was punished (which occurred in the presence of clicks at the rate of two per second) from the situation in which failure to make the avoidance response was not punished (which occurred in the presence of clicks at the rate of six per second). In this experiment, the discriminative stimuli functioned in terms of showing whether the avoidance contingency was operative or not, rather than signalling the imminent presentation of shock.

What is known about the conditions which affect the extent of stimulus control over avoidance responding?

Sidman (1966) notes that, while it is generally possible to train an animal to make avoidance responses in the presence of a stimulus signifying that shocks will be received for failure to perform the responses, and to refrain from responding in the presence of another stimulus signifying the absence of this contingency, this may be difficult where the animal is performing so well that it rarely fails to make the avoidance response. In such circumstances, the animal has few opportunities to learn that non-performance of the avoidance response, in the absence of the warning signal, does not lead to shock.

An experiment by Hoffman, Fleshler and Jensen (1963) examined under two conditions the generalization of the emotional response to a warning signal, thought to be important in the acquisition and maintenance of avoidance responding by some workers. In one condition, shocks were delivered between presentations of the stimuli, in the other they were not. It was found that both the emotional response to the warning signal, and the generalization of this to similar stimuli were greater in the shock condition. It could be said that the animals were 'sensitized' by the shock and responded to a wider range of stimuli.

d) *The higher the rate at which the warning signal is presented in discriminated avoidance, the greater the frequency of the avoidance response.* This is an obvious consequence of the previously noted observation that, in discriminated avoidance, the warning signal gains considerable stimulus control over the performance of the avoidance response.

e) *In free-operant avoidance, the frequency of avoidance responding is a function of the programmed interval between shocks, and of the interval between performance of the response and presentation of the next shock if no further response is made.* The relevant evidence is presented by Sidman (1966). The interaction of these two intervals yields a complex relation between the length of either and the frequency of avoidance responding. In some circumstances, reducing either interval increases the rate of avoidance responding.

f) *Administration of 'free shock' or other stresses increases the frequency of avoidance responses, and their resistance to extinction.* Sidman (1966) and Morgan (1968) cite a number of experiments in which the administration of 'free shock' (i.e. occasional unavoidable shocks) to an animal performing on a free-operant avoidance schedule had the effect of increasing the frequency of avoidance responding, and increasing the resistance to extinction.

Solomon, Kamin and Wynne's (1953) finding that, in their traumatic avoidance procedure, punishing the avoidance response by shock failed to extinguish the avoidance response, but in fact led to faster and more stereotyped responding, could also be seen as an example of the effects of 'free shock'; the inter-trial intervals used were three minutes, so that the punishing shock for one avoidance response could act as the 'free shock' for the next one.

Fonberg (1956) established avoidance responses (e.g. lifting a foreleg) in dogs using electric shock or a strong puff of air as the noxious stimulus. An 'experimental neurosis' was then induced in the dogs by subjecting them to a very difficult discrimination problem. With the onset of the neurosis, the previously established avoidance responses returned, although the warning signals to which they had previously been conditioned were not present. Variations in the degree of neurotic disturbance were accompanied by corresponding variation in the intensity and frequency of the avoidance responses.

What hypotheses do such generalizations suggest about the nature of obsessional–compulsive rituals ?

Generalization (a)
The basis of the distinction between the acquisition phase and the extinction phase in experimental studies of avoidance learning is that failure to make the avoidance response in the acquisition phase results in an externally applied punishment, but it does not do so in the extinction phase. On this criterion, obsessional–compulsive rituals must be viewed as avoidance responses in the extinction phase. Alternatively, we could define the acquisition phase as that phase in which failure to make the avoidance response results in an aversive state for the organism, whether this be the results of external or internal stimulation. In this case, the frequently reported clinical observation that obsessional–compulsive patients become distressed when they do not perform their rituals in situations which would normally elicit them would suggest that one could view the obsessional rituals as avoidance responses in the acquisition or maintenance phase.

On this line of reasoning, one would argue that an important factor determining the greater frequency and persistence of ritualistic behaviour compared with similar non-ritualistic behaviour is the emotional consequence of the non-performance of the action. This appears to be more aversive in the case of ritualistic behaviour. This suggestion applied to Case 1 for example, would suggest that the greater frequency of hand-washing and cleaning in this patient than in most normals is related to the greater aversiveness of the consequences of not making this action in the obsessional. As applied to Case 2, it would suggest that the greater frequency of actions such as dressing and undressing, writing and rewriting etc., in the patient than in normals is related to the greater aversiveness of the consequences of not making such actions in the obsessional.

We are now of course presented with the problem of explaining why the consequences of the non-performance of certain motor actions are more aversive in obsessionals than in normals.

In Case 1, the greater than normal aversiveness of omitting to wash the hands or clean clothes seems related to an intense fear of dirt; the presence of this on the hands or clothes, if they are not washed, constitutes a phobic stimulus for the patient, her fear reaction being greater than normal. An attempt to explain the presence of such a dirt phobia will be deferred to the discussion of aetiology. For the moment, it can be noted that it may be related to the patient's belief that any contact with dirt would result in some disease for herself or her baby. By analogy, one would expect that application of a liquid, believed to contain cyanide, to the hands of a normal subject would generate a greater than normal rate of hand-washing.

On this model, an important difference between patients with phobias who have obsessional rituals and those who do not would be that, in the latter, the phobic stimuli can be avoided by suitable motor action removing the subject from their presence. In the former, however, the nature of the phobic stimuli is such that they cannot be avoided in this way (e.g. dirt, which is everywhere and beyond the patient's ability to avoid easily). This resembles a suggestion made by Meyer (1966).

In Case 2, the greater than normal aversiveness of not performing repeated activities seems related to the presence of a high level of anxiety, resulting from the occurrence of intrusive anxiety-provoking thoughts and the presence of a phobia related to sexually relevant stimuli. The importance of the intrusive thoughts in eliciting anxiety and consequent ritualistic behaviour is shown by the observation that Case 2 reported few intrusive thoughts, little anxiety, and little ritualistic behaviour when occupied with interesting and important tasks. Again, the obsessional patient appears to have anxieties related to stimuli from which it is difficult physically to remove oneself (intrusive thoughts, and widely generalized sexual fears).

Attempts to explain the presence of such intrusive thoughts and widespread phobias will be presented later.

In Case 1, it is fairly clear why the particular responses which constitute the ritual should be able to prevent the increase in anxiety which arises on their non-occurrence; washing and cleaning responses temporarily remove the phobic stimulus, dirt. In Case 2, it is not so clear why the particular behaviours which make up the ritual should be able to prevent the occurrence of anxiety. This problem will be returned to on page 43.

The essence of the hypothesis derived from the empirical generalization (a) is thus that the high frequency and persistence of obsessional-compulsive rituals is related to the aversive consequences of the non-performance of such rituals (which remains to be explained). Experimentally testable predictions can be derived from this hypothesis:

1. the consequences of preventing an obsessional performing a ritual in situations where it would normally occur are more aversive than the consequences of allowing the ritual to occur;

2. the consequences of preventing an obsessional performing a ritual are more aversive to the obsessional than the consequences of preventing a normal person performing the corresponding behaviour.

Generalization (b)

The hypotheses derived from this generalization would be very similar to those derived from generalization (a), namely that the greater frequency and persistence of ritualistic hand-washing, compared to normal hand-washing, for example, results from the greater aversiveness of the consequences of not hand-washing in certain circumstances in the former than in the latter. Again, it leaves to be explained why this greater aversiveness should exist. This hypothesis leads to an experimentally testable prediction similar to the second of those suggested in the preceding section.

Generalization (c)

In terms of the line of thought suggested by this generalization, obsessional ritualistic behaviour might be described as normal behaviour which is no longer under appropriate stimulus control, i.e. in Case 1, for example, frequent and persistent hand-washing and cleaning might be appropriate if the 'dirt' which it removed had the power of killing the patient or those close to her, but as it does not have this power it is inappropriate. In other words, the patient fails to discriminate those situations where the avoidance response would be judged appropriate by most people from those where it would normally be judged inappropriate. Mather (1970) has in fact suggested this as a description of obsessional behaviour.

From the experimental studies cited under generalization (c), one could view this lack of discrimination as a result of the high frequency of occurrence of the avoidance response (ritual) to a certain set of related stimuli, so that the patient does not have the opportunity to discriminate the conditions under which non-performance of the avoidance response is punished from those under which it is not. However, here some difficulties occur in the direct extrapolation from the results of animal experiments. To use the example of the greater thoroughness of washing by a normal person after he has dipped his hands into cyanide solution than after he has dipped his hands into pure water, it is possible to maintain that the lack of persistent washing in the latter case is based on the direct experience that no aversive consequences follow omission of thorough washing. However, the more persistent washing in the former case is not (usually) based on the direct experience of the aversive consequences of omitting such washing. Rather, it is based on the symbolic representation of the consequences of such omission, derived from information obtained via language about the unfortunate consequences to others of such omission. It seems necessary to suggest that the obsessional's symbolic representation of the consequences of failure to perform the avoidance response is attached to a wider range of stimulus situations than would be considered appropriate by most people. Obviously, continued performance of the avoidance response to such stimuli will prevent the obsessional learning by direct experience that omission of the avoidance response in certain circumstances does not have aversive consequences. Such persistence of the avoidance response could be explained by hypotheses derived from generalizations (a) and (b).

Mather (1970) has suggested that a characteristic of obsessional–compulsive behaviour may be the fact that the discrimination between appropriate and inappropriate stimuli is particularly difficult, e.g. given the belief that dirt may contain potentially lethal 'germs', it is very difficult to make the distinction between 'safe' dirt, from which they are absent, and 'dangerous' dirt, in which they are present.

The importance of erroneous anticipated consequences in developing and maintaining avoidance responding can be seen in the development and maintenance of tribal ritualistic and superstitious behaviour, e.g. offering sacrifices to the gods to avert the consequences of their wrath (Frazer, 1925). Indeed, a recent study (Geer, Davison and Gatchel, 1970) has experimentally demonstrated this effect. Subjects were given a reaction time task and told to make their reaction to the onset of a six-second shock. After ten trials, half the subjects were told that by decreasing their reaction time they would reduce shock duration. The remaining subjects were simply told that shock duration would be reduced. All subjects, regardless of group assignment or reaction time, received three-second shocks in the second half of the study. The 'avoidance response' for the erroneously informed group was thus a brief reaction time, and it was in fact found that the reaction time in the second half of the experiment was significantly shorter for this group than for the other group. Further, during the second half of the study, subjects who believed they had control over the shock showed fewer spontaneous skin conductance responses and smaller skin conductance responses to shock onset than subjects who did not feel they had control, suggesting that the erroneous belief about control of the shock reduced the autonomic response to the shock.

However, obsessional rituals differ in one important way from other superstitious behaviours designed to avert noxious events; having made the appropriate sacrifice to the gods, primitive tribes could usually then get on with their lives quite happily without frequently repeating the ritual (which might not then be due until the following year), whereas a feature of obsessional rituals is that they are repetitive. This could be seen as a result of, having washed the hands once to remove infectious dirt, it is not long before the obsessional again comes into contact with such dirt from his surroundings. Alternatively, one could view the difference as one of lack of feedback that the avoidance response has been successful; in the case of the tribal ritual, the masses who have made the sacrifice may be assured by the priest that they have done all that is necessary and that the gods will be appeased for another year; in the case of a hand-washing ritual, it may be very difficult to observe that all 'germs' have been successfully removed from the hands by the washing procedure. Rescorla and LoLordo (1965) have demonstrated that presenting stimuli correlated with the absence of shock ('safety signals') has the effect of depressing the rate of a well-established avoidance habit. It could be said that obsessionals repeat their avoidance responses as a result of the absence of such 'safety signals'. However, it might then be asked why the obsessional continues to make the response at all in such circumstances; Bolles (1970) has suggested that receipt of such 'safety signals' is an important element in the reinforcement of avoidance responses, and, similarly, Meyer (1966) has questioned why, if they are 'unsuccessful' in achieving a safe state, obsessional rituals should persist. Perhaps one answer would be to suggest, with Meyer (1966), that the ritual is successful in producing a 'safety period' but that this is relatively short due to the presentation, relatively quickly, of more 'danger signals', in the form of frequently occurring stimuli (e.g. dirt, or anxiety-evoking intrusive thoughts). From animal studies, such a situation would be expected to generate a high frequency of response.

In terms of the effect of free-shock on the extent of stimulus generalization to a warning signal (Hoffman, Fleshler and Jensen, 1963), one could suggest that the poor discrimination, shown by obsessionals between appropriate and inappropriate stimulus situations for the performance of avoidance behaviour, is the result of increased 'arousal', 'emotionality' or 'sensitization', whichever term one happens to use to describe the effects of shock. It could be suggested that obsessional patients differ from normals in having an unusually high chronic level of arousal. A difficulty with this suggestion would be that it would suggest that obsessional patients should show a poor discrimination in all avoidance learning and thus have a far wider range of obsessional symptoms than they appear to have. It seems necessary to suggest that if heightened arousal is an important factor in making obsessionals poor in discriminating appropriate from inappropriate stimulus situations then the heightened arousal must be to some degree specific to the situations associated with the obsessional behaviour.

What then are the hypotheses that might be derived from generalization (c), and what experimentally testable predictions would be derived from them?

1. Obsessionals show a higher frequency of certain behaviours than normals as a result of their failure to discriminate between what most people would regard as appropriate stimulus situations for their occurrence and what most people would regard as inappropriate situations for their occurrence. This hypothesis could be tested simply by observing the situations where the obsessional rituals occur and getting normal people to rate them as appropriate or inappropriate. It is really unnecessary to do this experiment, as it could be suggested that this is one of the defining features of obsessional–compulsive behaviour.

2. The high frequency of occurrence of the ritualistic behaviour in certain inappropriate stimulus situations prevents the obsessional learning by direct experience the discrimination between appropriate and inappropriate stimulus situations. It would be predicted that preventing the occurrence of the rituals should eventually lead to the learning of the discrimination between appropriate and inappropriate stimulus situations.

3. The inability of the obsessional to discriminate between appropriate and inappropriate stimulus situations is related to the high arousal (emotionality, sensitization) at the time the discrimination is required. This would predict that measures of arousal would be higher in the obsessional in the situations in which the ritual normally occurs than in normals in the same situation.

Generalization (d)

The suggestion that the higher frequency of certain avoidance responses in obsessionals than in normals is related to the higher rate of occurrence of warning signals has been considered in the previous section. There it was suggested that this was related to the presence of phobic responses to frequently occurring stimuli, or to the presence of recurring anxiety-evoking intrusive thoughts. Hypotheses to account for the presence of these two peculiarities will be presented later (p. 223).

Test of this hypothesis would require a count of the occurrence of phobic responses or anxiety-evoking intrusive thoughts in obsessionals and normals.

Generalization (e)
The hypothesis suggested here is very similar to that suggested in the preceding section, namely, that if the ritual is not made, obsessionals would suffer aversive stimulation more frequently than normals due to the presence of phobic responses to frequently occurring external stimuli or to the presence of recurrent intrusive anxiety-evoking thoughts.

Generalization (f)
Generalization (f) can be concisely stated as follows: an already established avoidance response will occur with greater frequency and persistence if the animal is subjected to a state of noxious stimulation or stress, whether that noxious state is the one the avoidance response was originally learned to avoid or not.

The ritualistic washing and cleaning shown by Case 1 would be seen as an intensification of an avoidance response, previously established to avoid the aversive consequences of dirt and contamination, as a result of an increase in noxious stimulation (or arousal) resulting from a contamination phobia.

In Case 2, the intensification of certain normal motor behaviours (dressing and undressing, walking up and down stairs) would be seen as occurring as a result of an increase in noxious stimulation arising from the recurrent anxiety-evoking thoughts. In this case, there is not such an obvious relation between the nature of the stress stimulus and the motor behaviour as there was in Case 1. One would have to suggest that dressing and undressing etc. are avoidance responses in the sense that they reduce the occurrence of intrusive anxiety-evoking thoughts thereby reducing the level of noxious stimulation from that which would have occurred in their absence. One could view this as the distracting effect of any motor activity; Antrobus (1968) has shown that the extent to which internally derived thought stimuli occur is reduced by increasing the attention to stimuli of external origin. The motor activities the patient engaged in would increase the stimulation derived from external sources, thereby reducing the occurrence of intrusive anxiety-evoking thoughts. Engagement in story-writing or teaching seemed to have similar effects to the repeated motor activities in this patient.

Again, the hypotheses advanced depend heavily on the increase in arousal attributed to phobic stimuli or anxiety-evoking recurrent thoughts. It would be predicted that the obsessional in the situation normally eliciting ritual behaviour would be at a higher level of arousal than a normal person in that situation, and that in the obsessional, rituals are more probable when the obsessional is at high levels of arousal than at low levels. Walker and Beech (1969) in fact present evidence suggesting that the greater the level of patient discomfort before the onset of a ritual, the longer the ritual continues.

Viewing the ritualistic behaviour as an avoidance response appears to be a useful approach in explaining the high frequency of occurrence, persistence and repetitiveness of the behaviour but two important factors, to which the discussion has repeatedly returned, need to be explained: the presence of phobic responses to frequently occurring stimuli, possibly related to erroneous beliefs, and the presence of recurrent anxiety-evoking thoughts.

2. *The stereotyped form of the behaviour.* It seems unnecessary to dwell long on this aspect of ritualistic behaviour. James (1890) has noted that any frequently repeated habit tends to take on a stereotyped form. Solomon and Wynne (1953) noted that the avoidance responses made by their dogs took on a stereotyped form, which would be consistent with viewing obsessional rituals as avoidance responses. Yates (1962) cites a number of studies supporting the generalization that increasing arousal reduces the variability of responding, which would again be consistent with the suggestions already made about the importance of heightened arousal in obsessionals.

3. *The subjective sense of compulsion to perform the behaviour overriding an internal resistance against the performance of the behaviour.* The two main elements in this feature of obsessional–compulsive rituals refer to internal subjective states. It is obviously impossible to obtain reports on such states from animals, and the majority of experimental investigations of learning in human subjects have concentrated more on observation of overt behaviour than on reports of subjective experience. However, it is possible to use the results of experiments on animal and human learning, if we can translate the subjective phenomena of compulsion to perform a behaviour and resistance against its performance into those of opposing response tendencies. In this way, we could say that the obsessional–compulsive patient is in a state of conflict between performing a ritual and refraining from its performance, which would lead us to examine the literature on experimental studies of conflict. Such studies (e.g. Yates, 1962) have distinguished three main types of conflict situation:

a) approach–approach conflict, in which the subject has to make a choice between two responses, both of which are positively reinforced

b) approach–avoidance conflict, in which the subject has to choose whether or not to perform a response which will be followed by both positive and negative reinforcement

c) avoidance–avoidance conflict, in which the subject has to make a choice between two responses, both of which are negatively reinforced.

In terms of the discussion of preceding sections, the avoidance–avoidance paradigm seems to be the most profitable to examine in terms of deriving hypotheses on the nature of obsessional–compulsive rituals. An hypothesis derived in this way would be that the obsessional–compulsive patient is in avoidance–avoidance conflict whether to perform his ritualistic behaviour or not; by performing the ritual he avoids the aversive consequences of its non-performance, but, it is hypothesized, performance of the ritual also produces aversive consequences, which could be avoided by the non-performance of the ritual; hence the conflict. The fact that the ritual is performed suggests that the overall aversiveness of the consequences of performance of the ritual is less than the overall aversiveness of the consequences of non-performance of the ritual, which is what was suggested by saying the ritualistic behaviour is an avoidance response. However, it does suggest a new feature of obsessional–compulsive ritualistic behaviour, namely, that the results of its performance are aversive, rather than neutral. One could suggest that this aversiveness is related to the reactions of others to the patient's apparently senseless behaviour, to the patient's own reaction to his bizarre behaviour, to the fact that performance of the ritual precludes the occurrence of other, positively reinforced-behaviour at the same time, etc.

A testable prediction from this hypothesis would be that the consequences of performance of ritualistic behaviour (e.g. ritualistic hand-washing) are more aversive to the obsessional–compulsive patient than the consequences of performance of corresponding normal behaviour (e.g. normal hand-washing) are to a normal person.

This hypothesis has further ramifications. There is evidence that the state of conflict in the avoidance–avoidance conflict situation is itself aversive or arousal increasing. Such arousal or noxious stimulation would augment avoidance responding. The aversiveness of the consequences of performance of one episode of ritualistic behaviour could also have an effect on the performance of subsequent avoidance responses in the same way.

Further, a feature noted in experimental investigations of the avoidance–avoidance paradigm is for the subject to oscillate between the two alternative responses before making one or the other of them. This could be seen as analogous to the doubt and uncertainty as to whether a ritual should be performed or not which has been noted in a number of clinical descriptions (e.g. Mather, 1970).

In experimental investigations of the avoidance–avoidance paradigm, a solution which can be taken by the subject, unless the experimenter arranges otherwise, is to avoid making either of the punished responses by withdrawing from the experimental situation. This solution is not open to the obsessional–compulsive patient; as has already been noted, the nature of the stimuli producing an aversive state if the ritual is not performed makes it difficult to withdraw from them, and the same could be said of the aversive state resulting from the performance of the ritual.

4. *The behaviour appears senseless to others and embarrassing to the patient.* In terms of the avoidance conditioning model that has been examined, this characteristic of obsessional–compulsive ritualistic behaviour could be described as the realization by others and, at some level, by the patient, that avoidance responding is unnecessary in as much as there is nothing, in the sense of some external event likely to cause harm to life or limb, to be avoided. Specifically, it could be said that the obsessional's ritualistic behaviour cannot be modified through information received through what Pavlov described as the 'second signalling system' or, more simply, language. A striking example of this resistance of the obsessional's behaviour to information received through language is a patient, described by Stafford-Clark (1967), whose rituals related to fears of pregnancy persisted after she had undergone a hysterectomy, making it physically impossible to conceive.

For the moment, this feature of obsessional behaviour will be noted, and added to the problems which are to be explained in the section on aetiology (p. 223).

ii) *Type B hypotheses*
One problem with working at the level of Type A hypotheses is that it is not always possible to derive simple empirical generalizations which are true of all the behaviour we may have classified as avoidance responding. For example, as noted on page 204, the effect of shock intensity on resistance to extinction of avoidance responses varies with the experimental situations in which it is studied. The purpose of developing Type B hypotheses is to attempt to improve the predictions that can be made about behaviour in different settings. Also, in the case of obses-

sional–compulsive behaviour, Type B hypotheses have been of historical importance in the development of behavioural methods of treatment.

The most widely known and accepted theoretical model of avoidance learning is the two-factor theory developed by Mowrer (Mowrer, 1960; Herrnstein, 1969). As applied to the shuttle-box training procedure, (p. 202, this model would be as follows: in the initial stages of learning before the avoidance response has emerged, the animal will experience repeated pairings of the warning signal with shock; by a process of classical conditioning, the warning signal will acquire aversive properties and the animal will experience conditioned anxiety on its presentation; by making the avoidance response the animal terminates the warning signal, thus reducing the anxiety it experiences; this reduction in conditioned anxiety, rather than the avoidance of the shock, is the reinforcement operating in the acquisition and maintenance of the avoidance response. On this view, the only difference between escape responses and avoidance responses is that the former lead to the removal of the animal from a source of unconditioned aversive stimulation (e.g. shock) whereas the latter lead to the removal of the animal from a source of conditioned aversive stimulation.

This model would apply as follows to the compulsive washing behaviour in Case 1: dirt on the patient's hands or clothing evokes a conditioned anxiety response; washing the hands or clothes removes the source of this conditioned anxiety, and the ensuing reduction in anxiety serves to reinforce and maintain the washing behaviour. As applied to the repetitive motor behaviour in Case 2, this model would be as follows: the intrusion of blasphemy-related thoughts evokes a conditioned anxiety response; repeating gross motor behaviours such as climbing stairs removes the source of this conditioned anxiety by the distraction process that was discussed on page 213; such behaviour is followed by reduction in conditioned anxiety, which serves as reinforcement to maintain the gross motor behaviour.

In many ways this model is attractive; it has considerable support (e.g. Mowrer, 1960), and appears to encompass the clinical data quite neatly. However, there are a number of problems with it. Firstly, as Morgan (1968), Herrnstein (1969) and Bolles (1970) among others have pointed out, the model has difficulties accounting for the results of a number of experimental investigations. Specifically, there is evidence that avoidance responses can be learned and maintained if they lead to a reduction in the frequency of shocks which would otherwise be received, in the absence of any effect of the response in removing sources of conditioned anxiety. Secondly, the model does not always tally with everyday experience; to take the example of putting on a raincoat before going out into the rain, donning the coat is not accompanied by a noticeable wave of relief as the preceding anxiety recedes. Thirdly, a clear prediction from the model when applied to obsessional–compulsive rituals is that anxiety levels should be less immediately after completing a ritual than before it. While this appears to be true in a number of cases (e.g. Case 2), there is clinical and experimental evidence (e.g. Walker and Beech, 1969) that anxiety may actually be increased above preceding levels by the performance of the ritual.

The position advanced by Herrnstein (1969) is that the reinforcement maintaining avoidance behaviour is in fact the avoidance of noxious stimulation, i.e. the extent of noxious stimulation is less following the performance of the avoidance response than the extent of noxious stimulation following the non-performance of the avoidance response. In this position, the main role given the warning signal is that of a discriminative stimulus, i.e. it signals the situation in which the avoidance response will be successful from those in which it will be unsuccessful.

Herrnstein's suggestion that the avoidance of a programmed shock is in fact the main reinforcement in avoidance learning has been explicitly rejected by Mowrer (1960) and Schoenfeld (1950), and Skinner has even maintained that to say that behaviour is influenced by the non-arrival of an event 'violates the fundamental principles of science' (Morgan, 1968). While it is difficult to encompass Herrnstein's suggestion in traditional stimulus-response theories of learning, it is quite possible to do so in more sophisticated theories of learning (e.g. Estes, 1969) without violating the fundamental principles of science. It thus seems unnecessary to reject Herrnstein's suggestion, on logical grounds, which is fortunate as it has considerable empirical support, is consistent with common-sense, and is consistent with much of the reasoning that has been used in the discussion of Type A hypothesis.

It might be as well to clarify the distinction between the positions of Mowrer and Herrnstein. For Mowrer, the state of the animal after the performance of an avoidance response has to be less aversive than the state of the animal immediately before its performance; for Herrnstein, all that is necessary is that the state of the animal after the performance of an avoidance response should be less aversive than the state of the animal if it had not made the response in that situation; the state of the animal might well be more aversive after the completion of the response than before, but still less aversive than if the response had not been made.

It is not proposed to give a detailed exposition of a theoretical model, such as Estes' (1969), which can accommodate Herrnstein's proposal;

rather, let it simply be said that Estes' model appears to be able to accommodate the empirical generalizations that have been proposed earlier.

Non-ritualistic behaviour

Case 3 is an example of an obsessional–compulsive disorder in which the abnormal behaviour appears to consist of a recurrent mental event, an impulse to strike people, which is not accompanied by overt ritualistic behaviour. In the discussion of ritualistic behaviour, it has been suggested that, in some cases, the ritual behaviour is related to the occurrence of such recurrent mental events, e.g. the 'blasphemous thoughts', in Case 2.

It is obviously impossible to investigate mental events in animals, and little has been done in the way of direct experimentation on such events in humans. For the purposes of generating hypotheses, I shall regard mental events as essentially similar to more easily observable overt behaviour, so that the former can be viewed in terms of what is known about the latter.

A characteristic of these mental events is that they elicit anxiety. Viewing them as responses which are always followed by an aversive event, the problem arises: why does the behaviour persist in the face of its aversive consequences when this constitutes a punishment procedure and should, on a simple reinforcement model, lead to a reduction in the intensity of the behaviour? One obvious answer to this question is that the mental events are not responses whose rate of occurrence depends solely on the reinforcement contingent on them, but are responses which are elicited by certain environmental stimuli, and which may be to some extent independent of the reinforcement contingent on them. Such responses may be broadly divided into two classes, those depending on the innate organization of the nervous system, and those depending on learning based on the innate organization of the nervous system.

In the first class the following types of response (among others) have been described in animals and humans:

i) Fear responses to certain classes of stimuli (e.g. Marks, 1969).
ii) Aggression to certain classes of stimuli (e.g. Argyle, 1969, p. 28).
iii) Orienting, alerting or arousal responses to novel stimuli (e.g. Sokolov, 1963).
iv) Frustration: Gray (1967) has suggested that there is an innate

basis for the response to failure to obtain an anticipated reward, and that this response is operationally indistinguishable from a fear response.

All the above four responses could be described as ones in which certain sets of stimuli elicit responses involving an increase in arousal, apparently based on some aspects of the innate organization of the nervous system.

The second class of elicited responses would be those in which, by a process of learning (usually thought of as classical conditioning) previously neutral stimuli acquire the ability to elicit responses similar to those in the first class.

The hypothesis to be considered is that the recurrent mental events experienced by obsessionals are similar to the elicited responses which have just been discussed. An essential and obvious test of this hypothesis is the prediction that the mental events are under stimulus control, i.e. it should be possible to identify some stimulus conditions in which the events will be elicited with a higher probability than in other stimulus conditions.

Can this hypothesis suggest reasons why there should be a greater frequency of recurrent mental events in obsessional patients than in normals? Viewing such events as elicited responses, the obsessional must be in a situation in which he experiences more stimuli capable of eliciting such responses than does the normal person. This could occur in a number of ways, which Case 3 will be used to illustrate:

a) The environment of the obsessional might contain more stimuli that would normally elicit a given type of response than the environment of the normal person. In Case 3, this would suggest that the environment of the obsessional was such that it would elicit more aggressive impulses than the environment of the normal person. On this suggestion, it would be predicted that the normal person would experience the same number of aggressive impulses if put in the same environment as the obsessional. This seems unlikely.

b) By virtue of previous learning experiences, some stimuli may elicit responses in an obsessional but not in a normal person. As applied to Case 3, this would suggest that the ability of strangers and workmates to elicit intense aggressive urges was the result of a generalization to these stimuli of the response originally elicited by the military police. Such an account is similar to one of the most popular learning accounts of the origin of phobias, and is discussed further in the section on aetiology.

c) As a result of a difference in state, the obsessional may respond more frequently and intensely than the normal person to the same stimulus environment, i.e. there is a lower threshold for the elicitation of the response in the obsessional. Such a phenomenon is apparent in Case 3; the case history suggests that at low levels of anxiety the patient responds in a relatively normal way, and that aggressive impulses are only elicited when the patient is anxious. If such changes in state within an individual can produce changes in responsiveness to eliciting stimuli, then it is possible that differences in responsiveness between obsessionals and normals may also be a result of such differences of state.

There is evidence that changes in state can effect the probability of a given stimulus eliciting the types of response that have been discussed above. Hill *et al.* (1952) present evidence that the fear response to painful stimuli is greater under anxiety-evoking than anxiety-reducing conditions, and the experiment by Hoffman *et al.* (1963) already mentioned (p. 205) demonstrated that the fear response to a conditioned aversive stimulus was enhanced by preceding electric shocks.

Ulrich, Hutchinson and Azrin (1965) have shown that administering electric shock to animals will increase their tendency to show aggressive responses.

The effect of preceding electric shock in intensifying the response to novel stimuli is so well known as to have a specific descriptive term 'pseudoconditioning' (e.g. Kimble, 1964). The work of Lader and co-workers (e.g. Lader and Mathews, 1968) provides further evidence for a relationship between level of arousal and extent of orienting responding.

Gray (1967) presents evidence showing the effects of sedative drugs, such as amylobarbitone, reduce the response to frustrative non-reward, again suggesting that the extent to which the response is elicited depends on the state of the animal, perhaps its arousal level.

From such observations, one could propose the hypothesis that the greater frequency of certain types of mental events in obsessionals is the result of the greater responsivity they exhibit to certain eliciting stimuli as a result of a difference in state of arousal. This hypothesis would predict that in situations where obsessionals respond to a certain stimulus situation with a mental event of the type under discussion and normals do not, measures of arousal will be higher in the obsessional than the normal. Possible sources of this difference in arousal will be discussed in the section on aetiology.

It has been suggested that the mental events discussed so far are elicited by environmental stimuli and, to that extent, under stimulus control. However, there appears to be another class of recurrent mental event which does not seem so obviously under stimulus control. The 'blasphemous thoughts' of Case 2 would be examples of this class; it is reported that the thoughts were more pronounced when the patient was on her own, and that she felt continually afraid waiting for the thoughts to 'strike her'. If these are not elicited responses, but subject to the normal law of reinforcement, how is their persistence in the face of the anxiety they evoke to be explained?

From the earlier discussion in this chapter, it could be suggested that such mental events are maintained on an avoidance conditioning paradigm. The suggestion would be that 'having a thought' is an avoidance response and that the consequences of 'having a thought' in certain situations is less noxious than not having one. In Case 2, it would be suggested that the continuance of the fearful state of waiting for a thought to strike is more noxious than the actual consequences of having a thought. An experimental analogue of the situation described would be for a subject to be provided with two switches, depression of one of them producing an immediate aversive event and depression of the other producing the same event after some delay. Here, the aversive event would be equivalent to the thought and the pressing of the switch which produced it immediately rather than after a delay would be equivalent to the response of having a thought rather than sitting waiting for it to strike. It is in fact found (Badia, McBane, Suter and Lewis, 1966) that subjects placed in this situation learn to press the button producing the aversive event immediately.

It is less easy to test the avoidance paradigm in this situation than in previous cases. It is difficult to see how one could prevent the occurrence of a thought which would normally occur without changing the situation so that it would not normally occur, which would be required in order to demonstrate the reduced aversiveness of the consequences of having a thought compared with the consequences of not having a thought. A possible approach would be to obtain a measure of discomfort immediately before and after the occurrence of a thought; obtaining a reduction in discomfort by the performance of the thought would confirm the avoidance hypothesis, but failure to do so would not refute it.

In this section we have again deferred discussion of certain problems to the next section on aetiology. These are:

a) Why are the recurrent thoughts anxiety-evoking?
b) How do elicited responses become attached to new stimuli (the

problems posed by phobias, and generalized aggressive responses) and why do they not extinguish?

c) What is the cause of the heightened arousal in obsessionals in certain situations?

d) Why does the anxiety evoked by the thoughts not extinguish?

THE AETIOLOGY OF OBSESSIONAL–COMPULSIVE BEHAVIOUR

The discussion of the maintenance of obsessional ritualistic behaviour suggested that the origin and maintenance of the obsessional motor behaviour could be satisfactorily explained if the following features of obsessional–compulsive behaviour could also be explained:

a) The presence of phobias of objects of widespread occurrence (possibly related to erroneous beliefs), such fears being resistant to extinction, and to correction by information imparted by language.

b) The presence of recurrent, intrusive anxiety-evoking thoughts, the anxiety being resistant to extinction.

c) The presence of high levels of arousal in obsessionals in the situations in which the obsessional–compulsive behaviour normally occurs.

These are similar to the problems which arose from the discussion of non-ritualistic obsessional behaviour in the previous section, and this discussion of aetiology will concentrate on attempting to offer explanations for the origins of these three phenomena.

a) *Phobias of objects of widespread occurrence.* The aetiology of phobias is a topic that could be discussed at length (e.g. Rachman, 1968; Marks, 1969), and the discussion here must necessarily be brief. One of the more popular learning models of their genesis (e.g. Eysenck and Rachman, 1965) is that they represent conditioned anxiety responses. The suggestion here is that originally neutral stimuli, by temporal association with fearful events, themselves acquire the ability to elicit fear responses, by a process of classical conditioning. In terms of this model, the conditioned anxiety attached to the phobic stimuli does not extinguish, as a result of repeated experiences with the stimuli unpaired with fearful events, because motor behaviour develops to avoid contact with the phobic stimuli. Thus little chance for extinction by repeated or prolonged exposure to such stimuli exists.

This model, later modified (Rachman, 1968), has been criticized by a number of writers (e.g. Watts, 1971). A major problem is that it is rarely possible to identify in the case history some event in which the phobic stimulus was actually paired with a traumatic event. Another problem is that phobias tend to develop to only a restricted range of stimuli, rather than to a more or less random sample of all stimuli, as the simple conditioning model would require. Further, stressful events often appear to precede the development of a phobia rather than to occur in association with the phobic stimuli.

As an alternative, Watts (1971) proposed a sensitization theory of phobias. This theory suggests that the genesis of phobias is the result of some stress event sensitizing the subject to stimuli that have an innate tendency to elicit a fear response, e.g. he suggests that social anxieties in man are the result of a sensitization-induced amplification of the normal innately based response found in other primates to being looked in the eyes. This suggestion is obviously related to the discussion on page 221 of the increased responsiveness to a variety of eliciting stimuli which results from the application of electric shock or some other stress, and to the previously noted effects of free shock in enhancing avoidance responding.

To explain the persistence of phobias in the absence of any sensitizing stressor, Watts adopts a suggestion of Eysenck's (1968) that the presentation of a conditioned stimulus in the absence of an unconditioned stimulus results in two opposing trends – one to response decrement (extinction) and one to response enhancement. This is very similar to the theory of habituation proposed by Groves and Thompson (1970), for which they present quite compelling evidence for the existence of two distinct mechanisms, one of response enhancement, the other of response decrement. To explain the persistence of phobias, Watts suggests that conditions are such that the tendency for response diminution does not outweigh the tendency for response enhancement and so extinction does not occur. It is obviously necessary to specify what these conditions should be, and at the moment relatively little is known about what determines the relative magnitude of these two opposing tendencies. However, in the area of habituation of the orienting reflex, Lader and co-workers (e.g. Lader and Mathews, 1968) have demonstrated that habituation is slower the higher the level of arousal, as indicated by PGR measures, suggesting that the response-enhancement tendency may become relatively more powerful than the response-decrement tendency at high levels of arousal.

Perhaps it would be as well to give some illustration of these theoretical speculations by making suggestions as to the aetiology of the dirt phobia shown by Case. 1. This seems to be a good example of a case where no obvious association between the phobic stimulus and some traumatic event marked the inception of the phobia. Rather, it appears that the stressful event (associated with the birth of the baby) preceded the onset of the phobia. On the sensitization theory, this stress would strengthen an existing response tendency. Watts's theory would suggest that this was an innate response tendency, but as sensitization phenomena also appear to exist for learned anxiety responses, there is no reason why one should not suggest that the existing response tendency (fear of dirt) was the result of earlier learning. If this were the case, it is necessary to explain why all mothers do not become obsessional in the same way following the birth of a child.

One suggestion to account for the difference in behaviour between Case 1 and most other mothers would be that Case 1 had a greater than average response to the stress experience as a result of some relatively permanent characteristic which made her unusually sensitive to stresses of this kind. This would suggest some difference in premorbid personality between obsessionals and normals. This area is fully discussed in Chapter 4. Here, only one suggestion will be considered. That is that the greater responsivity to stress situations involving fear is related to high scores on neuroticism and introversion (Gray, 1970). The prediction would be that obsessionals as a group tend to be neurotic introverts, for which there is some evidence (Chap. 4). This would also imply their being high on measures of arousal (Eysenck, 1967b).

Another suggestion, and one that seems necessary to explain why sensitization should result in an exaggerated fear of dirt rather than a wider range of other behaviour anomalies, is that the existing response tendency to fear dirt is higher in Case 1 than in most mothers. This could be the result of unusual early learning experiences (parents unusually preoccupied with cleanliness) or a greater than average tendency to learn from average experiences (as a result of personality differences similar to those already described), or both.

These two suggestions (greater sensitivity and effects of earlier learning) are obviously not exclusive and probably both contribute to the development of obsessional behaviour.

Having appeared as a result of the sensitization arising from the stresses associated with the birth of the child, the tendency to give exaggerated responses to dirt stimuli would continue so long as this stress remained. However, it is necessary to give some explanation for the persistence of the phobia over a very long period. If a state of high arousal is an important factor in preventing the extinction of the phobic response (Lader and Mathews, 1968), it is necessary to find other sources of increased arousal once the original source of stress has disappeared. It is possible that the phobia could itself maintain the state of high arousal necessary to its own perpetuation; dirt is a fairly widespread feature of the environment and the repeated elicitation of the phobic response could maintain a sufficiently high level of arousal to prevent its own extinction. This suggestion is very similar to that of Lader and Mathews (1968). This process could be extended by the wide stimulus generalization which appeared to take place in this case, and which might itself be related to the high level of arousal (Chaps. 5 and 6). One could suggest further sources of increased arousal: the stress of having a phobia and obsessional rituals, related to the patient's own reaction to her apparent foolishness, and to the reaction of others (Chap. 6), and the arousal induced by the conflict of whether to perform the obsessional ritual or not (Chap. 6).

In this way, the patient could find herself in a self-perpetuating vicious circle.

The problem of why such fear reactions should be beyond the subject's cognitive control (i.e. resistant to information received via language about the actual contingencies operating) has been previously discussed by the author (Rachman and Teasdale, 1969) and will not be dwelt on here. It does seem to be the case that there are classes of fear responses which are not modified by information from the 'second signalling system', and phobias seem to be one of them. In fact, one could suggest that the patient's erroneous beliefs about the consequences of contact with dirt are an important factor in maintaining and extending the phobic behaviour.

b) *Recurrent, intrusive anxiety-evoking thoughts.*[1] For those anxiety-evoking thoughts which appear to be elicited by environmental stimuli, an aetiological model essentially similar to that proposed for the origin of phobias of widespread stimuli could be proposed. Where the thought is elicited by stimuli which have acquired phobic qualities, the thought itself is part of the total phobic response, and thereby anxiety-evoking. In the case of other types of mental event, e.g. the agressive impulses experienced by Case 3, it is suggested that the mental events themselves have acquired the properties of phobic stimuli in the same ways that external stimuli acquire such properties. In Case 3, it would be suggested that aggressive impulses acquired anxiety-evoking properties as a result of the traumatic experiences with the military police. The

---

[1] Since writing this passage, the author has become aware of the paper by Rachman (1971) in which he independently makes suggestions on the origin and maintenance of obsessional ruminations very similar to those discussed here.

subsequent appearance of the impulses eleven years later was the result of the sensitization resulting from the stress of the imprisonment and related events. In other cases, aggressive or sexual impulses might originally have acquired unusually great anxiety-evoking properties as a result of childhood learning experiences such as unusually severe parental punishment of such behaviour.

In the case of thoughts which are less obviously stimulus elicited, it would again be suggested that the thoughts acquire their anxiety-evoking properties in much the same way as external stimuli acquire phobic properties. In Case 2, for example, it would be suggested that the anxiety experienced when a 'blasphemous thought' occurred would be related to a more than usually strict religious upbringing in which great anxiety was associated with such thoughts, probably in a person with a personality peculiarly susceptible to fear (Gray, 1970). The anxiety evoked by 'waiting for the thought to strike' would probably be of importance in maintaining the state of sensitization in such cases.

THE TREATMENT OF OBSESSIONAL–COMPULSIVE BEHAVIOUR

Behavioural methods of treating obsessional–compulsive disorders are the subject of an entire chapter elsewhere in this book (Chap. 10), and so will not be discussed in detail here. Rather, the implications for treatment arising from the model outlined here will be briefly indicated.

Ritualistic behaviour

In terms of the avoidance model proposed to account for the maintenance of ritualistic behaviour, the reinforcement maintaining the behaviour is the fact that the discomfort experienced in certain situations is less following the performance of the ritualistic behaviour than following the non-performance of such behaviour. This model suggests that treatment should aim at eliminating the discomfort resulting from the non-performance of the ritual, thereby eliminating the reinforcement for the performance of the ritual, which should extinguish. It has been suggested that this discomfort is the result of anxiety related to phobias of widespread stimuli or the presence of recurrent anxiety-evoking thoughts.

Treatment requires the reduction of such anxiety, and the most obvious behavioural procedure to achieve this end is an extinction procedure in which the subject is repeatedly exposed to the threatening events without the occurrence of any externally imposed adverse consequences (Bandura, 1969, p. 386). The most common treatment procedures which seem to follow this extinction paradigm are systematic desensitization and flooding (see Chap. 10). Where the anxiety seems related to the presence of phobias of widespread stimuli, such procedures could be applied to these phobias in exactly the same way as in the treatment of phobias in non-obsessional patients, and this approach has met with some success (see Chap. 10). However, as the target of treatment is to eliminate the anxiety associated with the non-performance of the ritual, a more direct procedure would be to attempt to extinguish this anxiety as such. This would suggest a treatment technique in which the patient is repeatedly placed in situations which would normally elicit ritualistic behaviour and prevented from performing such behaviour, so that the anxiety associated with such non-performance would extinguish. Such a treatment technique has in fact been developed and appears successful (Chap. 10). It would be equally applicable to rituals in which the anxiety was related to recurrent anxiety-evoking thoughts as to cases where it was related to widespread phobic stimuli.

The prevention of the ritualistic behaviour with the subsequent extinction of anxiety related to its non-performance would result in the elimination of a number of sources of increased arousal, and thereby break in to the self-sustaining vicious circle by which it has been suggested the obsessional behaviour is maintained. Further, it would allow the patient to discriminate the situations in which avoidance behaviour was appropriate from those in which it was inappropriate.

Non-ritualistic behaviour

In terms of the suggestions made in the section on aetiology, the recurrent mental events which occur in non-ritualistic obsessional–compulsive behaviour can be usefully viewed as phobic stimuli. On this model, treatment would again be most usefully based on some form of extinction procedure. Where the events are elicited by external stimuli this procedure would consist of repeatedly placing the patient in situations which elicit the events, and attempting to eliminate the associated anxiety by an extinction procedure such as desensitization or flooding (Chap. 10). Where the mental events seem to be less under the control of eliciting stimuli, the patient would be asked repeatedly to experience the thought in some form of extinction procedure.

Rachman (1971) has made the very interesting suggestion that the demands for reassurance often made by obsessional–compulsive patients with no obvious ritualistic behaviour may serve the same function as motor rituals, i.e. they produce reassurance which avoids the increase in aversiveness which would occur if no reassurance were obtained. He suggests that treatment of such patients should include the removal of such reassurance, in exactly the same way as the treatment of patients with rituals should include preventing them performing their rituals.

CONCLUSION

Viewing obsessional-compulsive behaviour in the light of the results of experiments on animal and human learning appears to be useful in providing a conceptual framework in which to look at the problem, in generating experimentally testable hypotheses about the nature of the problem, and in suggesting possible methods of treatment.

This chapter has drawn on the work of other writers, noted in the text, and benefited from discussion with a number of colleagues, especially Drs Jack Rachman and Fraser Watts.

10

V. Meyer, R. Levy and A Schnurer

The behavioural treatment of
obsessive–compulsive disorders

INTRODUCTION

The term obsessive–compulsive has been applied to a large variety of disturbances of thought and behaviour encountered in psychiatric practice. These include the occurrence of prolonged periods of brooding, doubting and speculation with the inability of reaching a solution, the presence of strong urges or impulses to carry out acts which are unacceptable to the patient and which may give rise to feelings of guilt or anxiety, and the occurrence of sometimes elaborate rituals which are usually viewed by the patient as being senseless or embarrassing.

Numerous attempts to define this disorder have been made, but perhaps the most widely accepted formulation is that of Schneider. This is discussed at some length by Lewis (1936), who translates it as '. . . contents of consciousness which, when they occur, are accompanied by the experience of subjective compulsion, and which cannot be got rid of, though on quiet reflection they are recognized as senseless'. Lewis points out that the recognition of an obsession as senseless is not an invariable characteristic, but the feeling that one must resist the obsession is essential. It is this resistance that distinguishes compulsive phenomena from other psychopathological manifestations.

Lewis also criticizes the tendency to equate repetitive or stereotyped activities with obsessions, or to assume that any ritual or ceremonial is *ipso facto* obsessional. He points out that repetitive phenomena and stereotyped motor activity occurs in a wide variety of conditions such as schizophrenia, diseases of the basal ganglia, frontal lobe lesions etc., in which there may be no associated feelings of resistance.

In recent years there have been several follow-up studies (Pollitt, 1957; Ingram, 1961a, 1961b; Kringlen, 1965; Grimshaw, 1965) of obsessional patients, and although the prognosis is not felt to be as gloomy as is sometimes suggested in standard textbooks, it is generally agreed that treatment is extremely difficult and that results are often unrewarding. For example, the most comprehensive study of obsessional neurosis published in recent years (Kringlen, 1965) showed that of ninety patients followed up for 13–20 years only nineteen could be said to be much improved and when the follow-up period was shorter the results were even worse.

Although interest has been aroused by the use of behaviour therapy in these disorders, the results have generally been disappointing. The purpose of this chapter is to review and evaluate the various attempts to apply behavioural methods to the treatment of obsessive–compulsive disorders and to present some encouraging data resulting from the present investigators' application of a new method of treatment, 'apotrepic therapy'.

CASE STUDIES

Lack of adequate knowledge concerning the aetiology of many psychiatric disorders has not prevented behaviour therapists from attempting to treat them. Behaviour therapy rests on the assumption that the acquisition of abnormalities of behaviour can be understood on the basis of learning principles and that these same principles should be used in modifying such behaviour.

Most of the reports on the use of behaviour therapy in the treatment of obsessional neurosis concern single patients and there are no controlled studies. Thus, the existing reports offer illustrations of techniques rather than proofs of efficiency (see Paul, 1969). The methods have predominantly followed two strategies. The first is based on the theory of anxiety-reduction, and the principle of counterconditioning. The therapeutic change is achieved by inducing activities incompatible with emotional arousal, e.g. relaxation in the presence of gradually introduced anxiety-arousing stimuli; thus, classically induced conditioned effects (neutralization of the arousal evoked by threatening stimuli) exert control over instrumentally learned avoidance responses (Wolpe, 1958). The second strategy is to eliminate the habit which constitutes the obsessive–compulsive behaviour. The therapeutic change here is accomplished by a variety of techniques derived from the theory of extinction.

Cooper *et al.* (1965) included ten obsessional patients in their sample of neurotics assessed retrospectively on the basis of information extracted from case notes. As regards methods of treatment, these were described as 'a combination of graded practical retraining along the lines of Meyer and Gelder (1963)' and 'desensitization in imagination along the lines of Wolpe (1958)'. Three patients were reported as showing improvement at the end of treatment and after a one-year follow-up. This result was worse than that obtained in a control group treated mainly by supportive psychotherapy and drugs.

Amongst a large sample of neurotics treated by Wolpe, there were nineteen patients with obsessions. No information is provided as to how the obsessive symptoms were treated in each case. However, it appears that systematic desensitization (presentation of graded items to be imagined by a relaxed patient) was the method of choice. For some cases, 'training in assertion' was added; some had 'avoidance-conditioning' and 'thought-stopping'. In avoidance-conditioning electric shocks were paired with the imagined objects or situations that 'formed the substance of obsessions'. The thought-stopping procedure involved asking the patients to press a buzzer at the onset of the compulsive thoughts, whereupon the therapist would shout 'stop'. According to Wolpe repetition of this procedure eventually led to a habit of inhibiting disturbing thoughts. Unfortunately Wolpe did not give separate data on the results of therapy for his sample of obsessional patients. A limited amount of information (Wolpe, 1958; Table 1) suggests that he obtained better results than those reported by Cooper *et al.* (1965). The averages for therapeutic time and number of sessions, however, are well in excess of those given for this total sample.

More recently, Wolpe (1964) described in greater detail the treatment of one patient with compulsive hand-washing and cleaning rituals associated with fear of contamination by urine. Following about 100 sessions of systematic desensitization, transfer to real-life situations was not impressive and the patient then received desensitization *in vivo*. Considerable decrease in ritualistic behaviour was achieved and maintained for one year.

Walton and Mather (1963) distinguished between cases of recent onset where instrumental avoidance responses were elicited by 'CAD' (conditioned autonomic drive, i.e. anxiety) and chronic cases where instrumental avoidance responses became 'functionally autonomous' and independent of the chronologically earlier 'CAD'. They felt that, in the former, treatment should concentrate on the extinction of 'CAD' (i.e. reduction of anxiety) whereas in the latter both anxiety and motor behaviour had to be treated. Walton and Mather attempted to test this supposition, using six patients with severe obsessive–compulsive disorders, two of whom were of recent onset and the other four of long duration. The method of reducing anxiety consisted of systematic desensitization in imagination (in some cases intravenously administered sodium amytal was used to induce relaxation). Re-training to actual 'performance hierarchies' were employed to deal with maladaptive motor responses (avoidance responses and rituals).

In two cases of recent onset the reduction of the assumed 'CAD' by systematic desensitization was sufficient to produce elimination of ritualistic behaviour. On the other hand in two chronic patients this approach, though resulting in an apparent reduction of anxiety, left ritualistic responses relatively unaltered. Treatment of the motor component with a 'performance hierarchy' in the fifth, chronic, case effected a temporary remission of the motor compulsion, but anxiety increased. In the sixth case, also described as chronic, both systematic desensitization and retraining to 'performance hierarchies' were applied without success. Following leucotomy, which according to the authors decreased the intensity of the unconditioned autonomic reactivity, the same treatment was readministered and was effective.

The authors maintained that their results provided tentative support for their hypothesis. Apart from the fact that their highly speculative assumptions about some patients are hard to follow and accept, they do not consider any alternative explanations.

Bevan (1960) described a patient with obsessional ruminations who was treated by 'reciprocal inhibition'. The patient was required to engage in those activities which evoked anxiety and ruminations but was sedated with 100 mgms of Chlorpromazine. It appears that she had eight sessions over a period of four weeks and was reported to have improved. She then relapsed somewhat as regards the obsessions and exhibited bouts of renewed 'depression'. The latter was treated by the method of anxiety-relief (Wolpe, 1958). She was then seen by a psychiatrist as an out-patient for about fourteen months and at one stage was given Chlorpromazine. The final clinical assessment revealed that the patient was free of her ruminations.

A patient with four different rituals was treated by Walton (1960). We need not concern ourselves here with a rather complex and speculative Hullian theoretical formulation put forward by Walton to account for the disordered beheaviour and the rationale of treatment. The two most incapacitating rituals (1) clearing roads, passages, corridors of stones and pieces of paper lest people might fall, and (2) washing because of a fear of germs and dirt, were treated successfully in eighteen sessions. As regards the first ritual the patient was required to follow the therapist along a graded series of walks while under 75 mgms of Chlorpromazine.

The treatment of the second ritual was carried out as follows: The patient was given Chlorpromazine and then asked to approach a washing bowl without washing. Following this treatment two minor rituals improved although they were not directly treated. Seven months later the patient was readmitted complaining of excessive hand-washing and of general slowness (he had to do things thoroughly). Therapeutic efforts this time concentrated on the development of alternative adaptive responses to deal with stressful situations and assertive behaviour. The patient responded to this treatment and four months later the improvement was maintained.

A young woman with compulsive rituals linked to a fear of broken glass was treated by Haslam (1965). Her symptoms persisted despite fourteen hospital admissions and a leucotomy. Haslam used 'reciprocal inhibition techniques' which comprised 'reduction of hunger, sedation with Chlorpromazine and empathy with the doctor as the mechanisms whereby deconditioning and anxiety reduction might be achieved'. The gradual presentation of anxiety-evoking stimuli was *in vivo*. After fourteen sessions she was discharged and considered 'free of symptoms'. This outcome was maintained after a year's follow-up.

Worsley (1968) reported four patients who were treated mainly with 'desensitization by habituation'. The procedure required the patient to practise the avoided activities in a graded way. A patient who avoided writing letters because it evoked checking rituals, was required to progress from meaningless scribbling to loosely formed symbols and then to clearly defined ones and eventually to letters and words. Ritualistic washing and cleaning were dealt with by instructing the patient to reduce gradually the number of sheets of toilet paper and washing time. Considerable improvement was achieved in seventeen weekly sessions and it was apparently maintained over a two-year follow-up period. Another case suffered from a fear of contamination which prevented her from carrying out various activities. In this case a gradual approach programme was designed for each stressful situation and the patient carried it out herself under supervision. She made progress in five of the six activities during three or four weeks of the programme. At five months and three years follow-up she was able to carry out the five activities without anxiety but had made no progress with the sixth one. The third case presented a complex picture but it was felt that his anxiety was related to his 'compulsive' need to make himself responsible for organizing work and domestic circumstances. He was simply instructed to gradually delegate these responsibilities to other people.

After five weeks of practice and three visits to the clinic he improved and this improvement was sustained during the eighteen months follow-up period. The last patient was unable to read because of compulsive checking of the meaning of the ordinary words she read. In this case, she was requested to read two or three words without checking their meaning and if anxiety did not occur, to progress gradually to larger numbers of words. Another behaviour abnormality which consisted of compulsive house cleaning was treated with systematic desensitization. While relaxed, she imagined situations comprising an increasing amount of dust for increasing periods of time without indulging in cleaning activities. She made rapid progress and was discharged from hospital after four weeks of treatment. Two years later she was apparently still well.

Several therapists have used various forms of punishment in the attempt to eliminate compulsive behaviour. The general rationale of the approach is that if performance of a compulsive act is associated with the elicitation of anxiety instead of reduction of anxiety the ritual should disappear. Thorpe *et al.* (1966), for example, used an aversive relief method in the treatment of an obsessive–compulsive patient whose rituals were triggered off by the name of a deceased relative for whose death she felt unjustifiably responsible. The technique involved the presentation of the deceased relative's name. Each time the name appeared the patient had to read it out aloud whereupon she received a shock. At the end of twenty-three presentations a 'relief stimulus' which was not followed by a shock was displayed. After an initial improvement, she relapsed and declined further treatment. Solyom (1969) applied a modified version of this method to a 49-year-old housewife with many obsessive thoughts and rituals. Apparently a good outcome was obtained after seventy sessions over a period of nine months. No follow-up data is reported.

The treatment of a patient with an obsessive–compulsive neurosis whose identical twin brother had a similar disorder is described by Marks *et al.* (1969). The disorder consisted of a fear of contamination by dogs which produced extensive avoidance behaviour and ritualistic washing. The patient had sixty-two sessions of systematic desensitization in imagination and some of these sessions were combined with 'aversion-relief'. An attempt was also made to restrict the frequency, and duration of rituals and some avoidance behaviour. The aversion-relief technique consisted of making electric shocks contingent upon washing rituals and stopping the shocks when the patient touched 'contaminated' objects. A marginal improvement was achieved. 'Difficulties included very slow progress in desensitization, lack of transfer of improvement from one situation to another, and resistance by the patient to changing his complex habits.'

Leitenberg *et al.* (1970) investigated the relevance of practice as a therapeutic agent using five patients two of whom presented with strong impulses to hurt people with knives. Repeated practice of looking at and holding knives has been demonstrated to be of therapeutic value. However, in only one case was this treatment method continued and eventually led to considerable improvement.

Hersen (1968) reported the case of a 12-year-old boy with an elaborate set of some fourteen rituals. Additional complaints consisted of severe pains in the testicles, and tendency to contract 'viral infections' and 'school phobia'. Originally, the patient had psychoanalytically orientated psychotherapy for six months and he reported relief of his pain in the genital area. Other complaints remained unchanged and they were then dealt with by behaviouristic approaches. As regards the 'school phobia' the mother was instructed not to permit the boy to remain at home on school days. After ten counselling sessions with the mother, the patient's school attendance became normal and remained so for six months follow-up.

The patient's rituals were treated by 'implosive therapy' which involved repeated imagination of himself refraining from carrying out any rituals until his anxiety was extinguished. The items for visualization were arranged in a hierarchical order, starting from the one which evoked least anxiety. After nine sessions, during which seven items were successfully eliminated, the patient reports that he had successfully given up all rituals. Nine months follow-up revealed no relapse. However, following the termination of the treatment programmes for ritualistic behaviour and the 'school phobia' the patient had an additional three months of treatment in order 'to help him with difficulties he was having with his father'. This psychotherapeutic approach appears to have been employed during the period of follow-up for behaviour therapy so that the results are difficult to interpret. Although the method is described as 'implosion' it is in fact midway between desensitization and true implosive therapy.

Two patients with long-standing compulsive hand-washing rituals and obsessional fears of contamination from insecticides were treated by 'systematic desensitization' (Furst and Cooper, 1970). In the first case the patient reported consistent difficulty in imagining scenes in the hierarchy and experienced various degrees of anxiety throughout. The second case was given a trial of 'systematic desensitization' and 'desensitization' *in vivo*. The latter technique produced anxiety which did not extinguish in two sessions. Both cases are considered to demonstrate 'no change for the worse or the better'. It seems quite clear that this technique as described by Furst and Cooper (1970) demonstrates the failure of *unsystematic* implosive therapy rather than systematic desensitization.

Lazarus (1958), treating a complex case requiring a combination of therapeutic procedures, used the following technique for dealing with checking and re-checking rituals. The patient, while relaxed under hypnosis, was required to imagine carrying out his checking behaviour. During the third presentation of the scene the therapist induced anxiety in the patient by means of verbal suggestion. After nine sessions considerable improvement was reported.

This method has been named 'covert sensitization' (Cautela, 1966, 1967). Using this method the patient is required to imagine stimuli leading to abnormal behaviour and to associate these with the imagination of unpleasant experiences (e.g. nausea, vomiting). The major advantages of this approach are that it has no adverse side effects, it is highly adaptable, and patients can be taught to administer the therapy to themselves in everyday life, enabling them to exert self-control. So far the method has been applied on a limited basis to powerful appetitive behaviours, but it obviously could be used for compulsive–obsessive disorders.

Cautela (1966) reports the application of the technique to treatment of 'compulsive behaviour'. However, the cases used were suffering from obesity due to overeating which did not seem to fulfil the criteria which are usually associated with the term 'compulsive'.

Recently Cautela (1970) has described a new procedure called covert reinforcement (COR). Here as in the above the term 'covert' is used to indicate that both the response and reinforcing stimulus are presented in imagination. The author states that the COR procedure was apparently successful when applied to the compulsive behaviour of a male patient 'who felt compelled to check the gas jets, the locks on the car doors, and the water faucets'. When thoughts are antecedents of compulsive behaviour, the author suggests the combined use of thought-stopping and COR and offers the example of a female patient who felt that 'if she expressed resentment toward someone, their dead ancestors would punish her'. The patient was instructed to say 'stop' when the thought occurred, and 'reinforced' for thinking her thought was foolish. The author does not indicate whether or not the latter patient improved with treatment, nor is any mention made of assessment techniques used, duration of treatment, or follow-up as regards either of the two patients described above.

Both covert sensitization and covert reinforcement have been combined in the treatment of a patient who felt compelled to fold clothes over and over again (Wisocki, 1970). In the treatment the patient was instructed to imagine aversive situations (nausea and vomiting) occurring while she imagined herself performing her ritual. The patient was also instructed to imagine folding each item of clothing once and then putting it aside. After the patient signalled that she had completed the scene the therapist said, 'reinforcement' and the patient immediately imagined sipping tea. Progressive relaxation, systematic desensitization, assertive-training and thought-stopping were also employed with this patient who showed considerable improvement which was maintained at follow-up twelve months later.

Other attempts have also been made to apply operant methods to the modification of compulsive disorders. Wetzel (1966) reported a successful elimination of 'compulsive stealing behaviour' in a 10-year-old boy by rewarding him with social approval whenever he did not steal and when he carried out 'constructive behaviour'. The treatment was carried out by non-professional staff in a residential home for mildly disturbed children. There was all-round improvement in the boy's behaviour, and bedwetting, which he also suffered from, disappeared. The duration of the treatment was $3\frac{1}{2}$ months. However, it is not at all certain that the stealing was compulsive in the sense in which the present authors are using the term.

Weiner (1967) treated a 15-year-old boy with a one-month history of pervasive compulsive rituals involving a variety of activities. The therapist endorsed the positive value of the patient's ritualistic acts and encouraged him to perform them but at a frequency in line with realistic necessity. Treatment was given at eight weekly sessions and follow-up over seven months revealed that he remained 'essentially symptom free' and abandoned most of the 'substitute rituals' that were encouraged during therapy.

Bailey and Hutchinson (1969) reported the application of reinforcement principles in a 33-year-old deaf mute with 'epilepsy and psychotic reaction' who had 'compulsive' hand-washing and washed anything within reach. First of all a base line of the patient's hand-washing routine was obtained by a time-sampling technique. The attendants observed the patient once each hour and recorded their findings on a chart. Two base lines, one for the morning and one for the afternoon shift were taken. Treatment was introduced during the afternoon shift after one week of base-line observation. It consisted of rewarding desirable behaviour with brief attention and snacks, or with a part of his weekly allowance. Also the patient was praised (with sign language) for not engaging in washing. This reinforcement was at first applied only during afternoon shifts. However, after twenty-eight days of observation the same reinforcement was added to the morning shift. The percentage of observations of the washing in the afternoon shift dropped from 71 per cent during base-line assessment to 21 per cent. The treatment had no effect on the morning shift washing. The latter result, as the authors pointed out, undermines the confidence in the procedure. However, certain features of the morning ward routine might have prevented an adequate administration of the procedure, thus accounting for the discrepancy obtained.

Mather (1970) states that 'it would be logical to institute some form of discrimination learning in the treatment of obsessionals and to reinforce a response by a consistent programme of reward and punishment'. A case study is reported of a middle-aged female with a number of crippling obsessive-compulsive habits which had developed insidiously over an eleven-year period. The patient's compulsive behaviour was apparently contingent upon specific stimuli associated with diseases. The patient's treatment consisted of the 'blocking' of rituals which were dealt with in hierarchical order. The method of interruption was by verbal instruction. The patient was then exposed to various unhygienic stimuli – any decisive, immediate and non-repetitive response was reinforced by verbal social approval from the therapist (thought-stopping was also suggested to the patient at the end of therapy). The patient improved markedly during treatment (ten months) and was considered symptom free by one year (follow-up two years).

A similar technique has been employed by Rachman *et al.* (1970). As in the above, ritualistic responses were prevented during treatment sessions ($\frac{1}{4}$–3 hours) while the patient was taken through an *in vivo* hierarchy with the help of therapist modelling. The patient is reported as significantly improved after treatment and at a 6-month follow-up.

According to Taylor (1963) compulsive acts are maintained by positive reinforcement and the emotional arousal (anxiety) is not 'an integral feature of the primary behavioural error' but a consequence of the compulsive actions. For this reason any direct attempt to eliminate anxiety would leave the compulsive habit intact. Instead, appropriate treatment would subject the compulsive habit to negative reinforcement. These considerations led Taylor to apply a treatment programme for a patient with a trichopilomania of thirty-one years duration. The patient was simply instructed to say 'no, stay where you are,' or words to that effect, as soon as she became aware of the impulse to pluck her eyebrows. According to the report she was cured in ten days and no relapse occurred after three months' follow-up. No new symptoms developed and the itch in the eyebrows, which had always preceded depilation, disappeared.

A modification of this procedure is offered by Cautela (1969). The patient is required to think deliberately of the disturbing thought and then to signal with his index finger when he begins to have the thought. At the signal the therapist shouts 'stop'. Following this the patient is instructed to pair an image of saying 'stop' to himself with the thought. Eventually the patient learns to control the thought by saying 'stop' to himself whenever the thought occurs. Cautela states that this technique is particularly valuable in treating cases of obsessional thinking, hallucinations and compulsive behaviour.

A 27-year-old man who for the past 8–10 years had suffered from compulsive rechecking behaviour and 'preoccupations and fears' that his daily activities were incorrectly performed was treated with the above thought-stopping techniques, relaxation training as described by Wolpe & Lazarus and methohexitone sodium (Stern, 1970). It is reported that the patient was able to use this technique to control symptoms in his life situations (no follow-up data reported).

The above review covers sixty-two patients treated with methods based on learning principles. Lumping all cases together, a very rough assessment of efficiency (using an improved–unimproved dichotomy) indicates that about 55 per cent of patients were judged as improved. In one report (Cooper *et al.*, 1965), where the possible therapist bias was reduced by using independent raters, the figure drops to 30 per cent. One should bear in mind that the criteria of improvement are not comparable from report to report, assessment of changes in target behaviour are often anecdotal, and there is a total lack of no-treatment controls and in general, inadequate follow-up.

The sample of patients can hardly be regarded as homogeneous. Important differences such as duration, severity, type of disorder, presence of other complaints are evident. It is also doubtful whether some of the cases reported merit the diagnosis of obsessive–compulsive disorder.

Furthermore, a great variety of behaviour therapy methods have been applied, either separately or in combination and sometimes in association with other methods.

In view of this, although it appears that a behavioural therapy approach can be applied to obsessive–compulsive disorders, nothing can be said about its efficacy or its relevance to aetiology.

As one would expect, a great variety of procedures have been introduced even by therapists who adopted the same theoretical model and used the same learning principles. Even therapists who apparently subscribe to the anxiety-reduction hypothesis have used punishment indiscriminately, ignoring the evidence that in some cases punishment leads to an enhancement of the punished responses (e.g. Church, 1963; Martin, 1963; Sandler, 1964; Solomon, 1964).

The conditions under which punishment would be expected to produce paradoxical effects, that is, an increase instead of reduction in response frequency have been reasonably delineated (Church, 1963; Azrin and Holz, 1966). An increase in response will most likely occur when punishment is applied to escape or avoidance behaviour, especially if the aversive stimulus has the same physical properties as that employed to establish escape or avoidance behaviour (e.g. Sidman *et al.*, 1967, Brown *et al.*, 1964). These considerations led Kushner and Sandler (1966) to design aversion therapy procedures which should enhance the punishment effect.

Some therapists have concentrated their efforts on dealing with the assumed anxiety underlying the behaviour of compulsive patients, whereas others have directed their efforts at the motor phenomena. The distinction may be more apparent than real in that both approaches attempt to 'countercondition' anxiety and confront the patient with gradually more stressful situations while requiring him to refrain from carrying out rituals. The difference is that in achieving these aims one method deals directly with anxiety and introduces hierarchies in imagination, whereas the other does not systematically and deliberately control anxiety and uses real situations.

Finally, some therapists' treatment has been restricted to the main complaint, whereas others adopted a broader approach and attempted to deal with additional complaints.

APOTREPIC THERAPY

Rationale of treatment

Wolpe (1964) has argued that in the treatment of obsessional neurosis and phobic states the deconditioning of 'neurotic anxiety' is the most important factor. According to this view systematic desensitization by 'reciprocal inhibition' is the therapeutic method of choice for behavioural disorders mediated by anxiety. So far, this has been borne out by the results in relation to phobias but it has not been true of compulsive phenomena (Meyer and Chesser, 1970). There are plausible reasons for this difference in response to treatment. A phobic patient can withdraw completely from anxiety-provoking situations whereas the recurrent and pervasive nature of the ones evoking rituals in the obsessional prevent him from acquiring any successful avoidance behaviour. For a successful outcome of treatment it seems important to control disordered behaviour not only during the treatment sessions but also between them. The recurrence of abnormal responses between sessions is detrimental because the behaviour continues to receive its usual reinforcement. Such control is relatively easy to achieve in patients with phobias but extremely difficult, if not impossible, in a patient with persistent ritualistic actions (Meyer and Crisp, 1966). Secondly, the compulsive patient's concern with untoward consequences of failing to perform his ritual may hamper the response to treatment and be responsible for relapses.

These points indicated that one of the most important aims of the treatment should be the prevention of rituals for a long period of time while the patient is required to remain in the situations which normally evoke anxiety and ritualistic activities. It was postulated that such a procedure may be sufficient to obtain a beneficial outcome.

This procedure can be accommodated by different learning theories. For example, cognitive theories take into account the mediation of responses by goal expectancies developed from previous reinforcing situations. When these expectations are not fulfilled new expectancies may evolve which, in turn, may mediate new behaviour. Thus, if the obsessional is persuaded or forced to remain in feared situations and prevented from carrying out the rituals, he may discover that the feared consequences no longer take place. Such modifications of expectations should result in the cessation of ritualistic behaviour.

A number of animal studies provide support for the plausibility of this formulation (see Lomont, 1965). Prevention or delay of the escape from a feared situation hastens the extinction of the response.[1] It is

---

[1] Experimental studies exist which indicate that the efficiency of response prevention may depend on several factors, e.g. the intensity of the aversive stimulus during avoidance training (Baum, 1969); the extent to which the response has been over-trained (Baum, 1968); the amount of response prevention given (Baum, 1969). Lederhendler and Baum (1970) suggest that prevention is effective not because new responses (e.g. freezing) are learned on the basis of unextinguished anxiety, but because of the occurrence of non-feared behaviour during response prevention.

tempting to suggest that Maier's method of 'guidance' involved a similar procedure to the one the present authors describe below in that the rat was prevented from carrying out its repetitive behaviour (Maier and Klee, 1945) and physically guided towards the appropriate goal.

As we have seen, the relevant literature reviewed here fails to provide the behaviour therapist with a definite theoretical framework which can be used in planning effective treatment. Nevertheless, some of the observations described earlier led Meyer (1966) to develop a therapeutic programme which was successfully used to treat two patients with compulsive rituals. The results were sufficiently encouraging to study the effect of this technique in a consecutive series of obsessive–compulsive neurotics. The authors have renamed the method 'apotrepic therapy' (from ἀποτρέπω = to turn away, deter, or dissuade). This neologism has been adopted as it is purely descriptive and it does not carry any particular implications about aetiology or therapeutic mechanisms such as the term 'response prevention' which some might prefer.

Treatment

With one exception (case 6), all patients were admitted to a psychiatric ward. During the first week or two, their histories were taken and their behaviour observed and recorded. In taking case histories the emphasis was placed on behavioural analysis similar to the analysis technique described by Kanfer and Saslow (1969). Such analysis attempts to determine variables from the patient's history and those in his current situation which maintain his disordered behaviour. Determination of such variables from various areas enable one to design specific treatment procedures for each individual patient.

The treatment itself involved continual supervision during the patient's waking hours by nurses who were instructed to prevent the patient from carrying out any rituals. The nurses as well as the patients were instructed in the principles underlying the treatment procedures. The prevention of ritualistic behaviour was achieved in a variety of ways which included engaging the patient in other activities, discussion, sometimes cajoling and very occasionally – and only with the patient's consent – mild physical restraint. In cases where the rituals constituted the repetition of a normal and necessary activity, some judgement had to be exercised as to what was to be considered abnormal. The therapist visited the patient and staff daily for joint sessions lasting approximately thirty minutes. During the initial sessions the therapist instructed both the patient and the nurse to keep systematic records of the duration and/or frequency of ritualistic behaviour and to note and prevent any 'new' avoidance responses which had not been reported in the initial history. Where appropriate, situations described in the initial history which elicited either ritualistic behaviour or anxiety were arranged in a hierarchical order from the mildest to the most stressful. Patients as well as staff were given 'social reinforcement' in the form of praise by the therapist for accurate data collection as well as the elimination of ritualistic behaviour. In two cases (cases 4 and 7) small monetary rewards were used. 'Vicarious reinforcement' (Bandura, 1969) was also used for most of the patients by allowing them to meet and talk to patients who had previously been treated.

As soon as the total elimination of rituals under supervision was achieved, the therapist increased the stress where appropriate by confronting the patient with situations which normally elicited rituals. The therapist would frequently demonstrate the 'appropriate' behaviour in the stressful situation and then encouraged the patient to imitate his behaviour (Bandura, 1969). On a few occasions physical guidance was used, e.g. taking the patient's hand and placing it on a feared object. This is sometimes pompously referred to as 'contact desensitization' (Ritter, 1969). When total suppression had been maintained in spite of the stress, supervision was gradually diminished until the patient was totally unsupervised and was occasionally observed. He was instructed to ask for help when he felt he could not resist the compulsion. If a relapse occurred during this stage, supervision was reintroduced for a short period.

Following about a week without supervision, provided there was no evidence of compulsive behaviour, the patient was sent home for gradually increasing periods and when possible relatives were instructed on how to exert control over disordered behaviour. In cases of difficulty the patient was accompanied home by the therapist or by an experienced nurse. A recurrence of symptoms in the home situation was treated in the usual way.[2] When improvement was maintained at home the patient was discharged and followed up once a week at first and then at increasingly longer intervals.

All patients were asked to keep a daily record during the early part of the follow-up. They recorded the frequency of rituals and obsessional thoughts and any tendency to avoid situations which normally evoked them.

[2] Because of the distance between the patient's home environment and the hospital, case 9 was discharged home without accompaniment.

Methods of assessment

In addition to the observations outlined above patients were asked to rate their symptoms on a number of visual analogue scales (Aitken, 1969) which consisted of 100 mm lines, one extreme indicating maximum incapacity, the other complete normality. Ratings were obtained for 1) rituals, 2) anxiety, 3) depression, 4) work adjustment, 5) social adjustment, 6) sexual adjustment, 7) leisure activities.

The patients were also rated on similar scales by an observer. This rating was based on a psychiatric interview and supplemented by information obtained from relevant informants, e.g. nurses and relatives. Ratings were obtained for three stages: 1) before treatment, 2) immediately after cessation of treatment, 3) at follow-up (18 months–6 years). For cases 1 and 2 the ratings of the state before and immediately after treatment were retrospective.

Latterly we have used the Leyton Obsessional Inventory (Cooper, 1970) in addition to these ratings. This is a self-rating scale which gives 1) a symptom score, 2) a trait score, 3) a resistance score, 4) an interference score.

The patients

Fifteen patients were included in the main group on the basis of the following criteria:

1. They should suffer from true compulsive rituals and express resistance to the compulsion. Those with ruminative thoughts not associated with the rituals were not included as the method of treatment adopted would not be applicable.

2. The compulsive rituals should be the dominant incapacitating symptom and the diagnosis should be one of obsessive compulsive neurosis. Obsessional disorders occurring in the course of other conditions (e.g. schizophrenia, affective disorder, anorexia nervosa or organic disease) were not included although associated psychological difficulties which were always present were not taken as grounds for exclusion.

We should stress that although this account will lay particular stress on target symptoms we do not mean to imply that patients did not have other important problems. Indeed in one case (No. 11) discussed below the elimination of the target symptoms did not lead to any improvement in the patient's social adjustment and life situation.

3. No other treatment was to be given except for night sedation.

Where anti-depressants and tranquillizers were being prescribed these were stopped during the week preceding the onset of treatment.

The patients were followed up at monthly intervals during the course of the first year and approximately every six months thereafter.

One patient (case 10) who discharged himself from the hospital prematurely and failed to attend for follow-up was assumed to have relapsed. The last three patients had just completed treatment at the

TABLE 10.1 *Clinical characteristics of main group of patients*

Case	Age	Sex	Duration of symptoms (years)*	Type of symptoms
1	47	F	36	Repetition compulsion
2	33	F	6	Checking and washing
3	25	M	12	Hand-washing
4	23	F	11	Repetition compulsion
5	55	F	28	Repetition and hoarding
6	53	F	26	Hand-washing
7	30	F	8	Cleaning and dusting
8	20	F	9	Hand-washing
9	44	F	26	Cleaning and dusting
10	26	M	7	Repetition and hand-washing
11	35	M	10	Washing of hands, body and clothes
12	31	F	14	Repetition and hand-washing
13	26	F	4	Hand-washing
14	46	M	30	Repetition and checking
15	21	F	8	Repetition compulsion
	Mean 34·3	11F 4M	Mean 15·6	

* Many patients had transient episodes of obsessional behaviour in childhood which have been ignored in dating the onset of symptoms.

time of writing and no follow-up data was available. Some of the clinical characteristics of this group are given in Table 10.1.

In addition to the main group, four other patients who did not fulfil the full criteria were treated or partially treated by the method described above. These are referred to as a–d (Table 10.2).

Case a was referred very early in this study. He was receiving psychoanalytic treatment elsewhere and the performance of his rituals was taking so long that he was unable to attend for his sessions. The behavioural treatment was restricted to improving him sufficiently to allow him to continue with his analysis.

Case b was basically a case of anorexia nervosa with some compulsive rituals. She was having private psychotherapy outside the hospital and continues to do so. Her psychotherapist expressed the view that behaviour therapy had helped the patient to make better use of her psychotherapy sessions.

Case c was judged by the assessor to be suffering from a monosymptomatic delusion rather than from a compulsive disorder.

Case d came from abroad and spoke no English. Treatment in her home surroundings was thought essential and the referring psychiatrist in her country of origin was advised on how this might be carried out.

TABLE 10.2 *Clinical characteristics of subsidiary group of patients and reasons for exclusion from main group*

Case	Age	Sex	Type of symptom	Reason for exclusion
a	52	M	Washing and checking	Incomplete treatment aimed at enabling him to attend psychotherapist
b	22	F	Studying rituals and compulsive sunbathing and anorexia	Anorexia nervosa and concurrent psychotherapy
c	42	M	Washing forehead	Monosymptomatic delusion
d	34	F	Washing and repetition	Spoke no English

Results

With the exception of case 9, every patient showed a marked diminution in compulsive behaviour, sometimes amounting to a total cessation of the rituals. Patients occasionally experienced some increase in anxiety at the beginning of treatment but by the end of the course ratings for anxiety and depression had also diminished and there was usually a concurrent improvement in the other ratings except those for sexual adjustment which remained poor. In case 11 social adjustment and work adjustment, both of which were rated as very poor before treatment, remained so in spite of the total elimination of compulsive symptoms. In effect this patient was no better off in spite of the fact that he had lost his compulsive rituals.

Table 10.3 summarizes the changes in the observer ratings of rituals. On the whole, the other ratings changed in the same way except where indicated. 'Improved' refers to a fall in ritual score of 50 to 74 per cent, 'much improved' to a fall of 75 per cent or more, 'slightly improved' to a drop of 25 to 50 per cent and anything below 25 per cent is categorized as 'no change'.

It will be seen that at the end of treatment out of 15 cases in the main

TABLE 10.3 *Outcome of treatment based on observer rating of compulsive behaviour*

Case	Follow-up (in years)	Immediate outcome	Long-term outcome
1	6	Much improved	Much improved
2	6	Improved	Much improved
3	3	No symptoms	No symptoms
4	2	No symptoms	Much improved
5	2	Much improved	Improved
6	1·5	Improved	Improved
7	1	Improved	Much improved
8	1	Much improved	Much improved
9	1	Improved	Unchanged
10	—	Improved	? Unchanged
11	0·5	No symptoms	No Symptoms
12	0·5	Much improved	Much improved
13	—	Much improved	—
14	—	Much improved	—
15	—	Much improved	—

group 10 were either 'much improved' or totally asymptomatic. One was only slightly improved and the rest were 'improved'. During the period of follow-up 2 patients showed further improvement without treatment, 6 maintained their post-treatment level, 2 patients showed a slight tendency to a return in compulsive behaviour. One patient

TABLE 10.4 *Outcome of treatment in subsidiary group*

Case	Follow-up (in years)	Immediate	Long-term
a	3 (by letter)	Improved	? Slightly improved
b	1	Improved	Improved
c	0·5	Improved	Improved
d	0·5 (by letter)	No change	? No change

relapsed completely and one who failed to attend for follow-up is also assumed to have done badly.

Outcome in the subsidiary group was much less impressive. The results are given as a matter of interest in Table 10.4, although it is difficult to draw any definite conclusion from them.

ILLUSTRATIVE CASE HISTORIES

The following cases have been selected to show how varied the course of the condition could be following discharge and also in order to illustrate some of the problems encountered in organizing the treatment.

Case 1

A 47-year-old married woman with one child. She had a thirty-six-year history of obsessional thoughts and compulsive rituals. The thoughts at first consisted of intrusive swear words and later of ideas of a sexual nature evoking great anxiety which could only be allayed by performing various repetitive acts, e.g. dressing and undressing, writing and rewriting, walking up and down stair-cases retracing her steps. From the age of 29 she had had a variety of treatments including ECT, antidepressants, tranquillizers, a leucotomy at 32 and later eleven years of psychoanalysis. Her condition continued to deteriorate and just before her referral a second leucotomy had been considered. At the time of admission much of her day was taken up with the performance of rituals.

After two months in hospital, one month of which was taken up with close supervision and ritual interruption, there was a very marked diminution in rituals. Six years later she described her life as having been transformed by the treatment. She still had obsessional thoughts but these were less frequent and less intrusive. When they did occur they were far less likely to be followed by rituals. Since leaving hospital she had gone to a teachers' training college and was working full-time as a school teacher.

Case 6

A 53-year-old married woman with no children. She was of German Jewish extraction and very orthodox in her beliefs and religious observances. At the age of 27 she developed a fear of contamination by faeces which was only allayed by repetitive hand-washing which took several hours in the morning and later by ritual baths. The latter were judged by a rabbi to be vastly in excess of anything prescribed by the most orthodox form of Hassidic Judaism.

Initially she refused admission to hospital and was the only case treated as an out-patient. This meant that she was required to defaecate only in the hospital lavatory. She was then only permitted to wash for a specified time. This regime resulted in a marked reduction in hand-washing and although there was an increase after the supervision was stopped, this took her half an hour as compared with three hours before treatment. Since the follow-up ratings were completed she agreed to come into hospital for one week during which she had a further period of total supervision which resulted in a further reduction in rituals.

Case 7

A 30-year-old housewife with four children. The main complaint was of a 'craze for housework' of eight years' duration. She tended to clean her house from the time she got up until the time she went to bed. Although she stated that her behaviour was irrational she felt that the compulsion was 'too strong to fight'. Previous treatment included ten hospital admissions during which she received anti-depressants and tranquillizers, three courses of ECT, supportive psychotherapy and drug abreaction. During the few years before her admission she had not been out of hospital for more than a couple of months. She was referred from a long-stay psychiatric hospital where she was expected to remain. Treatment in hospital involved giving her a single room and making her responsible for its cleaning. This provoked her prolonged rituals which were then interrupted in the usual way. Although this achieved the desired effect in hospital, rituals returned when she was sent home for a few days. Domiciliary treatment was therefore arranged by having three nurses working in shifts and living in her house for a whole week. In spite of this only a modest diminution in symptoms was achieved and the prognosis was felt to be poor. However, a week after the end of treatment and without any assistance she decided that she 'had had enough' and she achieved a marked reduction in rituals without any help.

At follow-up she still had a tendency to excessive house cleaning but was working full-time as well as managing her house and had been out of hospital for a year with only the most tenuous of out-patient support.

Case 9

A 44-year-old married woman with no children who had a fear of con-tamination by dust. She had a disturbed family background and in childhood had suffered from stammering and food fads. Between the ages of 7 to 12 she had shown a tendency to repeatedly touch all her dolls and to hold her breath and count five. She had felt that unless she did this her parents would quarrel. Her parents separated when she was 13 and she went to live with her mother. At the age of 18 she was asked to leave her mother's house and soon after she developed her fear of contamination by dust. Her symptoms became worse after her marriage at the age of 20. She had elaborate rituals which involved extensive house-cleaning, dusting and the fanatical use of a vacuum cleaner which was employed to free both herself and her husband of dust. Two years before her admission she had been treated with imipramine and Promazine and had had a course of hypnotherapy. A year later she had had bilateral implantation of radioactive yttrium into the substantia inominata. This produced only a slight reduction in anxiety which was short-lived. Restriction of rituals was attempted in the usual way. She was given a single room and made responsible for keeping it clean but was only allowed to spend a few minutes a day to do so. She was then gradually exposed to dust, made to shake a duster out of her window and eventually in her room. Although during the preliminary interview it appears that she experienced a resistance to the compulsion, as treatment progressed she became more vehement in her protestations that she was being made to spread disease and the near-delusional quality of her beliefs became clearer. Inspection of her Leyton Observation Inventory showed her to have had an exceptionally low resistance score but a high symptom score. In spite of this she managed to control herself from dusting excessively in hospital.

She made three visits to her home. During the first two she was accompanied by a nurse and was able to refrain from dusting. However, her first weekend at home was marked by a return of the rituals which took her two hours. Her husband considered her improved and she asked to leave hospital. Intensive treatment at home was not attempted as she lived too far away. During the period of follow-up the rituals returned to their previous intensity except for the vacuum cleaning of her husband which did not recur.

DISCUSSION

It is clear that the study reported here is open to many of the criticisms that we have levelled at other studies. The ratings were crude, they were not carried out independently and there was no control group.

It does nevertheless comprise the largest group of patients treated by a behavioural method. Serious attempts have been made to include only true obsessional disorders and to follow up the patients systematically for very long periods. In addition, most of the patients were very severe cases who had had extensive and repeated courses of treatment by other methods which were given either separately or in combination. These included anti-depressants of both main categories, tranquillizers, ECT, leucotomy, psychotherapy, hypnosis and psychoanalysis.

Although comparisons with published figures for the prognosis of obsessional neurosis are not entirely legitimate they provide a tentative yardstick against which our results may be evaluated. Kringlen (1965) found that of 90 patients followed up for 13–20 years only 19 were much improved. Shorter periods of follow-up were associated with even worse results. He also found that an obsessional pre-morbid personality and the presence of severe symptoms both made for a bad prognosis. In the main group, 10 of the 15 patients would be judged as severe according to his criteria and all but 2 had obsessional pre-morbid personalities so that a bad outcome would be expected.

A more comparable group is provided by Cooper *et al.* (1965) in their retrospective study of neurotics treated by behaviour therapy. This included 10 obsessionals treated by a combination of 'graded practical retraining' and 'desensitization in imagination'. This group is very similar in age, sex and length of follow-up but had a shorter mean duration of symptoms (10 years). Of these 10 patients only 3 were judged to have improved, and none were rated as 'much improved'. The control group of 9 patients fared rather better in that 5 were improved and 2 were much improved after a year.

The results reported here are therefore encouraging and likely to have been related to the therapeutic intervention. The latter almost certainly consists of a number of components which are difficult to separate from one another.

1. *Therapist–patient relationship*

While this is likely to have been of some importance it should be remembered that the treatment was carried out largely by nurses who changed quite frequently. They were supervised by one or two psychologists and a psychiatrist. One might suppose that some of the ways in which this factor might have operated were by instilling confidence in the technique, by encouraging the patient to tolerate anxiety when it occurred but also by acting as a social reinforcer, i.e. successful resistance to the compulsion might have been rewarded by approval from the therapist.

2. *Alteration in the 'family dynamics'*

Careful interviewing of the patients and their immediate relatives usually made it clear that the latter had often adopted patterns of behaviour which reinforced the patients' symptoms. This well-known phenomenon is often described by therapists with a psychoanalytic orientation as 'colluding with the patient'. The treatment is likely to have produced an alteration in this situation, particularly as relatives were often made aware of the rationale of treatment and given some instruction on how to cope with any recurrence of rituals.

3. *'Modelling' or imitation learning* (Bandura, 1969)

This would almost certainly have been involved in dealing with avoidance behaviour, e.g. when a patient would not touch a particular object the therapist would repeatedly do so and urge the patient to imitate him.

4. *'Implosion' or 'flooding'* (Stampfl, 1968)

Although the method seems to bear some similarity to 'flooding' this is a superficial one unless one accepts the doubtful premise that rituals are always anxiety-reducing and that their prevention is always followed by a large increase in the level of anxiety. In fact, in most cases the procedure did not evoke anything more than mild tension and recordings of the galvanic skin response did not indicate any increase in spontaneous fluctuations (Levy and Meyer, 1971).

5. *'Response prevention'* and 6. *'Guidance'*

Experimental work in animals aimed at producing analogues of human compulsive behaviour (Metzner, 1963) and phobias (Baum, 1970) and then treating them have suggested that learnt avoidance responses originally evoked in traumatic situations are very difficult to extinguish unless the response is prevented. Although no experimenter has produced in animals a pattern of behaviour that is an acceptable model of human compulsive behaviour (Meyer and Levy, 1973) it has been shown that inappropriate and stereotyped behaviour patterns established in rats in frustrating circumstances are best eliminated by preventing the inappropriate response and guiding the animal towards the correct goal (Maier, 1949). This appears to be the paradigm which best fits the treatment described here.

There are also the related observations of Janet (1925) and Lewis (1936), who described obsessional patients who improved during military service. One might speculate on the role which 'response prevention' and 'guidance' might play within the rigid framework of service life.

No cross-validation of the method used has yet been reported although Rachman *et al.* (1970, 1971) appear to be attempting something similar. Rachman *et al.* (1971) compared the efficacy of 'modelling' and 'flooding' in the treatment of 10 chronic obsessive–compulsive patients. After a week of evaluation all patients were given a series of fifteen relaxation sessions over a three-week 'control' period. Half the patients were then treated by 'modelling' and the other half by 'flooding'. Each of the treatment periods consisted of fifteen sessions over three weeks. In 'flooding' the patients were exposed to the most disturbing situations and encouraged to refrain from carrying out any rituals for increasing periods of time after each session. 'Modelling' involved exposing the patients to the provoking situations presented in a hierarchical order starting with the least disturbing items. Each step in the hierarchy was first demonstrated by the therapist to the patient. Just as in the 'flooding' group the patients in the 'modelling' group were encouraged to refrain from carrying out rituals for increasing periods of time. The paper does not make clear how patients in whom a clear hierarchy could not be established (e.g. those with a tendency to checking) were treated. Assessments included clinical rating scales, attitude scales, avoidance tests, a 'fear thermometer' and various personality inventories. These measures were administered before treatment, after the three-week control period, after the three-week treatment periods and after three months follow-up. There was no significant difference between the two experimental groups although both showed significantly more improvement than in the control relaxation phase. Improvement was maintained during the three-month follow-up period although seven patients continued to have additional treatment.

This is the only controlled study on chronic obsessive–compulsive patients and although the sample appears similar to our own, the differences in the methods of assessment prevent any direct comparison of the results. Although they refer to their methods as 'modelling' and 'flooding' they point out the treatments contained several components and suggest that the lack of difference in the results obtained by the two methods might be due to the presence of a common factor.

We suggest that in so far as their methods were effective this was primarily because of the common element of response prevention. Our view is that it does not matter how the patient is exposed to the disturbing situations provided he or she is prevented from carrying out any rituals. We would expect that the more thorough the response prevention during and between treatment sessions, the better the outcome. This prediction is being tested in a study which is attempting to elucidate the importance of total supervision in between sessions. Various possible prognostic factors are also being studied. At first sight the length of the history, the age of onset of the symptoms, the severity of the condition and the age and sex of the patient do not seem to be reliable indicators of outcome. The type of symptom and how far it is situation-dependent may be of more significance although this is far from clear. On the other hand, the degree of subjective resistance which the patient experiences is rapidly emerging as an important element. Future work may well isolate subcategories of obsessional disorders with different natural histories and response to treatment in the way that it has already done in the case of phobias (Marks).

In summary, it would appear that recent behavioural methods and in particular those incorporating response prevention as an important component may have something to contribute not only to the treatment of obsessional disorders but to our understanding of the nature of this type of behaviour, to its classification and to its relationship to other psychological variables. The way seems open to a re-examination of many traditional ideas in this area of psychiatry.

Robert Cawley

Psychotherapy and obsessional disorders

INTRODUCTION

This chapter is written by a psychiatrist with no claim to special skill as a psychotherapist. It sets out to examine the proposition that psychotherapy is a useful method of treating obsessional disorders. In the author's judgement there is no adequate evidence either to give firm support to this view or to refute it. The question is more complicated than it seems at first sight, and the comments which follow will deal with the preliminaries to investigation rather than with established conclusions. To examine the matter in the depth it deserves, it will be necessary first to consider some of the issues central to modern concepts of psychotherapy, and then to review the nature of the problems of the obsessional patient which are amenable to different kinds of treatment. Some of the principal features in the dynamic psychopathology of these disorders will subsequently be summarized. These preliminaries will set the scene for considering the special problems in evaluating psychotherapy. The effects of this treatment will be assessed in the context of what is known in general about the outcome of obsessional disorders.

The whole matter of psychotherapy remains contentious, and among the reasons for this state of affairs it is possible to identify five inter-related themes.

Firstly, the concepts underlying psychoanalysis and psychotherapy are extremely difficult to comprehend, because their epistemological status is unclear. Looked at from one side, they are contemporary versions of issues which have occupied the attention of philosophers and metaphysicians for centuries. In more recent times Jaspers (1946) concerned himself with one of these issues when he described the distinction between the psychology of explaining (*erklärende Psychologie*), which is amenable to examination by the rules of logic and the methods of science, and the psychology of understanding or of meaningful connections (*verstehende Psychologie*) for which a systematic methodology is impossible. In his Ernest Jones lecture Hill (1971) discussed the place of psychoanalysis in regard to the need for distinguishing between the scientific methods appropriate for investigating and describing external reality and inner (psychic) reality. Perhaps for the wider field of psychotherapy even more than for the more restricted structures of psychoanalysis, the more closely one examines the salient issues – whether by theoretical review or practical investigation – the more elaborate is the necessary conceptual framework. Therefore the possibilities of succinctly formulating critical arguments and designing and executing crucial inquiries become more elusive. If conclusions are to be really useful they should consist of propositions which, though potentially refutable, are supported by convincing evidence. They should, moreover, be demonstrably relevant to the practice of medicine or clinical psychology. Debates about what is and what is not science have little to offer beyond the possibility of circular argument. We have not yet fully defined the canons of those disciplines which are necessary for the comprehensive investigation and understanding of human experience and behaviour. Nor have we established what kind of knowledge is necessary for the relief of certain types of human distress.

Secondly, unresolved and important semantic problems characterize much that has been written about psychoanalysis and psychotherapy, whether by its proponents or by its critics. Even matters which are irrational must be ultimately amenable to rational discourse. But sometimes what is written about these matters is obscure and lacking in linguistic clarity.

In the third place, no more than a very small proportion of the voluminous literature on psychoanalysis and psychotherapy is free from bias and pre-judgement. A disinterested and sceptical person, called upon to examine the evidence, might well dismiss most of it as inconclusive. In his strictures the writings of the critics would fare no better than those of the most convinced exponents. The biases take many forms. Sometimes they may be very simply characterized, for example, as explicit or inferred assumptions that scientific methods derived from the models of physics can be adapted, with little strain, to examine the claims of psychoanalytic theory and psychotherapy. At other times they can be intricate and involve complex variables concerned with ways of expressing and summarizing many of the most subtle and inconstant factors governing human experience and relationships.

Much has been written about the difficulties of empirical inquiry in psychoanalysis and psychotherapy. The many-sided nature of the disorders for which they may be employed; the absence of satisfactorily comprehensive criteria; the tendency for symptoms and other problems to alter or remit with the passage of time and with the play of intercurrent circumstance; the many variables, both specific and non-specific, involved in the treatment process; the long duration of treatment and the difficulty in following patients after its conclusion; and the lack of suitable bases for comparison – these and other formidable hindrances to conclusive experimentation have been described at length.

Finally, the value and tenets of a whole profession can be seriously threatened by the prospect of inquiry which is over-simplified though it may appear rigorous. The practitioners of psychoanalysis and psychotherapy have directed their emotional and financial resources over long years to a commitment to try to relieve particular types of human dilemma and suffering by the application of special techniques. Their professional standards and ideals might understandably seem to be assailed if supposedly objective assessments were made by investigators unfamiliar with these techniques. Likewise it may be that those whose careers are devoted to the more objective aspects of psychology are reluctant to concede that there may be information and techniques of treatment which lie beyond the reach of their science.

One aspect of the problem has been highlighted in a journal well known for its scientific rigour. A note in *Nature* (1968) referred to a blunt dismissal of psychotherapy and psychoanalysis by Professor Henry Miller (*Listener*, 1968), a neurologist, and commented that 'it is still respectable in Britain for distinguished men, doctors among them, to deny the intellectual foundations on which a great deal of psychotherapy is based'. To do justice to these intellectual foundations, scholarly examination and careful exposition would be more useful than denial or assertion.

The question at issue – the value of psychotherapy in the treatment of patients with obsessional disorders – has meaning only if we consider what is meant by psychotherapy, the nature of the problems presented by obsessional patients, and the criteria for evaluating treatment.

LEVELS OF PSYCHOTHERAPY

Numerous adjectives exist for describing types of psychotherapy – some eponymous, some indicating a certain style of treatment or a definition of aims, and some referring to the duration or intensity of the proposed treatment, its superficiality or depth, and its complexity or simplicity. The array is bewildering: a brief search of the literature, or informal conversations with a number of psychotherapists, will reveal that the typologies or classifications of psychotherapy are inefficient and in practice have negligible discriminating power. There is no consensus of opinion about the labelling; the classes are polythetic and not mutually exclusive; and there is seemingly as much variation within as between different classes. Nor is it possible to obtain a precise definition of common ground, beyond a vague statement to the effect that individual psychotherapy consists of a special kind of relationship between two people, one a patient (or client) and one a doctor or other trained professional, outwardly characterized by verbal interchanges, and directed towards helping the patient with psychological symptoms, illness or problems. Clearly it would be advantageous to adopt a set of operational definitions of types or levels of psychotherapy. These definitions should be as simple as possible and – if we are investigating the efficacy of the treatment – they must be followed by careful attempts to specify and characterize the many variables which operate when a course of psychotherapy is undertaken. Elsewhere (Cawley, 1971) the writer has argued that it is possible in operational terms to distinguish between three domains of psychotherapy.

(i) The most extensive meaning is synonymous with the doctor–patient relationship, and in this sense its history is as old, and its scope as wide, as medicine itself, and it is practised with more or less awareness by all doctors and by others involved in the treatment of patients. It does not derive from any formulated theory. Most would regard its value and importance as self-evident at this level, though it varies greatly in style and impact. It has something in common with other relationships of a professional but non-medical kind. It is not susceptible to rigorous evaluation, or indeed to any evaluation at all, except perhaps in those limited situations where therapeutic procedures can be automated. For operational purposes we can designate treatments falling under this heading as *psychotherapy in the extensive sense*.

(ii) In a stricter sense, psychotherapy comprises an assemblage of methods and skills which are central to psychiatric practice and which can be regarded as including (among others) the so-called supportive, directive, client centered, 'non-directive', counselling, and distributive forms of treatment. These methods lay emphasis on a number of more or less imponderable variables. Attempts can be made to specify these as, for example, friendly interest; unhurried concern; a non-censorious, helpful and sympathetic attitude; empathy; informed judgement; reflective advice; belief in the value of the patient's knowing what is ostensibly the truth and avoiding what is ostensibly self-deceit; all accompanied by a manifest respect for the patient's individuality, and for his rights and responsibilities in making his own decisions about his future. The putative value of these methods and objectives does not rely on any unified and coherent theory or set of theories, nor is it in general empirically demonstrable. However, it is possible to identify and isolate certain variables and styles of practice and to compare these, in controlled circumstances, with contrasting patterns. The relevant skills are widely applicable and patently diverse; their application may depend on numerous variables relating to the patient, the symptoms and other problems, the therapist, and the expectations and inter-relationships of the two participants. These forms of treatment can be designated for operational purposes as *informal psychotherapy*.

(iii) In its most restricted usage, psychotherapy denotes highly developed and skilled psychological techniques for treating certain patients with specified disabilities. These are the formal, analytic, exploratory or dynamic therapies – for present purposes the adjectives are used synonymously – which are practised by those with a special training, usually involving a personal psycho-analysis. There are many varieties of dynamic psychotherapy, each based on its own theoretical postulates. Our present designation for this class is *formal psychotherapy*.

These three domains of psychotherapy may be distinguished from each other by the contexts in which they are practised, and by their contrasting manifest purposes. Formal psychotherapy may be distinguished from informal psychotherapy (and more conspicuously from psychotherapy in the extensive sense) in two ways. Firstly, there are definable differences in application and technique – for example the establishment of a transference relationship, and the offering of interpretations concerning affinities between conflicts in current relationships, conflicts in previous relationships, and conflicts which emerge in the transference relationship. Secondly, those who practise this form of treatment have participated in a special form of training and experience which both in content and technique is distinct from the training received by other doctors or therapists. Treatments classed as formal psychotherapy may be withheld absolutely whilst a patient is being treated medically or by other psychological means, whereas various components of the first two domains of psychotherapy, as here defined, are inevitable whenever a therapist meets a client or patient. Therefore the efficacy of formal psychotherapy can – at least theoretically – be assessed as a kind of treatment which may or may not be employed in defined circumstances.

It must be conceded, however, that these three levels of psychotherapy share much common ground. Both the language and the concepts of psychoanalysis may enter at each level, as psychoanalysis has become so firmly established in Western societies as one of the models for understanding and discussing human experience, relationships, and development. For example, the notion of the dynamic unconscious has achieved common currency. The work of Freud and his successors has had pervasive and stimulating effects on much of our thinking about these matters, as well as on literature, art, and other creative endeavour extending far beyond the scientific field. In W. H. Auden's words, it has created 'a climate of opinion'. The assimilation of psychoanalytic concepts into the prevalent culture has muddled the question of the epistemological status of psychoanalytic theory. It has also clouded the issue of whether techniques of treatment which depend on application of the principles of psychoanalytic theory have specific value in treating defined groups of patients. That is why, when we are concerned with questions of the specific effects of treatment, we must be as rigorous as possible in defining questions. There is some advantage in separating the issue of specificity from the general themes which have had such far-reaching impact in so much of psychology and psychiatry. These considerations are especially important in investigating a treatment which, if demonstrably effective, should be widely available.

Formal psychotherapy, as here defined, is prescribed most extensively for sub-groups of patients suffering from neurotic disabilities. The phenomena of such disorders include a wide range of symptoms which are seen as psychogenic though they may have somatic as well as psychic expression. The disorders are also characterized by problems of living – affecting personal adjustment, attitudes and relationships – and by other suffering which can be described at an experiential rather than objective level. Many of the problems are secondary, in the sense that one kind of problem usually leads to others, and disturbances in personal relationships lead to discord which exacerbates and distorts the primary disturbances. In addition – and this is crucial to formal psychotherapy – the symptoms and overt evidences of maladjustment can be seen as deriving from a more central disorder involving forces below the surface which can be conceptualized as *intrapsychic disturbances*. These underlying variables are by their very nature inaccessible to direct expression and measurement. But they, rather than symptoms, are the immediate targets for treatment by formal psychotherapy.

In attempting to define levels of complexity, or specificity, of psychotherapy, mention must be made of an important distinction between two aspects of what we have here designated as formal psychotherapy. Psychoanalysis, in the stricter sense, is distinguishable from other, usually briefer, forms of analytical psychotherapy in its aims, its indications, its techniques, its time-relationships, and sometimes its theoretical sub-structure. The distinctions are rather complex and have been explored by several authors (see for example Bibring, 1954; Wallerstein, 1969; Adler, 1970; Tyson and Sandler, 1971). In these communications and in discussions at the International Psycho-Analytical Congress at Rome in 1969 (reported by Adler) attempts were made to conceptualize the more loosely defined area of psychotherapy as compared with the highly structured and delineated field of psychoanalysis. Attention was called to the lack of clinical data in this area of psychotherapy, and many disagreements and uncertainties were highlighted. To some psychoanalysts the really important distinction is between full psychoanalysis and other forms of psychotherapy.

It must be acknowledged that the operational distinction between formal psychotherapy and other forms of treatment is arbitrary. Some authors (e.g. Hill, 1969; Wolff, 1970, 1971b) have written compellingly about the importance of psychotherapeutic methods to general psychiatry. It can be argued that the borderland is extensive, and that there are many gradations from formal psychotherapy to the application of certain principles which should be common to all forms of psychiatric treatment, so that the distinction is intangible, and indeed should become more so. These are important viewpoints. The present contention is that, for clarity of discussion, we should contrast on the one hand what can be achieved by formal psychotherapy, using interpretative methods in the context of a transference relationship with specially trained personnel, and on the other hand what can be done by general psychiatrists using an array of other methods and techniques which can be called psychotherapeutic in an informal sense but which do not depend directly on applications of formulated psychodynamic theories.

If we adopt this distinction as operationally valid for present purposes, a related issue will call for separate examination elsewhere. The techniques of general psychiatry (or informal psychotherapy) may be made more effective by a training procedure and a limited apprenticeship in the practice of formal psychotherapy. In other words, the educational value, for general psychiatrists, of a knowledge of formal psychodynamic theories and their applications is an important matter which can conveniently be considered separately from the question of the efficacy of formal psychotherapy in defined circumstances.

THE OBSESSIONAL PATIENT: AIMS OF TREATMENT

The claims sometimes made for psychotherapy are so far-reaching and so important in their implications for the nature of obsessional disorders that it is necessary to itemize the several aspects of these disorders which are, potentially at least, amenable to treatment.

Like patients with other types of neurotic disability, those classed as suffering from obsessional illnesses or obsessional personalities experience difficulties which may be categorized as follows:

   (i) Symptoms
  (ii) Signs – physiological concomitants of anxiety
 (iii) Abnormalities in behaviour
 (iv) Problems of living: personal maladjustment
  (v) Subjective discomfort
 (vi) Intrapsychic disorder: dynamic psychopathology

The *symptoms*, the *physiological concomitants of anxiety*, and the *abnormalities in behaviour* characteristic of obsessional illness and obsessional personalities are discussed elsewhere in this book. They can all be elicited or observed with a fair degree of reliability. It is here necessary only to emphasize that obsessional symptoms in the strict sense rarely occur in isolation. Obsessional experiences and behaviour are commonly associated with other symptoms, e.g. pervasive anxiety, social anxieties, anxiety related to other objects and circumstances, depressive symptoms, lassitude and depersonalization. Sometimes these manifestations can be seen as deriving from the obsessional symptoms and sometimes the relationship between different manifestations are obscure, so that uncertainty may surround the question of whether the obsessional symptoms are primary or secondary. Occasionally it may be impossible to make the distinction.

Problems of living are almost invariably experienced by patients with obsessional disorders. Their presence and nature can be inferred more or less directly by what the patient says and what is said about him by those involved in his life. Maladaptive obsessional personality traits of two types have been described – one including obstinacy, rigidity, moroseness and irritability, and the other consisting of uncertainty, indecisiveness, and over-submissiveness. People having these attributes will tend to encounter difficulties of many kinds in their interactions with others. They may also experience difficulties in the pursuit of their occupation, and in ordering the daily routine of their life and leisure time. The adaptive efficiency of the patient with an obsessional disorder becomes reduced, restrictive patterns of living become established, and difficulties are commonly generated in many departments of life. Like all maladaptive behaviour patterns, problems of one kind lead to problems of another kind, which in turn have their repercussions; so that we are commonly faced with an intricate network of difficulties for which the common origin may be difficult to discern. The sequence of events is dependent upon many variables concerned with the illness or disability, the other features of the patient's personality, his particular interpersonal relationships and his life situation. In addition there may be iatrogenic influences. The resulting processes can be summarized under such headings as social, marital, familial, sexual and occupational difficulties. They inevitably change in pattern and emphasis with the passage of time, and with events.

Subjective discomfort is a term used here to represent experiential data to some extent overlapping with symptoms as elicited and to some extent accessible to the observer only by what the patient says or by acts of intuition and empathy. Subjective discomfort is difficult to observe, describe, and measure. In many people suffering from mental and emotional disorders and indeed in many ostensibly healthy people, considerable personal distress with no particular reference is an episodic or constant experience. This type of distress is not quantifiable, and indeed can be communicated only incompletely and with difficulty. It may be described as feelings of despair, tension or uneasiness, or it may attach to inability to communicate feelings, self-accusation or feelings of personal defeat and humiliation. The process of eliciting subjective discomfort at this level is prone to many distortions, most prominently those induced by direct questioning and the expectations of the observer.

Intrapsychic disorder is the most problematic class of difficulties experienced by obsessional (or other) patients, because it encompasses concepts of a second order, which have been referred to briefly above. To some, the very idea of discussing problems or disorders occurring within the mind, at an unconscious level, is anathema. To others, it is central to any attempt at understanding and relieving symptoms, since these are seen as no more than the external and perhaps transitory and shifting manifestations of conflict at another level. Whilst experimental psychology accepts the notion of extra-conscious mechanisms involved in learning, and the idea of investigating how current responses are influenced by previous experience, it does not accept the concept of the dynamic unconscious. The dynamic psychopathology of obsessional disorders is the focus for their treatment by formal psychotherapy, and will be reviewed briefly in the next section.

TABLE 11.1 *Principal relationships postulated between type of treatment and targets for treatment in obsessional disorders*

Principal targets of treatment	MAIN TYPES OF TREATMENT				
	Behaviour therapy	*Psycho-tropic drugs*	*Psycho-therapy in extensive sense*	*Informal psycho-therapy*	*Formal psycho-therapy*
Symptoms	×		×		
Physiological disturbance		×			
Abnormalities in behaviour	×		×		
Personal mal-adjustment			×	×	
Subjective discomfort				×	
Intrapsychic disorder					×

The six categories of difficulty experienced by patients with obsessional disorder may be seen as providing the possible targets for treatment. Different methods of treatment have different explicit aims, and it is all too easy to overlook this fact when attempts are made at comparing the results of contrasting treatment regimes. Table 11.1 demonstrates in an approximate way the main targets for each of the principal methods of treatment.

The statements embodied in this schematization are provisional, and the matter is here necessarily simplified, perhaps greatly over-simplified. For example, no mention is made of the roles of different personnel – nursing staff, occupational therapists, social workers, psychologists and psychiatrists – in executing the various forms of treatment. Also in practice different forms of treatment may be exhibited simultaneously – as when a programme of behaviour therapy includes the use of drugs and requires an effective working relationship between the therapist and the patient. But it seems necessary at this stage to emphasize that contrasting forms of treatment are directed towards different targets, and that their methods are fashioned accordingly; the treatments differ according to what is regarded as the appropriate target, or the key problems of the obsessional patient. For any treatment the general assumption is that if the defined aims of that treatment are achieved, the other features of the disorder will turn out to be non-existent or of subordinate importance, and will therefore recede.

With this categorization of problems presented by patients with obsessional disorders the claims of different forms of treatment can be defined more precisely. In prescribing psychotropic drugs, for example, it might be postulated that arousal levels would be lowered, anxiety symptoms relieved, and at the same time there would be a lessening of obsessional symptoms and associated problems of living. As far as formal psychotherapy is concerned, there are three related claims: (i) that formal psychotherapy reduces the extent and/or the intensity of the intrapsychic disorder, (ii) that when the intrapsychic disorder is to some degree relieved, personal maladjustment will diminish, and (iii) that symptoms will remit. Relief of symptoms is seen as the least important goal of treatment. Indeed, the patient's continued suffering is sometimes seen as providing motivation for persisting with treatment (Freud, 1913a). Treatment might be counted as partially successful if improvement were restricted to the intrapsychic disorder alone, in that future more serious disturbances would be averted. On the other hand it might be said that improvement in personal maladjustment was a necessary condition for ascribing limited success to the treatment. By contrast, the type of treatment defined as informal psychotherapy would be focused not on the symptoms nor on the intrapsychic disorder, but on alleviating the effects of the symptoms on the patient's day-to-day life, on his relationships and on his overt attitudes to himself and others. Given adequate criteria for these variables, some of the components of informal psychotherapy can be investigated though, as indicated in the previous section, the process *in toto* defies evaluation.

We shall now be concerned more exclusively with examining the claims of formal psychotherapy in the treatment of obsessional disorders. It will first be necessary to say more about the postulated intrapsychic mechanisms.

THE DYNAMIC PSYCHOPATHOLOGY OF OBSESSIONAL
DISORDERS

Since classical psychoanalytic theory and derivative systems have had
so much to say about the origins and nature of obsessional symptomatology, they cannot be ignored in a book devoted to the subject.
From the foregoing it will be plain that much discussion of these matters
will be necessary in the future if the place of psychotherapy in the
treatment of these disorders is ever going to be made clear to those who
are not prepared to accept authoritarian viewpoints, whether advanced
by the exponents or by the adversaries of psychoanalytic theories
(Millar, 1969).

The comments which follow make no claims to completeness – they
refer only to some of the landmarks in the mainstream of psychoanalytic thinking about the subject.

The development of Freud's thinking on obsessional disorders may
be traced over a period of thirty years (Freud, S., 1896, 1907, 1908,
1909, 1913a, 1913b, 1913c, 1916, 1926). At the end of that time, in
Inhibitions, Symptoms and Anxiety he wrote that obsessional neurosis
was 'unquestionably the most interesting and repaying subject of
analytic research', but commented on the fact that the problem had not
been mastered. Forty years later, at the 24th International Psycho-
Analytical Congress in Amsterdam (1965), one aspect of the situation
was summarized by Sandler and Joffe (1965):

> In surveying the psychoanalytic literature on the obsessive compul-
> sion disorders one cannot fail to be impressed by the fact that there
> appears to be a continual need to re-examine this topic. Yet, in spite
> of this, over the years little essential change has taken place in our
> views on obsessional phenomena. There is no doubt that Freud's
> ideas on the subject have stood the test of time and of clinical experi-
> ence, and the fact that so many authors have arrived at formulations
> which are fundamentally identical with Freud's testifies to this; at
> the same time their very need to explore and re-explore obsessional
> disturbances bears witness to a feeling that the subject is still far
> from being well understood; a feeling which has found its main
> expression in the main topic of this Congress.

The psychoanalytic view of the origin of neurosis in general suggests
that, after the ego has developed to a stage where drives are at a relatively advanced (genital) level, an intolerable increase in anxiety or
conflict, related to the oedipal situation, leads to *regression* of drives to

earlier (pregenital) fixation points. Infantile, pregenital impulses of a sexual-aggressive kind then emerge. The superego has an important influence at this stage, evoking anxiety and guilt which cause further conflict within the ego; hence defensive mechanisms of various kinds are called into play. These contain the conflict or anxiety with varying degrees of success. Symptoms and character disorders are formed by various combinations and interactions of the initial intolerable anxiety, the regressed position and the primitive (id) impulses which derive from this, the anxiety and guilt evoked by the superego, and the ego defence mechanisms. The type of neurotic disorder which results depends on the extent of the regression (i.e. the level of the fixation point to which the drives are transferred), on the content of the re-jected impulses and fantasies, and on which particular defence mech-anisms are employed (Anna Freud, 1965).

In obsessional disorders, the regression of drives is to the anal sadistic level. This proposition is seen as the cornerstone of the develop-ment of obsessive–compulsive neurosis. The resulting 'anal sadism' combines with the oedipus hostility felt for the parent of the same sex, and this leads to increased ambivalence of object relationships and also to bisexual qualities in the drives. Ego defence mechanisms most prominently concerned are displacement, reaction formation, denial, iso-lation, undoing, rationalization and intellectualization. As a result of these defence mechanisms and of the altered drive impulses there are various changes in ego function. The defence mechanisms, though elaborate, are insufficient to prevent the conflict from increasing in its effects; and there is no stable compromise solution (as there is in conversion hysteria). A compulsive symptom may represent a condensation of primitive drives and defences against them. The superego becomes tyrannous and commanding. Secondary defensive conflicts appear, including further reaction formations and counter-compulsions, and there may be a tendency for symptoms to evolve from a defensive to a gratifying or self-indulgent function.

In his summary of the psychoanalytic theory of obsessive–compulsive symptom formation Fenichel (1945) stated that the regression of drives to the anal sadistic level, pathognomonic for symptom formation, depends on three variables – the pre-existing residues of the anal sadistic phase of libidinal development, the degree and style of phallic organization reached during the course of development, and the strength of the defending ego. In exceptional cases, obsessional dis-order may, according to Fenichel, be based not on regression but solely on a disturbance of development at the anal sadistic stage. But in general the great importance of the oedipus complex, and of castration anxiety in promoting regression, was regarded by this author (as by so many others) as well established.

In the classical psychoanalytic literature on obsessional disorders much is written about the function of the mechanisms of *isolation* of the ideational content from the emotional cathexis. This promotes a cleavage of ego functions into logical and illogical. Other recurring themes include the intellectualization of emotionally-charged drives and impulses; the consequent tendency of the obsessional individual to indulge in magical thinking and belief in the omnipotence of thought; the outstripping of libidinal development by ego development; and the emergence of precocious or sadistic features in the superego directed towards the ego as a result of reaction formation.

Discussion of current psychoanalytic views of obsessional neurosis was the main topic of the International Psycho-Analytical Congress in 1965; and these views are cogently summarized by Anna Freud (1966). As pointed out by Sandler, the main themes have remained unchanged for four decades, despite the large volume of detailed clinical material published in the form of individual case studies of adult and child patients in analysis. The one noteworthy development is in regard to views about ego functions. Sandler and Joffe (1965) develop the idea that regression of ego functioning accompanies the drive regression. Ego functioning relating to cognition, perception and control develops most prominently during the anal phase, and regression in these functions goes some way to explaining the nature of the defence mechanisms in obsessional neurosis. The result is a particular style of ego-functioning characterized by a tendency to use methods of cognitive and perceptual control which would be appropriate only at an earlier stage of ego development.

The method of psychoanalysis is to pursue each disorder or difficulty back to its origins, or earliest indications in the patient's life. By the nature of the elaborate defence mechanisms employed by the ego, this task is difficult in theory and certainly also in practice. Numerous individual case reports in the analytic literature testify to the practical difficulties. Fenichel (1945) considered that although 'compulsive neurosis is the second type of transference neurosis and the second great field in which psychoanalysis is indicated' (the first being hysteria), yet the difficulties are formidable. As the mechanism of isolation is so prominent in obsessional symptom formation, the technique of free association which is the main tool of the psychoanalytic method is hindered. The morbid ideas, stemming from traumatic earlier experiences, are present in consciousness, but they are intellectualized, and stripped of their original connection and of their emotional cathexis; therefore it is difficult or impossible for the analyst to identify them. Archaic and magical thinking obscure the situation further. Moreover the defensive style of obsessional patients may force them to prefer the *status quo*, to cling to their symptoms, and to develop numerous subordinate defences. Fenichel lists the special difficulties in the psychoanalysis of obsessionals to include regression, isolation, the role of the superego, the presence of anxiety, the particular ways in which thought and speech are affected, and the changes in object relationships.

Other systems of dynamic psychopathology, developed directly or indirectly from psychoanalysis, lay emphasis on different hypothetical intrapsychic structures and functions. For none is there the same agreement among different writers as is the case with the classical psychoanalytic model. No attempt will be made to summarize them here.

Analysts and others who practise formal psychotherapy of a kind which does not amount to full psychoanalysis use techniques which depart considerably from the classical psychoanalytic model. The writer's understanding of the situation is that they are more empirical, more oriented towards considering the dynamics of the individual in terms of both ego function and current interpersonal problems, and more flexible in their formulations of intrapsychic disorders. In short, they employ a wider range of models (developed *ad hoc* as well as on psychoanalytic principles), object relation theories and varying concepts of ego psychology. By the same token, however, they do not have the same definable framework for a unified dynamic psychopathology.

This formulation of the dynamic psychopathology of obsessional disorders makes no claim to be comprehensive or definitive; and it is certainly not authoritative. It is a simplified interpretation of the present state of affairs as seen by a non-specialist. How the main elements are related to symptoms and have come to be regarded as the underlying mechanisms for which the symptoms are merely emblems is fairly plain. The seemingly trivial content of many obsessions, and their repetitiveness, may understandably be interpreted as displacement. The common concern of obsessional patients with aggressiveness, hostility, uncleanliness, sex and religion are consistent with the anal sadistic idiom and the idea of a conscience or superego fighting against the unwanted drives. The necessity for resisting obsessions and compulsions, felt so characteristically by patients with these illnesses, suggests an ego fighting for survival against forces within and surrounding itself. The term 'undoing' might be used deliberately by a compulsive patient unsophisticated in psychiatric jargon. Likewise 'isolation' is an easily understandable term for describing how objects become separated from their appropriate affect, or how inappropriately strong affect attaches to trivial objects in obsessional disorders. It is easy to see how much of the terminology of dynamic psychopathology developed as an attempt to systematize the observations made on patients, and how the structure of the theory advanced as a set of unifying concepts. It is easy to recognize the brilliance of the attempt to construct a useful model from fragments of evidence, and it is clear that a high capacity for conceptual thinking, associated with perceptive and intuitive understanding of the experiences of patients, can lead to some very sophisticated theoretical reasoning. The content and perhaps the form of obsessional symptoms are explicable in terms of personal history and individual experience; but an aetiological theory should surely distinguish between circumstances which cause and those which shape events. It is in the extent to which it claims to be an aetiological theory concerned with mechanisms, the extent to which it is concerned with causation, and the extent to which it regards this distinction as meaningless, that the claims of psychoanalytic theory seem hardest to define and examine.

The psychoanalytic theory of obsessional disorder, like the psychoanalytic view of neurosis in general, seems to have become more elaborate than the phenomena it sets out to elucidate. Its logical status is precarious. It is in part an attempt at systematizing a natural history, in part a metaphor that has become reified, and in part a semantic hypothesis or framework for interpreting observations and constructing models (Rycroft, 1966; Hill, 1971). It is sad that so important a topic has not found its appropriate public language. For present purposes five conclusions about the propositions of psychoanalytic theory and other psychodynamic formulations of obsessional disorders seem justifiable: (i) they are not *ipso facto* correct; (ii) their credibility cannot rest on the fact that they derive ultimately from observations on patients because the patients come from a biased sample and the same clinicians act as both observers and interpreters; (iii) therefore they must stand or fall by their heuristic value and their therapeutic potential; (iv) rigorous methods for assessing their heuristic value and/or their therapeutic potential do not seem to have been developed; and (v) there is much scope for clearer practical exploration of these issues by collaborative efforts between psychoanalysts and others who stand outside the subject and feel concerned that the credentials of psychoanalysis shall be stated in such a way that they can withstand rigorous examination.

PROBLEMS IN ASSESSING THE EFFICACY OF PSYCHOTHERAPY
IN OBSESSIONAL DISORDERS

Among the many underdeveloped domains of psychiatry, one which calls for disciplined examination is concerned with the functional relationships between academic knowledge and theoretical systems on the one hand, and the processes of decision-making in clinical practice on the other. One may safely predict that inquiry into this field will call into question the common assertions that practice consists of direct applications of theoretical knowledge, and that the growth of knowledge is promoted by the results of clinical experience. Theoretical formulations, and even firm knowledge, at an academic level, cannot by themselves support the claims made for derivative forms of treatment. All treatment must prove itself in practice before it can be accepted as useful; it must be subjected to empirical test, and be judged by its results. Theoretical considerations may be expected to say something about the circumstances in which particular methods might be tried out, and about ways of doing so. But they can be no substitute for the trial of treatment. In one sense every time a patient is treated, an experiment is undertaken, as a result of which it is hoped that certain effects will be apparent: first and most important, that the patient will not be damaged; that he will benefit; that the therapist may learn something; that he may be able to apply what he has learned to the treatment of other patients; and lastly that he may be able to communicate what he has learned, for the ultimate benefit of patients treated by other people. It is important to recognize that, where treatment is concerned, experimentation is inevitable. Therefore it is appropriate sometimes to control variables in order to optimize the heuristic potential. It is unethical to continue to practise a form of treatment the efficacy of which is not under continuous reappraisal. It follows that the accumulation of clinical experience does not conflict with the deliberate undertaking of therapeutic experimentation. They are merely different stages of the same process. The more heterogeneous a group of patients, the more necessary is a disciplined approach aimed at understanding the salient variables and their interrelationships; and the more important it becomes to know the limits within which generalization is permissible.

All plans for treatment begin by postulating a relationship between a type of treatment and the relief of a particular condition. The postulate may be explicit or merely implicit; it may be an assertion (as in instances where the therapist for one reason or another feels certainty), or it may be a conjecture or hypothesis. Where uncertainty is admitted, the meanings behind the terms *relationship, type of treatment,* and *relief of a particular condition* must be examined.

To establish that there is a *relationship* between giving treatment and achieving the desired result it is clearly necessary to do more than demonstrate that one follows the other. To establish the specificity of the association, it is necessary to know whether the patient would have got better anyhow, without treatment; whether he would have got better as quickly, or more quickly with some other treatment; whether the recovery was complete and lasting; whether the treatment had unwanted effects, and so on. To be able to show that a relationship exists there must be some comparison between results with the treatment on trial and those with no treatment (or a standard form of treatment), as well as some indication of the constancy of the relationship, and of the conditions in which it is more predictable or less predictable.

The *type of treatment* may be simply a course of medication, or it may consist of a very elaborate procedure, involving many variables, as in dynamic psychotherapy. In either case it can be expected that the treatment will include *specific* and *non-specific* factors. Specific factors (such as a pharmacological preparation; a pattern of interpretations within a transference relationship) are seen as central to the treatment. The non-specific factors include many variables associated with the treatment, subordinate to it, but of possible therapeutic significance (for example the size, shape and colour of the tablets, what the patient expects of them, what he is told; the number, frequency and duration of the interviews, and the patient's and the therapist's expectations). In recent years much attention has been focused on the non-specific, 'placebo' and psychosocial correlates of treatment, especially in the field of pharmacology (see for example Klerman, 1963; Honigfeld, 1964). If the non-specific effects with drugs are elaborate and therapeutically significant, it is *a fortiori* likely that this is true also for psychotherapeutic procedures. In these, the interplay of possible specific and non-specific factors has been explored with particular cogency by Frank (1961, 1971).

Relief of a particular condition. It is not necessary to emphasize that the criteria of type and severity of illness, and of change, should be comprehensive and adequately specified. This may be a simple matter or it may call for complex procedures.

There are several approaches to the problem of estimating the efficacy of any treatment. One is to study an individual case, or a small number of cases, in detail, and to generalize from this experience, perhaps with the help of theoretical reasoning. Another is to seek consistencies or agreements between experienced clinicians. These methods, and others like them, are however no more than preliminary explorations leading to crucial investigations which satisfy the appropriate rules for demonstrating whether or not a given stimulus (treatment) is followed by a given response (improvement of some kind) in given circumstances (specifications of characteristics of patients and treatment). Methods adequate for deciding whether psychotherapy is a useful treatment for obsessional disorders need to be more complicated than those for deciding whether implosion is a useful treatment for a specific phobia, much more complicated than those for deciding whether imipramine is a useful treatment for depressive illness, and very much more complicated than those for deciding whether streptomycin is a useful treatment for tuberculous meningitis. In assessing treatment, methodological and practical problems are introduced by variability or uncertainty in the course of the illness. Further problems are introduced when the criteria of type and severity of the disorder are elaborate; and still further problems enter when the treatment process itself is many-sided and difficult to dissect.

Earlier in this chapter it has been suggested that it would be profitable to define three classes of psychotherapy: (i) psychotherapy in the extensive sense, (ii) informal psychotherapy, and (iii) formal psychotherapy, including psychoanalysis. Within each of these classes there is much variation; for example, formal psychotherapy varies according to the duration and frequency of interviews, total duration of treatment, theoretical assumptions, defined objectives of treatment, form and content of interviews, personality characteristics of the therapist, expectations of the therapist and patient, the quality of the relationship which becomes established between the therapist and patient, and many others. Some of these variables may be regarded as non-specific to the treatment (e.g. duration and frequency of interviews) and others as specific, to a varying extent, to the treatment in general or to the individual treatment situation.

It was also suggested earlier that obsessional disorders can be characterized by several sets of variables, including symptoms and signs, focal behaviour disturbances, maladaptive patterns of living and relationships, and (where these are held to be meaningful and relevant) intrapsychic disturbances. For each of these sets of variables, multiple criteria are necessary, and must be subjected to tests of reliability and validity.

Since different forms of treatment have different targets – explicitly stated or implicit in their claims – it was suggested (p. 268) that a table of provisional hypotheses could be drawn up. For formal psychotherapy, some such hypotheses might be more fully stated as follows.

(i) Formal psychotherapy is associated with identifiable and favourable realignments in intrapsychic functions, i.e. with sought-after dynamic changes.

(ii) Dynamic changes brought about by formal psychotherapy are associated with improved interpersonal relationships and diminished psychosocial maladjustment.

(iii) Dynamic changes are associated with symptom removal without symptom substitution.

It would be only too easy to extend this list to comprise scores of preliminary hypotheses, of a kind which could be tested (albeit with difficulty) and the support or refutation of which would constitute an advance in therapeutics. For it is clear that in assessing treatment the hypotheses must be meaningful *within the terms of what is claimed for the treatment in question*. It is with these prior considerations in mind that we can turn to the literature to see what evidence has, in fact, accumulated to support the claims of psychotherapy in obsessional disorders; what evidence there is to refute these claims; and what reasoning, different from that above, can be invoked to suggest that these formulations of the questions we have to ask are incorrect or inappropriate.

THE OUTCOME OF OBSESSIONAL DISORDERS

When the results of a given form of treatment are being evaluated, a knowledge of the outcome of events in people suffering from untreated obsessional disorders of different degrees of severity would serve as a basis for comparison. Not surprisingly, such knowledge is lacking. Like other neurotic syndromes, obsessional disorders come to the notice of the medical and paramedical professions only when they reach a certain degree of severity, in terms of being to some extent intolerable or incapacitating. Many people, it may be supposed, experience symptoms or other difficulties and do not seek any sort of professional advice; and others may obtain treatment of an unorthodox kind from practitioners of 'fringe medicine'. Of those who seek medical help, an unknown proportion are treated in general practice and others, presumably those most severely affected, are referred to psychiatrists, psychologists or psychotherapists. Whether or not a request is made for medical help in general, or specialist help within the framework of medicine, is likely to depend not only on severity but also on a number of psycho-social, cultural, subcultural, and administrative variables. These may include aspects of the individual's personality, life situation, the avail-ability of treatment of various kinds, and public attitudes and expecta-tions with respect to these treatments. Some of them may alter with the caprices of fashion. It may be that there is a relationship between the prestige of a form of treatment and the demand for it – i.e. the number of individuals who take on the role of patient. The matters are largely intangible, but it seems important to recognize that when we study obsessional disorders – or other types of neurotic disability – we are seeing only one part of the field. And our sampling frame may be chang-ing with time in an unpredictable fashion. These *caveats* apply to all our reasoning about aetiology, phenomenology, and diagnosis, as to other aspects of the so-called natural history of illness.

Even for those who seek psychiatric help the course of the untreated disorder remains uncertain. The practice of medicine and psychiatry is such that, even in the absence of treatment of demonstrable efficacy, something has to be done to try to help the patient. So factual data about the outcome of obsessional disorders can be available only with respect to patients who have been treated. Therefore any review of the prognosis of obsessional illness is subject to limitations due to incom-plete sampling, to the fact that patients have, of necessity, received some form of treatment, and to assumptions about reliability and homo-geneity of diagnosis.

There are reports of the outcome of obsessional disorders at, or shortly after, termination of treatment. But as the treatment is com-monly sought only after some years' experience of symptoms, as the disability may fluctuate in severity or show a phasic course, and as almost any therapeutic intervention in any neurotic disorder can have short-term non-specific effects, we need to turn to studies in which patients have been followed for some years after their initial referral.

A number of such studies exist, and some of their results have been summarized by Goodwin *et al.* (1969). Some consistent patterns emerge, although there is a good deal of variation from one to another. This is not surprising, for there is no uniformity of method. Some investiga-tions (Langfeldt, 1938; Müller, 1957; Hastings, 1958; Ingram, 1961; Kringlen, 1965; Greer and Cawley, 1966; Noreik, 1970) included in-patients alone. Others (Lewis, 1936; Rudin, 1953; Pollitt, 1957; Balslev-Olesen and Geert-Jørgensen, 1959 and Lo (1967) reported on samples consisting of in-patients and out-patients in varying proportions, whilst Grimshaw (1965) followed up a series consisting only of out-patients. Thus the severity of the illness at the start of treatment presumptively varied considerably from one sample to another. Different investigators followed their patients over differing periods of time, using a variety of methods for obtaining follow-up data. Most of the inquiries were concerned only with obsessional disorders but Hastings (1958), Greer and Cawley (1966) and Noreik (1970) reported on larger groupings of patients, and the outcome for obsessional illness could be compared with that for other disorders. The criteria of good or bad outcome also varied from global estimates to more specific mention of presence or absence of symptoms, severity of symptoms, and social maladjustment. Müller (1957), Pollitt (1957), Ingram (1961), Grimshaw (1965), Greer and Cawley (1966) and Lo (1967) assessed both symptoms and social adjustment in terms of work and social life. Examination of this literature provides a salutary reminder of the difficulties of conducting large-scale inquiries into long-term outcome. None of the studies was comprehensive in terms of recording manifestations of obsessional disorder in the six categories outlined on page 266; indeed, all studies were purely descriptive, making no reference to possible psychodynamic changes. It is hard to see how these could have been included in any valid way.

A detailed discussion of the results would be out of place here. They differ in part because of inconsistencies in sampling and in method and duration of follow-up. But on the average – and recognizing that the variability is high – it seems fair to make a generalization. If a series of patients with obsessional illnesses, severe enough to be treated at some time in hospital, is looked at after about five years have elapsed, it can be expected that about one quarter will have recovered; about a half will have improved a good deal though they will still experience symptoms, possibly incapacitating; and the remaining quarter will be unchanged or worse. Of the last sub-group a few will have come to be regarded as schizophrenic. For a series not having needed hospital admission, about two-thirds will be much improved in terms of symptom relief and social adjustment, whilst the remainder will have improved to a lesser extent, or be unchanged or worse. These remarks apply to patients treated by the routine methods which have been available at various times over the last thirty years or so.

Comparisons of different treatments in the series of patients here discussed are of little value because in no case was treatment randomized. Patients were treated according to the ideas then prevailing, according to the facilities available, and according to the persuasions of the psychiatrist concerned. In some studies (Pollitt, 1957; Balslev-Olesen and Geert-Jørgensen, 1959; Ingram, 1967; and Noreik, 1970) comparisons are made between leucotomized and non-leucotomized patients with respect to long-term outcome. The leucotomized patients did better. This is likely to be a comment on the selection procedures for leucotomy rather than on specific effects of the operation – though Pollitt (1957) makes a modest claim, from his series, that leucotomy was the only treatment which in some cases influenced the natural course of events. On the other hand Lewis (1936) reported that of his 50 patients, 17 had received intensive psychotherapy of an analytic kind, and a majority of these did badly 'not because of any insufficiency in the method or its application, one may suppose, but because the most difficult and demanding cases were referred for this treatment'. But in the series of neurotic patients investigated by Greer and Cawley (1966), patients who had formal psychotherapy fared better than those having other forms of treatment; however, this group of patients also scored favourably on all the demographic, social and clinical variables associated with a good prognosis, so that it seems that the patients most favoured in certain respects were selected for psychotherapy. Similarly Ernst (1959) and Noreik (1970) found that patients selected for psychotherapy had a better long-term prognosis, whilst Grimshaw (1965) reported that, of his 100 patients, 14 had 'systematic psychotherapy using psychodynamic theories to give insight into the mechanisms of the illness', usually in weekly interviews for a year or more. These patients fared no better and no worse than others in the series. Thus no conclusions about the comparative efficacy of different forms of treatment can be drawn from this series of investigations. All in all, the statement by Lewis (1936) about his series seems equally true in general today, as far as follow-up studies of obsessional illnesses are concerned: 'attempts to distinguish between the value of one form of treatment and another are futile because there is no rigour of method and sometimes the change in the patient had less apparent connection with the medical treatment than with external happenings. . . .'

When outcome of obsessional disorders is compared with that of other neurotic disabilities, there is some conflict of evidence. Hastings (1958) found no difference in the proportions – nearly 50 per cent – having a good outcome. Grimshaw (1965) on the basis of his work with outpatients and from his review of the literature found no reason for attributing a more unfavourable prognosis to obsessional disorder than to other neurotic states. But Eitinger (1955) reported that in his series obsessional neuroses were the most chronic. Likewise Greer and Cawley (1966) found that for all neurotic disorders in their series of 146 patients, 78 (51 per cent) had recovered or much improved after five years; the corresponding figure for patients with obsessive–compulsive reactions was only 8 out of 21 (38 per cent).

No data are available for determining the long-term prognosis of people with obsessional personalities. There is a general consensus that such individuals are especially prone to depressive illnesses (see for example Kendell and DiScipio, 1970) as well as to obsessional illnesses. Furthermore the presence of anancastic personality traits is not a necessary precondition for developing an obsessional illness. But like other disorders of personality, the patterns of maladjustment are related to external variables in a complex way. How these patterns determine vulnerability to one or other kind of illness remains uncertain. Moreover, many individuals with anancastic personalities become identified as patients only when they develop florid symptoms of one kind or another.

RESULTS OF PSYCHOTHERAPY IN OBSESSIONAL DISORDERS

Operational definitions of types or levels of psychotherapy have been proposed (pp. 262–6) and a scheme has been put forward in outline for categorizing the targets for treatment in obsessional patients (pp. 266–9). By taking into consideration the strategies of different forms of treatment, and by recognizing that each treatment is directed at different targets, it is possible to construct a framework (p. 268) for formulating hypotheses postulating specific relationships between a particular treatment and a particular response. Second-order hypotheses can then be set up to investigate the relationship between the particular response and overall improvement.

Using this approach for examining the claims of formal psychotherapy, we should now search the literature for evidence to support or refute either or both of the two propositions:

   (i) that formal psychotherapy brings about intrapsychic (dynamic) changes of a beneficial kind;

   (ii) that the intrapsychic changes evoked by formal psychotherapy are accompanied by improvements in personal adjustment, by diminution in subjective discomfort, by improvement in respect of the patient's symptoms and signs and focal disorders of behaviour, or by some combination of these three classes of variables.

The distinction between these may be considered pedantic by some and slipshod by others. So for the sake of completeness we should also search for evidence which short-circuits it:

(iii) that formal psychotherapy brings about improvement in symptoms and signs of obsessional illness, diminution in subjective discomfort, and improved personal adjustment.

In our search of the literature purporting to examine any or all of these three propositions, it will be necessary to recall the prerequisites for regarding evidence as acceptable, namely, the explicit recognition that a statement about the usefulness of treatment is a comparative statement; and the necessity for adopting adequate and communicable criteria descriptive of the patients, the disorders to be treated, and the form of treatment.

An extensive literature gives an affirmative answer to the first of the three propositions set out above. It consists of studies of single cases or small groups of cases, and the data are generally reported along with discussion of their implications for psychoanalytic or other psychodynamic theories. On this reckoning the data seem potentially useful. But they cannot be accepted as serious evidence for a variety of reasons. Of these the most prominent are as follows:

(a) The criteria of intrapsychic disorder are expressed in a private language. There is no certainty that people who use this language are using concepts consistently and within the same patterns of meaning, and no attempt is made to set out the propositions in a way which is fully understandable to an outside observer.

(b) There is no recognition of the principle that useful statements about treatment are comparative statements. Even the possibility of using one period of a patient's experience (without treatment) as a control for another period is not exploited in a disciplined way.

(c) There is an admixture, sometimes impossible to unravel, of observations (or reports of observations) of a patient's behaviour, including his verbal behaviour, the therapist's interpretations (to his audience) of these observations, and theoretical reasoning and generalization.

(d) The reports usually concern only a fragment of analysis or psychotherapy.

The reader who doubts the fairness of these judgements may turn to the reports of the discussions on obsessional disorder at the 24th International Psycho-Analytical Congress (1965). If, like the writer, he is eager to find evidence that psychoanalysis and psychotherapy are advancing to the stage in which their credentials as treatment can be examined rigorously and without fear, he will be sadly disappointed. Much of the Congress was devoted to further consideration of Freud's Rat Man (e.g. Zetzel, 1966; Kestenberg, 1966; Grunberger, 1966), to discussion of a patient who had been analysed for three years in childhood and who subsequently returned to analysis as a young adult, providing opportunity for confirmation of arguments which, in the strict sense are circular (Ritvo, 1966; van der Leeuw, 1966; Nacht, 1966). There was a lengthy report about the supposed interplay between the character formation and bowel motions of a four-year-old boy (Ramzy, 1966). The conclusion is that, despite the dedication, often the high ability, and sometimes the charisma of those who write about psychoanalysis, they are unable or unwilling to bring their concepts and methods into public symposium. As a result, it is not possible to confirm or refute the hypothesis that psychoanalysis or other forms of dynamic psychotherapy bring about intrapsychic changes of a useful kind. The appropriate investigations have not been carried out; or else they have not been reported in convincing terms. Likewise, no evidence is available relevant to the other two propositions mentioned above. No controlled studies have been undertaken.

If unbiased data are unavailable, there may be something to be gained by examining biased data. There are various reports of the outcome of psychotherapy in selected series of patients. These are of limited value because of the very fact that the patients selected for this form of treatment were generally – and quite properly – those thought most likely to benefit by it. Luff and Garrod (1935) carried out a follow-up study ($\geqslant 3$ years) of 500 patients who had been treated by formal psychotherapy at the Tavistock Clinic. The criteria for assessment were comprehensive, including not only symptoms but also life situation, employment, attitudes, and capacity for withstanding stress. Of the 60 obsessionals, 34 (59 per cent) were rated as much improved or improved on discharge from treatment and 31 (52 per cent) were similarly rated at follow-up. These figures are slightly lower than those for the series as a whole (66 per cent and 55 per cent respectively). The best results were obtained for patients diagnosed as having anxiety states and those with sexual difficulties. The results of Luff and Garrod's study are inconclusive because factors influencing selection for treatment are unknown and because there is no basis for direct comparison. The outcome of the disorder in their obsessional patients is of the same order as that for patients having miscellaneous kinds of treatment, reported above (pp. 279–82). Knight (1941) compared the results of psychoanalytic treatment at various Institutes. The numbers of patients treated for 'compulsion neurosis' varied from one clinic to another. For the Berlin Institute of Psychoanalysis it was 106 in 11 years; for the London Clinic of Psychoanalysis it was 17 in 11 years; the Chicago Institute of Psychoanalysis took 8 such patients in 6 years, and the Menninger Clinic took 7 patients in 5 years. Results of treatment differed little from one Institute to another. In all, 138 patients were taken on for treatment at all centres at the stated times. 37 (27 per cent) of these broke off treatment during the first 6 months. Of the remaining 101, 27 were regarded as 'apparently cured' and 36 as 'much improved' at the end of treatment, i.e. 63 per cent were thought to have gained substantial benefit from their treatment. For the 396 patients with all other psychoneuroses, 114 patients (30 per cent) broke off treatment. Of the remaining 282, 98 were regarded as 'apparently cured' and 81 as 'much improved' at the end of treatment, i.e. 64 per cent seemed to have gained substantial benefit. Obsessional patients therefore were not conspicuously more inclined than other neurotics to persevere with treatment; those who did so were equally likely to be seen as having been helped substantially, though a smaller proportion of obsessionals were rated as fully 'cured'.

These figures were taken by Knight from the decennial and other reports of the various centres; they represent (presumably) the therapists' own ratings, and there were no follow-up data. We therefore have a short-term success rate of just under two-thirds for selected patients judged by obviously (and understandably) biased observers. In the circumstances this is not strikingly better than the estimates of longer-term prognosis reported earlier (pp. 279–82). Cremerius (1962) (cited by Rachman, 1971a) compared the results of different treatment regimes, including psychoanalytic treatment, in 605 neurotic out-patients. Treatment was not randomized so the comparison is of limited value. Overall the 56 patients selected for psychoanalytic treatment had fared no better by the end of treatment, and only a little better 8 to 10 years later. Obsessional patients did less well than the others. Unpublished studies in the United States suggest that some cases are cured by psychoanalysis, and that short-term treatment is not very helpful. These studies also indicate that methods of diagnosis and evaluation of results are not standardized, so that valid conclusions cannot be reached.

From such evidence as is available, there are no grounds for feeling optimistic about the place of psychoanalysis or other types of formal psychotherapy in the treatment of obsessional disorders (Cameron, 1968). On the other hand, the problem has not been investigated by methods which really do justice to the claims of formal psychotherapy or to commonly held views of what constitutes acceptable empirical evidence.

There is now a very large American literature on the evaluation of psychotherapy in general (see for example Truax and Carkhuff, 1967; Strupp and Bergin, 1969). Among the enormous number of investigations which have been undertaken to this end, two principal themes can be discerned. One is concerned with the outcome of events among heterogeneous groups of patients who have received broadly defined types of psychotherapy, comparing it with the outcome for patients treated otherwise. The second theme, overlapping with the first, focuses attention on the possibility of identifying critical variables in the patient, the therapist, and the therapeutic relationship. From the first theme the conclusion has emerged that the amount of variation among patients treated by psychotherapy is greater than that among those not so treated. Hence, it is argued, psychotherapy is beneficial to some patients and possibly harmful to others; whilst its average effect is negligible, there are people who stand to benefit, and the problem becomes one of deciding which patients, in which circumstances, will gain from particular types of therapy given by therapists with particular characteristics. From the second theme, efforts are made to validate measurement of those properties of a doctor or psychologist which make him a good therapist. Qualities of 'genuineness', 'empathy', and 'non-possessive warmth' are held to be amenable to quantification, and also to be demonstrably influential in determining therapeutic success. It would be inappropriate to review this literature in the present context. It has become very complicated and it throws little light on the question of whether obsessional disorders are helped by one or other kind of psychotherapy. Diagnostic categories are held to be less important as indications for treatment and as prognostic indicators than other variables concerning the patient, his personality, and his life situation.

SUMMARY AND CONCLUSIONS

The question of whether psychotherapy is a useful form of treatment for patients with obsessional disorders is one which raises formidable issues. It would be impossible to answer the question, or even to set out the issues, in a way which would give satisfaction to all those with wide experience of obsessional disorders or to all those who have pondered deeply on questions central to psychotherapy. It would be impossible even to review succinctly all the literature relevant to the theme. The writer is very much aware that he has produced only one of many possible formulations of the problem. Nevertheless it is suggested that an appraisal of the present situation permits three summary statements: (i) provisional conclusions, (ii) implications of these for future investigation, and (iii) implications for clinical practice.

Provisional conclusions

Psychotherapy is a term used to cover a very wide spectrum of methods of psychological treatment. More specific definitions of different types of psychotherapy or of possible components of psychotherapy are needed if it is to be investigated, practised, or taught effectively. One approach to the problem, adopted by many American investigators, is to try to identify as many as possible of the salient variables which operate during the course of different forms of psychotherapy. An alternative approach, favoured by the writer, is to distinguish the more specific from the less specific types of psychotherapy by defining three levels: (i) psychotherapy in its widest sense, co-extensive with the doctor patient relationship; (ii) informal psychotherapy, a wide range of techniques which can be described rather than defined; and (iii) formal psychotherapy, conducted by specialists and having as a central feature the development of a transference relationship within which the therapist offers to the patient a series of interpretations relating the transactions within this relationship to present and to past experiences. It is argued that this way of looking at different aspects of psychotherapy is useful because it distinguishes operations carried out by people with different types of skill. Also it distinguishes a set of techniques which may or may not be invoked from a different though overlapping set of techniques which are always involved to some extent by doctors and others responsible for treating people who are emotionally disturbed. It is further argued that of the questions which can readily be answered the most prominent is whether formal psychotherapy has any value in treating obsessional patients.

Obsessional disorders have wide-ranging features which can be conveniently though arbitrarily arranged under six headings: symptoms; signs; focal disturbances in behaviour; problems of living of many kinds which can be designated as maladjustment; personal suffering; and hypothesized intrapsychic disturbances. If the disorder is formulated in this manner, various targets for treatment can be identified under the six headings. The aims of different modalities of treatment – drugs, behaviour therapy, and the three types of psychotherapy here defined – can then be stated more clearly. As a result there is a framework for constructing hypotheses linking particular forms of treatment with particular effects. In this way each type of treatment can – at least theoretically – be assessed according to criteria based on its own stated aims and methods.

Psychiatrists and psychologists see only a selected sample of obsessional disorders – presumably the most severe – and it is therefore impossible to make general statements about the outcome of untreated disorders. Follow-up studies which have been carried out on samples of former in-patients suggest that in general it may be expected that five years after treatment about a quarter of patients will have recovered; about half will have improved to some extent but will have residual symptoms and social incapacity to a varying extent; and a quarter will be no better, and perhaps worse. Patients treated only as out-patients have a rather better prognosis.

There is no evidence to support or refute the proposition that formal psychotherapy helps patients with obsessional disorders. The hypothesis has not been examined by methods which could produce valid evidence.

Implications for further investigation

The distinction, or overlap, between the three defined types of psychotherapy could with advantage be further explored. Psychoanalysts and others practising formal psychotherapy could clarify the situation if they could devise a set of agreed general statements describing the hypothetical intrapsychic processes and their deviations in obsessional illness in terms which are (a) self-consistent, (b) related in an understandable way to possible therapeutic interventions and (c) able to lead to specific hypotheses which can be supported or refuted by the outcome of events in treatment. This task will be extremely difficult; psychoanalytical theory and its derivatives are concerned with representations of a world where logical connections may appear to be upside-down or otherwise distorted. But it is surely possible to devise a language and syntax for describing the irrational in rational and communicable terms. The matter of informal psychotherapy likewise calls for further specification, with attempts to identify salient variables. It should (in the writer's opinion) be investigated as a set of problems separate from formal psychotherapy.

The nature of the functional disturbance in obsessional disorders – the relationships between symptoms and the other kinds of dysfunction – may be clarified with the help of suitable descriptive indices. It would then be possible to formulate hypotheses with greater precision, and to indicate topics on which therapeutic research (not only in psychotherapy) should be focused.

Implications for practice

The problems of patients with obsessional disorders are in general unlikely to be helped on any large scale by formal psychotherapy. In a small proportion of such patients it may become fairly clear on clinical investigation that the obsessional symptoms are subordinate to identifiable interpersonal or intrapsychic problems. If it is judged that these patients are likely to be able to withstand, and profit from, a process of exploration directed at uncovering deeper problems, formal psychotherapy should be considered. There is no evidence that it will succeed: but the clinician is continually confronted with the necessity for making decisions on inadequate evidence. Therefore any available source of help should be exploited providing there is reason to believe that it will do no harm and as long as suitable targets for treatment can be identified.

In the writer's opinion, all other patients with obsessional disorders for which specialist help is sought should receive informal psychotherapy. The specification of this form of treatment is diffuse (p. 263) and the details of the procedures actually adopted will depend on many variables concerned with the disability, the patient's personality, his life situation, the appropriateness and availability of help from other forms of treatment including drugs and behaviour therapy, and the amount of time available. Informal psychotherapy may be time-consuming and demanding, and it may call for considerable skill. This skill may (as mentioned earlier) be helped by a period of training and supervision in formal psychotherapy, or it may not. It may depend more on qualities of personality than on training. It seems fair to assume that, up to a point at least, competence grows with experience. In the practice of informal psychotherapy (as for other types of treatment) it will generally be profitable to set clearly defined targets.

Finally it should be emphasized that, in the present state of our knowledge, the treatment of obsessional disorders is a multi-disciplinary affair. The diagnostic category alone is insufficient to serve as a basis for decisions regarding treatment. What is required is a careful formulation, setting out the symptoms and signs, the various types of maladjustment, the life situation and the important interpersonal problems. From this a programme of treatment should follow logically, the targets for each component being operationally defined. Tranquillizing or anti-depressant drugs may be indicated. There may be problems which can be attacked by a psychologist or other person sophisticated in the methods of behavioural manipulation. The social worker may have an important role in exploring and attempting to manipulate some of the salient variables in the patient's interpersonal relationships and social environment. For in-patients the part to be played by nursing staff and occupational therapists will need to be thoroughly explored. Within this context it will become apparent that informal psychotherapy is a necessary but not sufficient component of treatment.

M. Sternberg

Physical treatments in obsessional disorders

INTRODUCTION

The subject of this chapter is the effect on people with obsessional symptoms of drugs, electricity or surgical brain lesions. The number of recorded observations is small and most of them were not made under controlled conditions. The work of different doctors is seldom comparable in this field. Such knowledge as exists seems often to be based more on the persuasiveness and prestige of the investigator than on repetition of the result by independent observation or experiment. However, the way for orderly scientific advance has been prepared by the pioneers. Only organization, money and will are still lacking.

Names

Since Morel used the term 'obsession' in 1891 the following synonyms have become attached to this group of symptoms: obsessive compulsive reaction, neurosis, obsessive behaviour, obsessionalism, manie or folie de doute (Janet, 1903) Zwangskrankheit, or compulsion insanity (Kraepelin, 1921), obsessive tension states, anancastic disorder (Jaspers, 1946; Rados, 1959). These names have been used in the research on which this paper is based. 'Compulsive gambling', 'compulsive lying' and 'compulsive theft' have not been included in the study. Neither has the concept of 'obsessional personality' or 'anancastic personality' been considered.

Definitions

Most authors agree with Sir Aubrey Lewis (1934) that three essential characteristics must be described with an obsessional symptom:

1. The experience of an inner compelling force.
2. Internal resistance to it.
3. Retention of insight.

To this might be added:

4. Suffering – for many patients experience phenomena with the above characteristics and yet are not seriously upset or disabled. Feeling a hurt or being prevented from working may make a symptom out of a mental event. As in so many psychiatric disorders, those around the patient may suffer more than the patient. Their pressure may propel the person towards the doctor and into the position of patient. This has an important bearing on any treatment, particularly treatment in hospital and treatment with drugs. The prescriber and the patient must be considered. A mechanistic restriction to pharmacology and dose will not suffice here even if one nods in acknowledgement towards the placebo effect.

Natural history

Whilst this is not the place to discuss the natural history in detail, some indications concerning the course of the illness and of outcome without treatment are needed in order to be able to judge the efficacy of physical intervention. Greenacre (1923), Bumke (1921), Lewis (1936), Ibor (1952) and Pollitt (1956) considered that the majority of obsessive compulsive illnesses were phasic. Pollitt (1957) found that the mean number of attacks was two and that 88 per cent of his patients had only three attacks. Ingram, however, found that only 13 per cent had a phasic illness and that in 54 per cent it pursued a constant course (1961b); but it should be noted that his patients were drawn from a different population. An episodic course makes it difficult to judge any treatment. The patients' reluctance to continue with medication, or indeed help, is another complicating factor. In these circumstances large numbers of patients need to be observed for long periods in order to arrive at any definitive conclusions. The relative rarity of obsessive compulsive neurosis may be responsible for the paucity of investigations.

Luff and Garrod (1935) found that nearly 52 per cent of their selected and possibly atypical obsessional patients improved after psychotherapy alone (followed up for three years).

39 per cent of hospital patients followed up for nearly six years had improved symptomatically without leucotomy. 66 per cent were work-

TABLE 12.1 *Outcome in obsessional disorder without the intervention of leucotomy*

| | SAMPLE CHARACTERISTICS | | | | CONDITION OF FOLLOW-UP | | |
Investigator	Place	Patient source*	Number†	Follow-up to nearest year	Asymptomatic	Improved	Unimproved
Balslev-Olsen et al. (1958)	Denmark	o	52	0–8	6	58	37
Grimshaw (1965)	UK	i	97	1–14	40	24	35
Hastings (Goodwin, 1969)	USA	i	23	6–12	13	40	47
Ingram (1961)	UK	i	46	1–11	9	30	61
Kringlen (1965)	Norway	i	85	13–20	4	45	45
Langfeldt (1938)	Norway	i	27	1–11	26	41	33
Lewis (1936)	UK	i o	50	>5	32	34	34
Lo (1967)	Hong Kong	i	87	1–14	20	36	44
Luff et al. (1935)	UK	i o	49	3	39	27	34
Müller (1953 & 1957)	Switzerland	i	57	15–35	28	50	22
Pollitt (Goodwin, 1969)	UK	i o	66	0–15	24	48	28
Rennie (Goodwin, 1969)	USA	i	47	20	36	38	26
Rüdin (1953)	Germany	i	130	2–26	12	26	61

* i = inpatients   o = outpatients

† The number excluded leucotomized patients and those dead on follow-up. (from Goodwin *et al.*, 1969.)

ing. These results were reported by Ingram at a time when few treatments were available (1961).

Pollitt found that most of his patients were better after four years, and were better without leucotomy (1957). He noted that the symptoms gradually lessened until they became unobtrusive and only present when the patient was fatigued or anxious. Recovery was seldom smooth and even. Ingram, however, considered spontaneous recovery rare and felt that the outcome could hardly be worse than that found in his severely ill patients in hospital: 39 per cent constant and worsening; 15 per cent constant and static; 33 per cent fluctuating but never free; 13 per cent phasic.

The predictors of good outcome according to all authors are similar to those that are associated with favourable response to any treatment and are listed by Goodwin *et al.* (1969) (see Table 12.1) as:

1. Mild or atypical symptoms. Absence of compulsions (motor symptoms); phobic symptoms and ruminations predominate.
2. Short duration of symptoms prior to treatment.
3. Good previous personality.

Lewis (1936) noted that the specific content of the obsessions had no prognostic significance.

It is of some interest that brain damage may precede the onset of obsessional symptoms as in encephalitis (Szilard and Stutte, 1968), when antibiotics may be useful and a good outcome is to be expected. Gunshot wounds and the degenerations due to ageing (Slater and Roth, 1969; Krakowski, 1965) are other examples of brain cell death which may be associated with obsessional symptoms. Yet ageing and brain destructive operations often have a beneficial effect on patients with obsessive–compulsive neurosis (Slater and Roth, 1969; Kringlen, 1965). Remission of obsessional symptoms has been noted with semi-starvation in prisoners of war and with vomiting and with physical debility (Sargant and Slater, 1950).

CHEMOTHERAPY

1. *The Mono Amine Oxidase Inhibitors* combined with a minor tranquillizer will often cause depression to lift and tension to lessen or even disappear. They will not help pure obsessional states (Dally, 1967; Kalinowsky and Hippius, 1969; Van Renynghe de Voxvrie, 1968; Annesley, 1969). Isocarboxasid 10 mgm and chlordiazepoxide 5 mgm three times daily would be a suitable dose. The patient must be warned

about the necessary dietary restrictions and should be given a warning card to carry.

2. *Tricyclic anti-depressants* are usually unsuccessful except for trimipramine and clomipramine (van Renynghe de Voxvrie, 1968; Breitner, 1960; Laboucarie *et al.*, 1967; Maillet-Jurquet *et al.*, 1970). Clomipramine can be given as an intravenous infusion starting with 25 mgm in 250 ml dextrose saline and given over two to three hours. One infusion is given each day. The patient is closely observed. Regular recordings are made of blood pressure and pulse at ten-minute intervals. The dose is built up to obtain maximum benefit. If unpleasant effects intervene the dose is lowered and maintained. Early signs of excess are tremor, ataxia, dizziness due to hypotension. There may be difficulty in micturition. Treatment is best on an inpatient basis, but can be given to out-patients if adequate time and space for supervision are available. The maximum dose reached is usually about 200 mgm clomipramine in an infusion. The next day the dose is reduced and the decrease made up by a similar oral dose. The substitution from infusion to oral medication proceeds by steps and is complete after five to seven days. The patient is then maintained on his maximum dose of clomipramine for at least three months during which time he is discharged from hospital and resumes his work. In two patients observed by the author the results were dramatic and the cure complete. In neither patient had there been any clinical evidence of depression. Van Renynghe de Voxvrie (1968) treated fifteen patients with clomipramine, but only one with intravenous infusion method. These few results are only suggestive and no double blind trial has been published to date. However, a complete removal of obsessional symptoms is of interest even if it has only been observed in a few patients.

Doxepin and amitriptylene were found to benefit patients in a double blind trial carried out by Bauer and Novak (1969). The drugs are similar chemically and allow of flexible dosage, but their cholinergic side effects may be troublesome to obsessional patients.

3. *Tranquillizers*

Trifluoperazine has little effect (Kalinowsky and Hippius, 1969). Neki and Kishore found that the obsessional symptoms improved when they treated a patient's tropical eosinophilia with the piperazine diethyl carbamazapine (1962).

Chlordiazepoxide is considered ineffective by Kalinowsky and Hippius (1969), but satisfactory by Breitner, who found that six out of his seven patients responded well to treatment (1960). Hess (1968) also obtained good results with 60–80 mgm chlordiazepoxide daily in divided doses. Dally (1967) recommends it in combination with an anti-depressant drug and, if necessary, ECT.

Diazepam was helpful in relieving anxiety in 40 to 50 per cent of Bethune's 140 patients (1964), but only one of these patients had suffered from a long-standing obsessional disorder. She did, however, obtain 'complete relief'. While the details are lacking in Bethune's paper, Venkoba Rao gave a careful account of 16 obsessional patients, 8 of whom were treated with placebo and 8 with diazepam (1964). The trial was not double blind and he followed the patient's progress for only six weeks. He found that the patients treated with diazepam improved compared with those treated with placebo. Compulsions, however, remained even in the treated patient.

Orvin compared *Oxazepam* to chlordiazepoxide and placebo in a double blind crossover trial (1967). He found that 68 per cent of his 24 patients with obsessional symptoms improved significantly on oxazepam as compared to 13 per cent on chlordiazepoxide and none on placebo.

Perphenazine in low dosage (2 mgm three times daily) may help some patients (Dally, 1967). *Triflupromazine – Vesprin* is said to be helpful (Kalinowsky and Hippius, 1969).

Methylperidol (luvatren), 15 to 40 mgm, gave improvement in half of a series of six patients, without weight gain and without side effects (Reiter, 1969).

Cholorpromazine relieved the obsessional's tension but did not affect his mode of thought (Garmany *et al.*, 1954).

Levopromazine up to 1700 mgm daily, combined with LSD and psychoanalysis was used to achieve first regression and then retraining, with success, on one patient, a doctor (Nishizono, 1969). Three other patients failed to respond.

4. *Narcotherapy* using short-life barbiturates, such as *thiopentone* or *methohexitone*, may be helpful in the treatment of anxiety in obsessional patients (Kalinowsky and Hippius, 1969). Administration of barbiturates by mouth is undesirable because of the danger of addiction and the suicide risk. *Meprobamate* was considered to be no better than barbiturate for these patients. Prolonged sleep induced by barbiturates caused confusion (Sargant and Slater, 1950).

5. *Carbon dioxide abreaction*, using Meduna's method makes obsessional patients worse (Sargant and Slater, 1950) or at best is ineffective (Slater and Roth, 1969). *Lysergic acid diethylamide* may produce long-lasting obsessional ruminations and has no effect on the compulsions.

Many patients are worse after this attempt at treatment (Dally, 1967).

Methyl amphetamine abreaction is occasionally helpful (Slater and Roth, 1969), but there is a serious risk of addiction if the treatment is often repeated.

Intravenous acetylcholine in doses of up to 0·2 g and given over 20 to 30 seconds was used on 81 patients by Lopez Ibor (1952). 60 per cent rapidly recovered, but many relapsed and needed repeat courses of treatment. Sargant treated 70 patients with the same method, but these were people suffering from 'mild obsessional personality with anxiety and some obsessional symptoms' and not afflicted with obsessional neurosis (1952). 25 per cent were greatly helped and 20 per cent improved.

7. *Insulin.* Long-standing neuroses are not improved or relieved by insulin subcoma treatment ('modified insulin'). There is, however, a decrease of anxiety in 60 per cent of patients treated with mild hypoglycaemia over four weeks and as in-patients (Berbath, 1959).

8. *Stilboestrol* may decrease tension in male obsessionals at the same time as their libido is decreased. Wieczorek found *ovulation inhibitors* useful in some female patients with repeated depressions where there was a regular coincidence in time with a phase of the ovulatory cycle. Some patients, of course, became more depressed.

9. *Lithium salts* may be helpful when there is an association between obsessive symptoms and cyclical mood changes (Editorial, 1968).

10. Treatments which have been found ineffective are *reserpine* and *metrazole* (pharmacological convulsions) (Kalinowsky and Hippius, 1969).

ELECTROCONVULSIVE THERAPY

Obsessional symptoms are common in depression (Kendell and DiScipio, 1970; Gittleson, 1966b) and electroconvulsive therapy (ECT) is accepted as effective treatment for depression, even when it develops in a person who already had an obsessional disorder (Slater and Roth, 1969; Roth, 1965). The treatment is directed against the depression. As it lifts the obsessional symptoms may lessen or depart. The patient may attribute his depression to the obsessional disorder. When he is no longer depressed, he may again be able to tolerate the obsessional symptoms. Sargant and Slater (1950) warn of the harmful effects of

ECT when it is used to treat an obsessional disorder, presumably in the absence of depression. When the patient recovers from the treatment he returns to his old patterns of thought and behaviour, but has a residual memory impairment in addition to his original troubles. In some patients there is an outburst of aggression after the first one or two treatments. In others a state of depersonalization with anxiety develops which may persist for years. Kalinowsky and Hippius (1969) warn of the harmful regression which may occur in obsessional patients with intensive ECT.

ECT is only curative for some episodic obsessional disorders which are associated with depression and where the patient is free of all symptoms when he is not depressed. In the typical obsessive–compulsive neurosis ECT is best used with caution and only if depression develops and fails to respond to other measures. It would be necessary to admit the patient to hospital and assess him or her carefully after each treatment.

Stafford Clark (1954, 1965) reported one obsessional patient, a youth of 16, who was given twenty *electronarcosis* (Loukas *et al.*, 1965) treatments, with good results, but who relapsed at the end of a five-year follow-up. The treatment was given twice weekly, after muscle relaxant and general anaesthetic, at 250 volts maximum, 200–250 milliamps a.c., high frequency on a Shotter and Richs apparatus. The technique is described by Paterson and Milligan (1948). Garmany and Early (1948) considered the risk from this method to be more than the benefit and Gray Walter (1966) thought that 'electronarcosis' was a misnomer, the treatment being dependent on over-stimulation, exhaustion and reconditioning.

BRAIN SURGERY

1. *Standard leucotomy*

Willett, reviewing the subject in 1960, commented that 'a) Psychosurgery has been based upon a set of observations of dubious validity and on a tenuous rationale. b) The most responsible and best executed studies in the field have been most cautious in associating specific surgical procedures with clinical improvements.' He had carefully assessed the published animal and human studies to that date.

The possible benefit of leucotomy might be a reduction in anxiety tension and a lessening of reactive depression. Sargant (1962) found that tense, obsessive, ruminative people of good previous personality who had broken down after the age of 25 derived most benefit from leucotomy. There was a price to pay in the form of 3·1 per cent severe, permanent and undesirable side effects. His opinion was based on the 15,000 patients treated with leucotomy between 1942 and 1962 (two-thirds of whom had been treated between the years 1942 and 1954). Only a small proportion of these patients suffered from obsessional disorders. Indeed, his contra-indications to leucotomy included compulsions which were long-standing, a long history dating back to childhood, youth and lack of drive. Many of these features are common to obsessional patients. He favoured open operations and felt that multiple operations are sometimes indicated.

It would be difficult to decide upon leucotomy if one accepted Pollitt's (1957) view of the natural history of obsessional states with 68 per cent of his series of 150 patients starting their symptoms before the age of 25 years, most having a first attack between the ages of 11 and 15 and then pursuing an episodic course. He found the mean number of attacks was two. One might, however, hope for results like those of Freeman and Watts (1950), who considered 55 per cent were 'good' and 35 per cent 'fair' but did not describe in detail the patients, their symptoms or the means used to judge the results. They had operated on 85 people with obsessional tension states or obsessive–compulsive neurosis. *The ideas and compulsions continued* but feeling tone was lost. This seems a poor result from a serious operation. The decline in number of leucotomies carried out makes it likely that such is the opinion of the majority of clinicians.

Elithorn and Beck (1955) were of the opinion that 'anatomically similar lesions will not give the same result in different patients'. They based this opinion on a most careful clinicopathological report. It was not possible to produce anatomically similar lesions (Beck and Corsellis, 1960). Berliner *et al.* (1945) commented that they used 'the method of Freeman and Watts' and that it was 'almost blind'.

One had then an imprecise but 3 to 4 per cent lethal operation, the result of which was not to remove those symptoms which characterized obsessional disorder. From this point of view the effects were non-specific. They improved the patient's mood and relieved his tension and altered his personality. These changes, including the last, as Elithorn and Beck (1955) suggested, might, in about half the operated cases, lead to a 'cure' which seems to have been a general agreement that the patient was well; well enough to go home and resume his normal life. One must probably accept the judgement of experienced and learned psychiatrists that 'well' was just that, for all clinical purposes. Figure 12.1 shows some results.

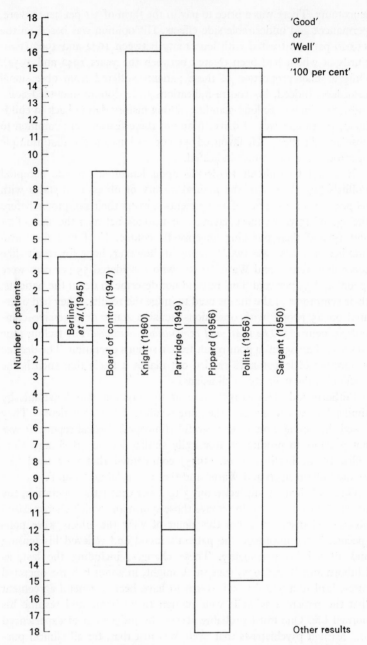

Fig. 12.1 Results of standard leucotomy in patients with obsessional symptoms.

2. *Other forms of leucotomy*

If standard leucotomy had as its original target the cure, or at least the amelioration of schizophrenia, and fell into disuse, then the descriptions of successor operations seem to be preoccupied with their own justification as regards accuracy and safety (Editorial, 1966).

Knight (1964) lists the following types of operation in historical sequence:

1. Moniz – alcohol injections.
2. Early operation destroying the central core of white matter.
3. Standard leucotomy of Freeman and Watts (1950).
4. Restricted lower segment version of Bauer and Novak (1969).
5. Scoville's orbital undercutting (1960).
6. Knight's modification of Scoville's operation of 1950 (Scoville, 1960).
7. Yttrium 90 seeds implanted stereotactically (Knight, 1964).

The titles of the first five may be taken as the surgeon's intention rather than what is actually done. Few pathological studies exist to show what the lesions were and the number of patients studied are very small indeed. Scoville, however, claimed that 'the technique can be exactly duplicated from patient to patient'. It does seem to be very difficult to make precise lesions at brain operations without the aid of stereotactic methods (Hassler, 1967). Knight (1964) claimed that 'only area 13' was affected by his method. The results of modified leucotomy on obsessional disorders seem less promising than those of standard leucotomy, as Figure 12.2 indicates.

Scoville (1960) comments that 'obsessive–compulsive psychoneurosis proved the most intractable' to treatment. It exhibited 'more variability and relapses' than the other psychoneuroses. Like the standard method, 'the benefit of selective leucotomy lies more in the blunting of the higher sensitivities than in a changing of disease patterns'.

The criticisms of Willett (1960) apply to all these papers.

It was not until Sykes' and Tredgold's work in 1964 that a proper and detailed study was made of the effect of leucotomy on patients with obsessional symptoms. The focus was on the patient and not on the operation. They confirmed that improvement was associated with decrease in tension and in scrupulousness. The patient's standards were reduced and fell into line with those of society. Everyone treated showed benefit for a time, but only 50 per cent maintained significant improvement. In most, '*the (obsessional) symptoms persisted but were less*

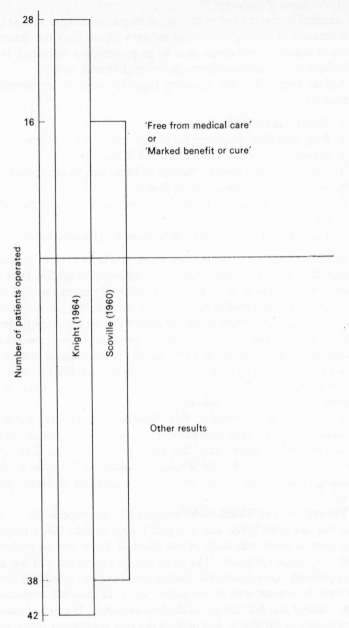

Fig. 12.2 Results of modified leucotomy.

disabling'. They made the useful distinction between ability to work and improvement as judged by the psychiatrist. They assessed capacity for leisure enjoyment and found it often reduced. There was a 1·5 per cent mortality in their series. 16 per cent of the patients had fits, maximum number 12. 5 per cent of patients had an adverse change of personality. This was commoner in patients under 40 with previously poor personality. Lack of consideration, lack of insight, release of hostility, outspokenness, reduction of affect, reduction of standards and excessive volubility were the main adverse factors which were noted.

The factors associated with a favourable result to leucotomy may be listed:

good previous personality, responsive to environment with good drive;
stable home environment;
work available or waiting to be resumed;
over the age of 40 years;
recent onset of illness;
presence of reactive anxiety and tension and phobias and rumination;
absence of long-standing or well-established compulsive rituals.

Most of them are associated also with spontaneous recovery and response to other forms of treatment.

Unfavourable factors with regard to leucotomy of any kind are:

age under 40 years;
unmarried, particularly unmarried women;
lack of drive, lack of response to environment;
early onset of symptoms and their acceptance (five years or more of illness in Sykes' and Tredgold's series, 1964);
personality abnormalities, including aggressiveness, sexual deviations, unadaptability and inflexibility;
symptoms suggestive of schizophrenia.

The present situation, therefore, seems to be that while half the patients with obsessional disorders who have some form of leucotomy may be expected to benefit greatly, these are also the patients who have a better prognosis without leucotomy. Those undergoing operation run a 1·5 per cent to 4 per cent risk of dying. 16 per cent may be expected to have up to twelve epileptic fits. There may be wound complications. Improvement in the patient's condition is associated with personality change and this is paid for by a permanent brain lesion. The changed personality is dependent on social factors for a successful outcome. One may have to wait for years to see the improvement (Sykes and Tred-gold, 1964; Pippard, 1956). With all these provisos it is the patient who is being adjusted to live more comfortably with his obsessional disorder and not the obsessional disorder which is being treated (Hassler, 1967). The present knowledge may be helpful to a clinician and may benefit his patient, but it rests on scientifically shaky foundations. Having failed to produce more than one study of effects on personality and working capacity in leucotomy's twenty-year period of acceptance, the chance is now small of working with adequate number of patients (Bonis *et al.*, 1968; Northfield, 1960).

3. *Other forms of brain operation*

Whitty in 1955 reported a series of 10 patients suffering from ob-sessional symptoms in whom area 24 of Brodmann was ablated by suction. He followed these patients' progress for from between two months and six years. He found that 6 had greatly improved, 4 im-proved, of whom one died. Although he considered that the personality was less blunted than after leucotomy, the reported changes in per-sonality and operative sequelae seem much the same. Lewin (1960) felt that anterior cingulectomy was to be preferred to other brain operations for obsessional patients and particularly for professionals. Le Beau (1953) found that his 7 patients who had undergone anterior cingulectomy because of obsessional symptoms were not noticeably better than before the operation. Crow (1973) in Bristol has used multiple lesions made with wire insertions and reported excellent results.

COMBINATIONS OF TREATMENT

It would be fair to quote the last sentence of the book by Kalinowsky and Hippius (1969). 'At present, we can say only that we are treating empirically disorders whose aetiology is unknown, with methods whose action is also shrouded in mystery.' In such a situation it is necessary to do the best one can for the patient, relieving and comforting where cure may be elusive. The empirical physical and chemical methods can usually give some relief. The problem is to establish such a relationship with the patient that confidence can be maintained while the empirical search continues for their individual prescription. The search would be difficult to tolerate, even in a person whose illness did not produce doubt and rumination. Salzman clearly describes the patient's doubt, ambivalence, insecurity and need to control the situation (1966). Patients with obsessional symptoms are often unreliable with regard to taking their medication. Many resent having to take tablets and are quick to complain of side effects, using them as an excuse to cease treatment. They are secretive about their symptoms and try to cope without psychiatric help (Stengel, 1956). Pollitt found that it was $7\frac{1}{2}$ years on the average from the onset of symptoms before a doctor was seen (1956).

A start can be made with a small dose of piperazine tranquillizer, perphenazine 2 mgm three times daily, or trifluoperazine 1 mgm three times daily combined with an anti-depressant. Doxepin 10 mgm three times daily or only morning and midday with amitriptylene 10 or 25 mgm at night would be suitable. If there is no response within one or two weeks, the dose can be cautiously increased to double the above, stopping if there is a complaint of side effects. At low doses the side effects are usually drowsiness, dry mouth, dizziness (due to postural hypotension). If, after four weeks, the simple out-patient treatment has not relieved the patient, or if the symptoms were severe at the onset, then he would best be admitted to hospital for a trial of intravenous clomipramine, followed by clomipramine by mouth. If the onset of obsessional symptoms coincided with severe depression, or if depressive symptomatology is prominent, trimipramine may be needed in the maximum dose tolerated by the patient with perphenazine and also ECT.

When there is no obvious depression, and when the symptoms have resisted treatment with doxepin and perphenazine, later clomipramine, then it would seem reasonable to try isocarboxazid with chlordiazepoxide, as described above, observing all the precautions and ensuring that the patient also understands.

Should all the above fail and the ability to work and lead a normal life be lost and should no natural spontaneous remission occur for one year or more, then it is worthwhile discussing with the patient, his family, general practitioner and an independent psychiatrist the possibility of a leucotomy of some sort. A case for operation may then be submitted for consideration to a neurosurgeon who has experience in this field.

After the leucotomy vigorous rehabilitation is needed, starting in hospital. The best setting is the psychiatric unit where the patient was originally treated. In some people one of the other physical treatments only becomes effective after leucotomy, even when the operation by itself failed to give lasting relief.

A proportion of patients obtain no help from any physical treatment. The size of this moiety is not exactly known, since the numbers in all the series are so small. 5 per cent may be a fair estimate.

CONCLUSION

Physical treatments have not yet been properly evaluated in the treatment of obsessional disorders. The most thoroughly investigated form of treatment has been leucotomy. The result is an even (50 per cent) chance of significant improvement.[1] There are observations which make worthwhile the study of trimipramine and particularly clomipramine as used in obsessional disorders. Patients with these disorders are usually intelligent and incapacitated in their prime (Pollitt, 1956; Rosenberg, 1967). If one had to draw up a list of priorities for nation-wide research in psychiatric illness, obsessional disorders and their treatment would surely deserve a high place. Study would have to be simultaneous in many centres, but centrally coordinated, and a Medical Research Council Centre for such study would be appropriate. The numbers for scientific investigation could only be obtained by joint effort.

[1] It may well be that Crow's methods hold some promise for the future (Crow, 1973).

References

ADER, R. (1964) Gastric erosions in the rat: effect of immobilization at different points in the activity cycle. *Science*, **145.**

ADER, R. (1971) Experimentally induced gastric lesions. *Adv. Psychosom. Med.*, **6,** 1–39.

ADLER, M. H. (1970) Report of panel on 'Psychoanalysis and psychotherapy'. *Internat. J. Psychoanal.*, **51,** 219.

AITKEN, R. C. B. (1969) Measurement of feelings using visual analogue scales. *Proc. Roy. Soc. Med.*, **62,** 989–93.

ALAPIN, B. (1972) Personal communication.

ANDERSON, E. W. (1971) No other English work of its kind. *Brit. J. Psychiat.*, **118,** 357–60.

ANDREW, R. J. (1956) Some remarks on behaviour in conflict situations, with special reference to Emberiza Spp. *Brit. J. Anim. Behav.*, **4,** 85–91.

ANNESLEY, P. T. (1969) Nardil response in a chronic obsessive compulsive. *Brit. J. Psychiat.*, **115,** 748.

ANTROBUS, J. S. (1968) Information theory and stimulus-independent thought. *Brit. J. Psychol.*, **59,** 423–30

APPLEZWEIG, D. G. (1954) Some determinants of behavioural rigidity. *J. Abnorm. Soc. Psychol.*, **49,** 224–8.

ARGYLE, M. (1969) *Social Interaction.* London: Methuen.

ASCH, M. G. (1958) Negative response set bias and personality adjustment. *J. Cons. Psychol.*, **5,** 206–10.

AZRIN, N. H. & HOLZ, W. C. (1966) Punishment. In HONING, W. K. (ed.) *Operant Behaviour: Areas of Research and Application.* New York: Appleton-Century-Crofts.

BADIA, P., MCBANE, B., SUTER, S. & LEWIS, P. (1966) Preference behaviour in an immediate versus variably delayed shock situation with and without warning signal. *J. Exp. Psychol.*, **72,** 847–52.

BAILEY, J. & HUTCHINSON, T. (1969) The treatment of compulsive hand-washing using reinforcement principles. *Beh. Res. & Ther.*, **7,** 327–9.

BALKAN, EVA & MASSERMAN, J. H. (1940) The language of phantasy. III. The Language of the phantasies of patients with conversion hysteria, anxiety state, and obsessive–compulsive neuroses. *J. Psychol.*, **10,** 75–86.

BALSLEV-OLESEN, T. & GEERT-JØRGENSEN, E. (1959) The prognosis of obsessive–compulsive neurosis. *Acta Psychiat. Scand.* Suppl. 136, **34,** 232–41.

BANDURA, A. (1969) *Principles of Behavior Modification.* New York: Holt, Rinehart & Winston.

BANNISTER, D. (1960) Conceptual structure in thought-disordered schizophrenics. *J. Ment. Sci.*, **106,** 1230–49.

BANNISTER, D. (1962) The nature and measurement of schizophrenic thought disorder. *J. Ment. Sci.*, **108,** 825–42.

BANNISTER, D. (1963) The genesis of schizophrenic thought disorder: a serial invalidation hypothesis. *Brit. J. Psychiat.*, **111,** 377–82.

BANNISTER, D. & FRANSELLA, FAY (1966) A grid test of schizophrenic thought disorder. *Brit. J. Soc. Clin. Psychol.*, **5,** 95–102.

BANNISTER, D. & FRANSELLA, FAY (1967) *A Grid Test of Schizophrenic Thought Disorder.* Barnstaple: Psychological Test Publications.

BANNISTER, D. & FRANSELLA, FAY (1971) *Inquiring Man.* Harmondsworth: Penguin.

BANNISTER, D., FRANSELLA, FAY & AGNEW, JOYCE (1971) Characteristics and validity of the Grid Test of Thought Disorder. *Brit. J. Soc. Clin. Psychol.*, **10,** 144–51.

BARNES, C. A. (1952) A statistical study of the Freudian theory of levels of psychosexual development. *Genet. Psychol. Monogr.*, **45,** 109–74.

BARRETT, W., CALDBECK-MEENAN, J. & WHITE, J. G. (1966) Questionnaire measures and psychiatrists' ratings of a personality dimension. *Brit. J. Psychiat.*, **112,** 413–15.

BARRON, F. (1955) The disposition towards originality. *J. Abnorm. Soc. Psychol.*, **51,** 478–85.

BATES, H. D. (1970) Relevance of animal-avoidance analogue studies to the treatment of clinical phobias: A rejoinder to Cooper, Furst and Bridger. *J. Abnorm Psychol.*, **75,** 104–12.

BAUER, G. & NOVAK, H. (1969) Doxepin, ein neues Antidepressivum; Wirkungvergleich mit Amitriptylin. *Arzneimittelforsch.*, **19,** 1642.

BAUM, M. (1968) Efficacy of response prevention (flooding) in facilitating the extinction of an avoidance response in rats: The effects of overtraining the response. *Beh. Res. & Ther.*, **6,** 197–203.

BAUM, M. (1969) Extinction of an avoidance response prevention: Some parametric investigations. *Can. J. Psychol.*, **23,** 1–10.

BAUM, M. (1970) Extinction of avoidance responding through response prevention (flooding). *Psychol. Bull.*, **74,** 276–84.

BAUM, M. (1971) Extinction of avoidance response in rats via response prevention (flooding): A test for residual fear. *Psychol. Rep.*, **28,** 203–8.

BAUM, M. & MYRAN, D. D. (1971) Response prevention (flooding) in rats: The effects of restricting exploration during flooding and of massed versus distributed flooding. *Can. J. Psychol.*, **25,** (2).

BEACH, F. A. (1947) A review of physiological and psychological studies of sexual behaviour in mammals. *Physiol. Rev.*, **27,** 240–307.

BEACH, F. A. (1951) Instinctive behaviour: Reproductive activities. In STEVENS, S. S. (ed.) *Handbook of Experimental Psychology.* New York: Wiley.

BECK, E. & CORSELLIS, J. (1960) Pathological and anatomical aspects of orbital undercutting. *Proc. Roy. Soc. Med.*, **53,** 737.

BEECH, H. R. (1969) *Changing Man's Behaviour.* Harmondsworth: Penguin.

BEECH, H. R. (1971) Ritualistic activity in obsessional patients. *J. Psychosom. Res.*, **15,** 417–22.

BEG, R. R. & HASAN, K. Z. (1970) Gilles de la Tourette's Syndrome; a report of two cases from Pakistan. *J. Pakistan Med. Assoc.*, **20,** 330–5.

BELOFF, H. (1957) The structure and origin of the anal character. *Genet. Psychol. Monogr.*, **55,** 141–72.

BENAIM, S. (1956) *A Clinical Study of Obsessional Illness in Old Age.* Dissertation for the Academic Postgraduate Diploma in Psychological Medicine of the University of London.

BERBATH, A. K. (1959) Effects of mild hypoglycaemia. In RINKEL, M. & HIMWICH, E. (eds.) *Insulin Treatment in Psychiatry.* New York: Philosophical Library.

BERKSON, G., HERMELIN, B. & O'CONNOR, M. (1961) Physiological responses of normals and institutionalized mental defectives to repeated stimuli. *J. Ment. Defic. Res.*, **5,** 30–9.

BERLINER, F., BEVERIDGE, R. L., MAYER-GROSS, W. & MOORE,

J. N. P. (1945) Prefrontal leucotomy: Report on 100 cases. *Lancet*, **2**, 325.

BERLYNE, D. E. (1960) *Conflict, Arousal and Curiosity*. New York: McGraw-Hill.

BERMAN, L. (1942) Obsessive–compulsive neurosis in children. *J. Nerv. Ment. Dis.*, **95**, 26–39.

BETHUNE, H. C. *et al.* (1964) A new compound in the treatment of severe anxiety states: Report on the use of diazepam. *New Zeal. Med. J.*, **63**, 153–6.

BEVAN, J. R. (1960) Learning theory applied to the treatment of a patient with obsessional ruminations. In EYSENCK, H. J. (ed.) *Behaviour Therapy and the Neurosis*. Oxford: Pergamon Press.

BIBRING, E. (1954) Psychoanalysis and the dynamic psychotherapies. *J. Amer. Psychoanal. Assoc.*, **2**, 745–70.

BIERI, J. (1966) Cognitive complexity and personality development. In HARVEY, O. J. (ed.) *Experience, Structure and Adaptability*. New York: Springer.

BINDRA, D. (1959) *Motivation: A Systematic Reinterpretation*. New York: Ronald Press.

BINDRA, D. & SPINNER, N. (1958) Response to different degrees of novelty: The incidence of various activities. *J. Exp. Anal. Behav.*, **1**, 341–50.

BLACKER, C. P. & GORE, A. T. (1955) Triennial Statistical Report, Bethlem Royal and Maudsley Hospitals.

BLUM, G. S. (1949) A study of the psychoanalytic theory of psychosexual development. *Genet. Psychol. Monogr.*, **39**, 3–99.

BOARD OF CONTROL (1947) Results in 1000 leucotomies. London: HMSO.

BOLLES, R. C. (1960) Grooming behaviour in the rat. *J. Comp. Physiol. Psychol.*, **53**, 306–10.

BOLLES, R. C. (1970) Species-specific defence reactions and avoidance in learning. *Psychol. Rev.*, **77**, 32–48.

BONARIUS, J. C. J. (1970) *Personal Construct Psychology and Extreme Response Style*. Ph.D. thesis, Gronigen.

BONIS, A. *et al.* (1968) Indications for leucotomy. *Encephale*, **57**, 439–73, 525–63.

BOREN, J. J., SIDMAN, M. & HERRNSTEIN, R. J. (1959) Avoidance, escape and extinction as a function of shock intensity. *J. Comp. Physiol. Psychol.*, **52**, 420–5.

BRATFOS, O. (1970) Transition of neuroses and other minor disorders into psychoses. *Acta Psychiat. Scand.*, **46**, 35–49.

BREITNER, C. (1960) Drug therapy in obsessional states and other psychiatric problems. *Dis. Nerv. Syst.* (Suppl.) **21**, 31–5.

BRIERLEY, HARRY (1969) The habituation of forearm muscle blood flow in phobic subjects. *Neurol. Neurosurg. Psychiat.*, **32**, 15–20.

BROADHURST, P. L. (1957) Determinants of emotionality in the rat: I. Situational factors. *Brit. J. Psychol.*, **48**, 1–12.

BROADHURST, P. L. (1958) The contribution of animal psychology to the concept of psychological normality/abnormality. *Prox. XIII Congress Internat. Assoc. of Applied Psychol.* Rome.

BROADHURST, P. L. (1958) Determinants of emotionality in the rat: II. Antecedent factors. *Brit. J. Psychol.*, **49**, 12–20.

BROADHURST, P. L. (1960a) Abnormal animal behaviour. In EYSENCK, H. J. (ed.) *Handbook of Abnormal Psychology.* London: Pitman Med. Publishing Co.

BROADHURST, P. L. (1960b) Applications of biometrical genetics to the inheritance of behaviour. In EYSENCK, H. J. (ed.) *Experiments in Personality*, Vol. I. London: Routledge & Kegan Paul.

BROADHURST, P. L. (1967) Psychology in its natural habitat. Inaugural lecture, University of Birmingham.

BROWN, F. W. (1942) Heredity in the psychoneuroses. *Proc. Roy. Soc. Med.*, **35**, 785–90.

BROWN, J. S., MARTIN, R. C. & MORROW, M. W. (1964) Self-punitive behaviour in the rat: Facilitative effects of punishment on resistance to extinction. *J. Comp. Physiol. Psychol.*, **57**, 127–33.

BRUSH, F. R. (1957) The effects of shock intensity on the acquisition and extinction of an avoidance response in dogs. *J. Comp. Physiol. Psychol.*, **50**, 547–52.

BUMKE, O. (1929) *Lehrbuch der Geisteskrankheiten.* Leipzig: Springer. (3rd ed., Munich: Bergmann.)

CAINE, T. M. & HAWKINS, L. G. (1963) Questionnaire measure of the hysteroid-obsessoid component of personality. *J. Consult Psychol.*, **27**, 206–9.

CAINE, T. M. & HOPE, K. (1967) *Manual of the Hysteroid–Obsessoid Questionnaire.* London: University of London Press.

CAMERON, D. E. (1968) *Psychotherapy in Action.* New York: Grune and Stratton.

CAMPBELL, DOUGAL, SANDERSON, R. E. & LAVERTY, S. G. (1964) Characteristics of a conditioned response in human subjects during extinction trials following a single traumatic conditioning trial. *J. Abnorm. Soc. Psychol.*, **68**, 6, 627–39.

CAPSTICK, N. (1971) Anafril in obsessional states: A follow-up study. Vth World Congr. Psychiat., Mexico.

CARON, A. & WALLACH, M. A. (1959) Personality determinants of repressive and obsessive reactions to failure-stress. *J. Abnorm. Soc. Psychol.*, **59**, 236-45.

CARR, A. T. (1970) *A Psychophysiological Study of Ritual Behaviours and Decision Processes in Compulsive Neurosis.* Unpubl. Ph.D. thesis, University of Birmingham.

CASTLE, W. E. (1930) *Genetics and Eugenics.* Cambridge, Mass.: Harvard University Press.

CASTLE, W. E. (1940) *Mammalian Genetics.* Cambridge, Mass.: Harvard University Press.

CATTELL, R. B. & STICE, G. (1958) *Handbook of the 16 PF Test.* Champaign, Illinois: IPAT.

CAUTELA, J. R. (1966) Treatment of compulsive behaviour by covert sensitization. *Psychol. Record*, **16**, 33-41.

CAUTELA, J. R. (1967) Covert sensitization. *Psychol. Record*, **20**, 459-68.

CAUTELA, J. R. (1969) Behaviour therapy and self control: Technique and implications. In FRANKS, C. M. (ed.) *Behaviour Therapy: Appraisal and Status.* New York: McGraw-Hill.

CAUTELA, J. R. (1970) Covert reinforcement. *Beh. Ther.*, **1**, 33-50.

CAWLEY, R. (1971) Evaluation of psychotherapy. *Psychol. Med.*, **1**, 101-3.

CHAMPION, R. A. & JONES, J. E. (1961) Forward, backward and pseudo-conditioning of the GSR. *J. Exp. Psychol.*, **62**, 58-61.

CHOWN, S. M. (1959) Rigidity – a flexible concept. *Psychol. Bull.*, **56**, 195-223.

CHURCH, R. (1963) The varied effects of punishment. *Psychol. Rev.*, **70**, 369-402.

CLARIDGE, G. S. (1967) *Personality and Arousal.* Oxford: Pergamon Press.

CONGER, J. J., SAWREY, W. L. & TURRELL, E. S. (1958) The role of social experience in the production of gastric ulcers in hooded rats placed in a conflict situation. *J. Abnorm. Soc. Psychol.*, **57**, 214.

COOPER, J. (1970) The Leyton Obsessional Inventory. *Psychol. Med.*, **1**, 48-64.

COOPER, J. E., GELDER, M. G. & MARKS, I. M. (1965) Results of behaviour therapy in 77 psychiatric patients. *Brit. Med. J.*, **1**, 1222-5.

COOPER, J. & MCNEILL, J. (1968) A study of houseproud housewives and their interactions with their children. *J. Child Psychol. Psychiat.*, **9**, 173–88.

COOPER, J. E. & KELLEHER, M. Y. (1972) The Leyton Obsessional Inventory: A principal components analysis on normal subjects.

COURT, J. H. & GARWOLIE, E. (1968) Schizophrenic performance on a reaction-time task with increasing levels of complexity. *Brit. J. Soc. Clin. Psychol.*, **7**, 216–23.

CREMERIUS, J. (1962) *Die Beurteilung des Behandlungserfolges in der Psychotherapie.* (Cited by Rachman, 1971.)

CROW, H. J. (1973) Intracerebral polarization and multifocal leucocoagulation in some psychiatric illnesses. *Psychiat. Neurol. Neurolchir.* (Amsterdam), **76**, 365–81.

DALBIEZ, R. (1941) *Psychoanalytic Method and the Doctrine of Freud.* London: Longmans Green.

DALLY, P. (1967) *Chemotherapy of Psychiatric Disorders* (pp. 27, 80, 114, 125). London: Logos Press.

DELAY, J. (1966) Psycho-pharmacologie et psychiatrie. (Adresse présidentiale au Congrès Internationale de Neuropsychopharmacologie) *La Presse Médicale*, **74**, 1151–56.

DELIUS, J. D. (1970) Irrelevant behaviour, information processing and arousal homeostasis. *Psychol. Forsch.*, **33**, 165–88.

DELL, P., BONVALLET, M. & HUGELIN, A. (1961) Mechanisms of reticular de-activation. In WOLSTENHOLME, G. E. W. & O'CONNOR, M. (eds.) *The Nature of Sleep.* London: Churchill.

DOTY, R. W., BECK, E. C. & KOOI, K. A. (1959) Effect of brainstem lesions on conditioned responses of cats. *Exp. Neurol.*, **1**, 360–85.

DUFFY, E. (1962) *Activation and Behavior.* New York: Wiley.

DYKMAN, R. A., REESE, W. G., GALBRECHT, C. R., ACKERMAN, P. T. & SUNDERMANN, R. S. (1968) Autonomic responses in psychiatric patients. *Ann. N.Y. Acad. Sci.*, **147**, Art. 7, 237–303.

EDITORIAL (1966) Surgery for mental illness. *Brit. Med. J.*, **1**, 310–11.

EDITORIAL (1968) Supplementary information about Lithium treatment of manic depressive disorders. *Acta Psychiat. Scand.*, Suppl. 203, 149.

EITINGER, L. (1955) Studies in neuroses. *Acta Psychiat. Scand.*, Suppl. 101.

ELITHORN, A. & BECK, W. (1955) Prefrontal leucotomy: A clinico-pathological report. *Lancet*, **1**, 23.

ELKINGTON, J. St C. (1946) In PRICE, F. (ed.) *A Textbook of the Practice of Medicine* (7th ed.), p. 1717. London: Oxford University Press.

ELLIOTT, M. H. (1934) The effect of hunger on variability of performance. *Amer. J. Psychol.*, **46**, 107–12.

ERNST, K. (1959) *Die Prognose der Neurosen*. Berlin: Springer.

ESQUIROL, J. E. D. (1838) *Des Maladies Mentales*. Vol. II. Paris: Baillière.

ESTES, W. K. (1969) New perspectives on some old issues in association theory. In MACKINTOSH, N. J. & HONING, W. K. (eds.) *Fundamental Issues in Association Learning*. Halifax: Dalhousie University Press.

EYSENCK, H. J. (1947) *The Dimensions of Personality*. London: Routledge & Kegan Paul.

EYSENCK, H. J. (1957) *The Dynamics of Anxiety and Hysteria*. London: Routledge & Kegan Paul.

EYSENCK, H. J. (1958) Hysterics and dysthymics as criterion groups in the study of introversion–extroversion: a reply. *J. Abnorm. Soc. Psychol.*, **57**, 250–2.

EYSENCK, H. J. (1959a) Anxiety and hysteria: reply to Vernon Hamilton. *Brit. J. Psychol.*, **50**, 64–9.

EYSENCK, H. J. (1959b) The differentiation between normal and various neurotic groups on the Maudsley Personality Inventory. *Brit. J. Psychol.*, **50**, 76–7.

EYSENCK, H. J. (1959c) *Manual of the Maudsley Personality Inventory*. London: Methuen.

EYSENCK, H. J. (1960) *Experiments in Personality*. London: Routledge & Kegan Paul.

EYSENCK, H. J. (1962) Animals or humans: Some problems of comparative psychology. *Proc. Roy. Soc. Med.*, **55**, (7).

EYSENCK, H. J. (1965) A three-factor theory of reminiscence. *Brit. J. Psychol.*, **56**, 163–81.

EYSENCK, H. J. (1967a) *The Biological Basis of Personality*. Illinois: Charles C. Thomas.

EYSENCK, H. J. (1967b) Single-trial conditioning, neurosis, and the Napalkov phenomenon. *Beh. Res. & Ther.*, **5**, 63–5.

EYSENCK, H. J. (1968) A theory of the incubation of anxiety/fear response. *Beh. Res. & Ther.*, **6**, 309–21.

EYSENCK, H. J. & BROADHURST, P. L. (1964) Experiments with animals. In EYSENCK, H. J. (ed.) *Experiments in Motivation*. Oxford: Pergamon Press.

EYSENCK, H. J. & CLARIDGE, G. (1962) The position of hysterics and dysthymics in a two-dimensional framework of personality description. *J. Abnorm. Soc. Psychol.*, **64**, 46–55.

EYSENCK, H. J. & EYSENCK, S. B. G. (1964) *Manual of the Eysenck Personality Inventory*. London: University of London Press.

EYSENCK, H. J. & RACHMAN, S. (1965) *Causes and Cures of Neurosis*. London: Routledge & Kegan Paul.

FARBER, I. E. (1948) Response fixation under anxiety and non-anxiety conditions. *J. Exp. Psychol.*, **38**, 111–31.

FEDIO, P., MINSKY, A. F., SMITH, W. J. & PANNY, D. (1961) Reaction time and EEG activation in normal and schizophrenic subjects. *Electroenceph. Clin. Neurophysiol.*, **13**, 923–6. (See Stern & McDonald, 1965.)

FELDMAN, R. S. (1953) The specificity of the fixated response in the rat. *J. Comp. Physiol. Psychol.*, **46**, 487–92.

FELDMAN, R. S. & WALLER, H. (1962) Dissociation of electrocortical activation and behavioural arousal. *Nature*, **196**, 1320–2.

FENICHEL, O. (1945) *The Psychoanalytic Theory of Neurosis*. New York: W. W. Norton.

FERNANDO, S. J. M. (1967) Gilles de la Tourette syndrome: A report of four cases. *Brit. J. Psychiat.*, **113**, 607–17.

FINGERMAN, M. (1969) *Animal Diversity*. New York: Holt, Rinehart & Winston.

FONBERG, E. (1956) On the manifestation of conditioned defensive reactions in stress. Cited in Wolpe (1958).

FORBES, A. R. (1969) The validity of the 16 PF in the discrimination of the hysteroid and obsessoid personality. *Brit. J. Soc. Clin. Psychol.*, **8**, 152–9.

FOULDS, G. A. (1951) Temperamental differences in maze performance. Part I. Characteristic differences among psychoneurotics. *Brit. J. Psychol.*, **42**, 209–17.

FOULDS, G. A. (1959) The relative stability of personality measures compared with diagnostic measures. *J. Ment. Sci.*, **105**, 783–7.

FOULDS, G. A. (1965) *Personality and Personal Illness*. London: Tavistock Publications.

FOULDS, G. A. & CAINE, T. M. (1958) Psychoneurotic symptom clusters, trait clusters and psychological tests. *J. Ment. Sci.*, **104**, 722–31.

FOULDS, G. A. & CAINE, T. M. (1959) Symptom clusters and personality types among psychoneurotic men compared with women. *J. Ment. Sci.*, **105**, 469–75.

FOX, M. W. (1968) *Abnormal Behavior in Animals*. Philadelphia: W. B. Saunders.

FRANK, J. D. (1961) *Persuasion and Healing*. Baltimore: Johns Hopkins Press.

FRANK, J. D. (1971) Therapeutic factors in psychotherapy. *Amer. J. Psychother.*, **25**, 350–67.

FRANKE, K. H. (1968) Zur Behandlung von Phobien mit einem neuen Anxiolyticum. *Arzneimittelforsch.*, **18**, 1570–1.

FRANKL, V. E. (1960) Paradoxical intention: A logotherapeutic technique. *Amer. J. Psychother.*, **14**, 520–35.

FRANKL, V. E. (1969) Logotherapy. In SAHAKIAN, W. S. (ed.) *Psychotherapy and Counselling*. Chicago: Rand McNally.

FRANSELLA, FAY (1970a) Construing and the dysphasic. Unpubl. ms.

FRANSELLA, FAY (1970b) Measurement of conceptual change accompanying weight loss. *J. Psychosom. Res.*, **14**, 347–51.

FRANSELLA, FAY (1971a) The structure of construing in the anorexic patient. Unpubl. ms.

FRANSELLA, FAY (1971b) A personal construct theory and treatment of stuttering. *J. Psychosom. Res.*, **15**, 433–8.

FRANSELLA, FAY & CRISP, A. H. (1970) Conceptual organization and weight change. *Psychosom. Psychother.*, **18**, 176–85.

FRAZER, J. G. (1925) *The Golden Bough* (abridged ed.). London: Macmillan.

FREEMAN, W. & WATTS, J. W. (1950) *Psychosurgery* (2nd ed.). Oxford: Oxford University Press.

FRENCKEL-BRUNSWICK, E. (1949) Intolerance of ambiguity as an emotional and perceptual personality variable. In BRUNER, J. S. & KRECH, D. (eds.) *Perception and Personality*. Durham, NC: Duke University Press.

FREUD, ANNA (1965) *Normality and Pathology in Childhood*. New York: Internat. Universities Press.

FREUD, ANNA (1966) Obsessional neurosis. (Summary of psychoanalytic views as presented at 24th Internat. Psychoanalytic Congress, Amsterdam, July 1965.) *Internat. J. Psychoanal.*, **47**, 116–22.

FREUD, S. (1896) Further remarks on the neuropsychoses of defence. *Standard Edition of the Complete Psychological Works of Sigmund Freud*, **3**, 170. London: Hogarth Press and the Institute of Psychoanalysis.

FREUD, S. (1907) Obsessive acts and religious practices. *Standard Edition*, **9**, 118.

FREUD, S. (1908) Character and anal erotism. *Standard Edition*, **9**, 169.

FREUD, S. (1909) Notes upon a case of obsessional neurosis. *Standard Edition*, **10**, 221.

FREUD, S. (1913a) Further recommendations on the technique of psychoanalysis. On beginning the treatment. *Standard Edition*, **12**, 123.

FREUD, S. (1913b) The predisposition to obsessional neurosis. *Standard Edition*, **12**, 322.

FREUD, S. (1913c) Totem and taboo. *Standard Edition*, **13**, 88.

FREUD, S. (1916) Introductory lectures on psychoanalysis. *Standard Edition*, **15**, 259.

FREUD, S. (1926) Inhibitions, symptoms and anxiety. *Standard Edition*, **20**, 144.

FREUD, S. (1948) *Collected Papers*, Vol. III, ed. Ernest Jones. London: The Hogarth Press.

FREUDENBERG, R. K. (1966) The functions and attitudes of professional staff in psychiatric hospitals. *Proc. Roy. Soc. Med.*, **59**, 7, 591–4.

FRIEDMANN, M. (1914) Zur Auffassung und Kenntnis der Zwangsideen und der isolierten Überwertigen Ideen. *Z. ges. Neurol. Psychiat.*, **21**, 333–450.

FURST, J. B. & COOPER, A. (1970) Failure of systematic desensitization in two cases of obsessional–compulsive neurosis marked by fears of insecticide. *Beh. Res. & Ther.*, **8**, 203–6.

GAINSBOROUGH, H. & SLATER, E. (1946) A study of peptic ulcer. *Brit. Med. J.*, **2**, 253–8.

GAITANDE, M. R. (1958) Cross-cultural study of the psychiatric syndromes in out-patient clinics in Bombay, India & Topeka, Kansas. Paper presented at the 114th meeting of the American Psychiatric Assoc., San Francisco.

GARMANY, G. & EARLY, D. F. (1948) Electronarcosis, its value and its dangers. *Lancet*, **1**, 444–6.

GARMANY, G., MAY, A. R. & FOLKSON, A. (1954) The use and action of chlorpromazine in psychoneurosis. *Brit. Med. J.*, **2**, 439–42.

GASTAUT, H. (1957) The role of the reticular formation in establishing conditioned reactions. In JASPER, W. H. (ed.) *Reticular Formation of the Brain*. Boston: Little, Brown.

GEER, J. H., DAVISON, G. C. & GATCHEL, R. I. (1970) Reduction of stress in humans through non-veridical control of aversive stimulations. *J. Pers. Soc. Psychol.*, **16**, 731–8.

GERTZ, H. O. (1966) Experience with the logotherapeutic technique of paradoxical intention in the treatment of phobic and obsessive–compulsive patients. *Amer. J. Psychiat.*, **123**, 548–53.

GESELL, A. L. (1940) *First Five Years of Life*. New York: Harper. (1941, London: Methuen.)

GIEL, R., KNOX, R. S. & CARSTAIRS, G. M. (1964) A five-year follow-up of 100 neurotic out-patients. *Brit. Med. J.*, **2**, 160–3.

GITTLESON, N. L. (1966a) The effects of obsessions in depressive psychosis. *Brit. J. Psychiat.*, **112**, 253–9.

GITTLESON, N. L. (1966b) The phenomenology of obsessions in depressive psychosis. *Brit. J. Psychiat.*, **112**, 261–4.

GITTLESON, N. L. (1966c) The fate of obsessions in depressive psychosis. *Brit. J. Psychiat.*, **112**, 705–8.

GITTLESON, N. L. (1966d) Depressive psychosis in the obsessional neurotic. *Brit. J. Psychiat.*, **112**, 883–7.

GOODWIN, D. W., GUZE, S. B. & ROBINS, E. (1969) Follow-up studies in obsessional neurosis. *Arch. Gen. Psychiat.* (Chicago), **20**, 182–7.

GRANT, DAVID A. (1943a) Sensitization and association in eyelid conditioning. *J. Exp. Psychol.*, **32**, 201–12.

GRANT, DAVID A. (1943b) The pseudo-conditioned eyelid response. *J. Exp. Psychol.*, **32**, 139–49.

GRANT, DAVID A. (1945) A sensitized eyelid reaction related to the conditioned eyelid response. *J. Exp. Psychol.*, **35**, 393–402.

GRANT, DAVID A. & DITTMER, DANIEL G. (1940) A tactile generalization gradient for a pseudo-conditioned response. *J. Exp. Psychol.*, **26**, 404–12.

GRANT, DAVID A. & HILGARD, ERNEST R. (1940) Sensitization as a supplement to association in eyelid conditioning. *Psychol. Bull.*, **37**, 478–9.

GRANT, DAVID A. & MEYER, H. Z. (1941) The formation of generalized response sets during repeated electric shock stimulation. *J. Gen. Psychol.*, **24**, 21–38.

GRAY, J. A. (1967) Drugs and disappointment in the rat. *Advancement of Science*, March, 595–605.

GRAY, J. A. (1970) The psychophysiological basis of introversion-extroversion. *Beh. Res. & Ther.*, **8**, 249–66.

GREENACRE, P. (1923) A study of the mechanism of obsessive compulsive conditions. *Amer. J. Psychiat.*, **79**, 527–38.

GREER, H. S. & CAWLEY, R. H. (1966) Some observations on the natural history of neurotic illness. *Mervyn Archdall Medical Monogr.* No. 3, Australian Medical Association.

GRETHER, W. F. (1938) Pseudo-conditioning without paired stimulation encountered in attempted backward conditioning. *J. Comp. Psychol.*, **25**, 91–6.

GRIMSHAW, L. (1964) Obsessional disorder & neurological illness. *J. Neurol. Neurosurg. Psychiat.*, **27**, 229–31.

GRIMSHAW, L. (1965) The outcome of obsessional disorder: a follow-up study of 100 cases. *Brit. J. Psychiat.*, **111**, 1051–56.

GROVES, P. M. & THOMPSON, R. F. (1970) Habituation: A dual-process theory. *Psychol. Rev.*, **77**, 419–50.

GRUNBERGER, B. (1966) Some reflections on the rat man. *Internat. J. Psychoanal.*, **47**, 160–8.

GRYGIER, T. G. (1961) *The Dynamic Personality Inventory*. London: NFER.

GUILDFORD, J. P. (1959) Traits of creativity. In ANDERSON, H. H. (ed.) *Creativity and its Cultivation*. New York: Harper.

GURVITZ, M. S. (1951) *The Dynamics of Psychological Testing*. New York: Grune & Stratton.

GUTHEIL, E. (1950) Preface to STECKEL, W. *Compulsion and Doubt*. London: Peter Nevill.

HALL, C. S. (1934) Emotional behaviour in the rat. I. Defecation and urination as measures of individual differences in emotionality. *J. Comp. Psychol.*, **18**, 385–403.

HALL, C. S. (1940) The inheritance of emotionality in the rat. *Psychol. Bull.*, **37**, 432.

HAMILTON, D. L. (1968) Personality attributes associated with extreme response style. *Psychol. Bull.*, **69**, 192–203.

HAMILTON, J. A. & KRECHEVSKY, I. (1933) Studies in the effect of shock upon behaviour plasticity in the rat. *J. Comp. Psychol.*, **16**, 237–53.

HAMILTON, V. (1957a) Perceptual and personality dynamics in re-actions to ambiguity. *Brit. J. Psychol.*, **48**, 200–215.

HAMILTON, V. (1957b) Conflict avoidance in obsessionals and hys-terics, and the validity of the concept of dysthymia. *J. Ment. Sci.*, **103**, 666–76.

HAMILTON, V. (1959a) Eysenck's theory of anxiety and hysteria: A methodological critique. *Brit. J. Psychol.*, **50**, 48–63.

HAMILTON, V. (1959b) Theories of anxiety and hysteria: A rejoinder to Hans Eysenck. *Brit. J. Psychol.*, **50**, 276–80.

HARE, ROBERT D. (1968) Psychopathy, autonomic functioning and the orienting response. *J. Abnorm. Psychol.*, Monogr. Suppl. (June), **73**, 3, Part 2, 1–24.

HARLOW, H. F. (1939) Forward conditioning, backward conditioning, and pseudo-conditioning in the goldfish. *J. Genet. Psychol.*, **55**, 49–58.

HARLOW, H. F. (1958) The nature of love. *Amer. Psychol.*, **13**, 673–85.

HARLOW, H. F. (1959) Love in infant monkeys. *Sci. Amer.*, **200**, 68–75.

HARLOW, H. F. (1961) The development of affectional pattern in infant monkeys. In FOSS, B. M. *Determinants of Infant Behaviour.* New York: John Wiley & Sons. (London: Methuen.)

HARLOW, H. F. (1962) Development of the second and third affectional systems in Macaque monkeys. In TOURLENTES, T. T., POLLACK, S. L. & HIMWICH, H. E. *Research Approaches to Psychiatric Problems: A Symposium.* New York: Grune & Stratton.

HARLOW, H. F. & HARLOW, M. K. (1965) The affectional systems. In SCHRIER, A. M., HARLOW, H. F. & STOLLNITZ, F. *Behaviour of Nonhuman Primates,* Vol. 2. New York: Academic Press.

HARLOW, H. F. & TOLTZIEN, F. (1940) Formation of pseudo-conditioned responses in cat. *J. Gen. Psychol.,* 23, 367–75.

HARLOW, H. F. & ZIMMERMAN, R. R. (1959) Affectional responses in the infant monkey. *Science,* 130, 421–32.

HARRIS, J. DONALD (1941) Forward conditioning, backward conditioning, pseudo-conditioning, and adaptation to the conditioned stimulus. *J. Exp. Psychol.,* 28, 491–502.

HASELRUD, G. M., BRADBARD, K. & JOHNSTON, B. P. (1954) Pure guidance and handling as components of the Maier technique for breaking abnormal fixations. *J. Psychol.,* 37, 27–30.

HASLAM, M. T. (1965) The treatment of an obsessional patient by reciprocal inhibition. *Beh. Res. & Ther.,* 2, 213–16.

HASSLER, R. (1967) Sterotoxic treatment of compulsive and obsessional symptoms. *Confin. Neurol.,* 29, 153–8.

HASTINGS, D. W. (1958) Follow-up results in psychiatric illness. *Amer. J. Psychiat.,* 114, 1057–66.

HAWKS, D. W. (1964) The clinical usefulness of some tests of over-inclusive thinking in psychiatric patients. *Brit. J. Soc. Clin. Psychol.,* 3, 186–95.

HEBB, D. O. (1949) *The Organization of Behaviour.* New York: Wiley & Sons.

HEIM, ALICE (1970) *Intelligence and Personality.* Harmondsworth: Penguin.

HEIN, P. L., GREEN, R. L. & WILSON, W. P. (1962) Latency and duration of photically elicited arousal responses in the electroencephalograms of patients with chronic regressive schizophrenia. *J. Nerv. Ment. Dis.,* 135, 361–4. (See Stern & McDonald, 1965.)

HERRNSTEIN, R. J. (1966) Superstition: A corollary of the principles of operant conditioning. In HONIG, W. K. (ed.) *Operant Behaviour: Areas of Research and Application.* New York: Appleton-Century-Crofts.

HERRNSTEIN, R. J. (1969) Method and theory in the study of avoidance. *Psychol. Rev.*, **76**, 49–69.

HERSEN, M. (1968) Treatment of a compulsive and phobic disorder through a total behaviour therapy progress: A case study. *Psychotherapy: Theory, Research and Practice*, **5**, 220–5.

HESS, J. P. (1968) The treatment of obsessional and phobic states. *Dapim Refuiim.*, **27**, Nos. 7–8.

HILDEBRAND, M. P. (1958) A factorial study of introversion–extroversion. *Brit. J. Psychol.*, **49**, 1–12.

HILL, D. (1969) *Psychiatry in Medicine.* London: Nuffield Provincial Hospitals Trust.

HILL, D. (1970) Aggression: Innate drive or response? *Proc. Roy. Soc. Med.*, **63**, (2).

HILL, D. (1971) On the contributions of psychoanalysis to psychiatry: Mechanism and meaning. *Internat. J. Psychoanal.*, **52**, 1–10.

HILL, H. E., KORNETSKY, C., FLANARY, H. & WIKLER, A. (1952) Effects of anxiety and morphine on discrimination of intensities of painful stimuli. *J. Clin. Invest.*, **31**, 473–80.

HODGSON, R. J. & RACHMAN, S. (1972) The effects of contamination and washing in obsessional patients. *Beh. Res. & Ther.*, **10**, 111–17.

HOFFMAN, H. S., FLESHLER, M. & JENSEN, P. (1963) Stimulus aspects of aversive controls: The retention of conditioned suppression. *J. Exp. Anal. Behav.*, **6**, 575–83.

HOLLINGSHEAD, A. B. & REDLICH, F. C. (1958) *Social Class and Mental Illness.* New York: Wiley.

HONIGFELD, G. (1964a) Non-specific factors in treatment: I. Review of placebo reactions and placebo reactors. *Dis. Nerv. Syst.*, **25**, 145–56.

HONIGFELD, G. (1964b) Non-specific factors in treatment: II. Review of social–psychological factors. *Dis. Nerv. Syst.*, **25**, 225–39.

HUDSON, L. (1970) *Frames of Mind.* Harmondsworth: Penguin Books.

HUSSAIN, A. (1964) The results of behaviour therapy in 105 cases. In WOLPE, J., SALTER, A. & REYNA, A. (eds.) *Conditioning Therapies.* New York: Holt, Rinehart & Winston.

HUTT, CORINNE (1968) Exploration of novelty, i.e. children with and without upper CNS lesions and some effects of auditory and visual incentives. *Acta Psychologica*, **28**, 150–60.

IBOR, J. L. (1952) Anxiety states and their treatment with intravenous acetychlorine. *Proc. Roy. Soc. Med.*, **45**, 511.

IHDA, S. (1965) Psychiatrische Zwillingsforschung in Japan. *Arch. Psychiat. Nervenk.*, **207**, 209–20.

INGRAM, I. M. (1961a) The obsessional personality and obsessional illness. *Amer. J. Psychiat.*, **117**, 1016–19.

INGRAM, I. M. (1961b) Obsessional illness in mental hospital patients. *J. Ment. Sci.*, **107**, 382–402.

INGRAM, I. M. (1961c) Obsessional personality and anal-erotic character. *J. Ment. Sci.*, **107**, 1035–42.

INOUYE, E. (1965) Similar and dissimilar manifestations of obsessive compulsive neurosis in monozygotic twins. *Amer. J. Psychiat.*, **121**, 1171–75.

ISAACS, S. (1933) *Social Development in Young Children*. London: Routledge & Kegan Paul.

JACKSON, D. D. (1960) A critique of the literature of the genetics of schizophrenia. In JACKSON, D. D. (ed.) *Etiology of Schizophrenia*. New York: Basic Books.

JAHRREISS, W. (1926) Über einen Fall von Chronischer systematisierender Zwangserkrankung. *Arch. Psychiat.*, **77**, 596–612.

JAMES, W. (1890) *The Principles of Psychology*. New York: Henry Holt.

JANET, P. (1903) *Les Obsessions et la psychasthénie*. (2nd ed., 1908) Paris: Baillière.

JANET, P. (1925) *Psychological Healing*. Vol. II. London and New York: Allen & Unwin.

JASPER, H. H. (1954) Functional properties of the thalamic reticular system. In DELAFRESNAYE, J. F. (ed.) *Brain Mechanisms and Consciousness*. Oxford: Blackwell.

JASPER, H. H. (1961) Thalamic reticular system. In SHEER, D. E. (ed.) *Electrical Stimulation of the Brain*. Austin, Texas: University of Texas Press.

JASPERS, K. (1946) *General Psychopathology*. (7th ed.) Trans. by HOENIG, J. & HAMILTON, M. W. Manchester University Press.

JASPERS, K. (1963) *General Psychopathology*. Chicago: University of Chicago Press.

JAY, G. E. (1963) Genetic strains and stocks. In BURDETT, W. J. (ed.) *Methodology in Mammalian Genetics*. San Francisco: Holden-Day.

JEWELL, P. A. & LOIZOS, C. (eds.) (1966) *Play, Exploration and Territory in Mammals*. London: Academic Press.

JONES, L. C. T. (1954) Frustration and stereotyped behaviour in human subjects. *Quart. J. Exp. Psychol.*, **6**, 12–20.

JUDD, L. L. (1965) Obsessive compulsive neurosis in children. *Arch. Gen. Psychiat.*, **12**, 136–43.

KAILA, K. (1949) Über den Zwangsneurotischen Symptomenkomplex. *Acta Psychiat. Neurol. Scand.*, Suppl. 57.

KALINOWSKY, L. B. & HIPPIUS, H. (1969) *Pharmacological, Convulsive and other Somatic Treatments in Psychiatry*. New York and London: Grune & Stratton.

KANFER, F. H. & SASLOW, G. (1969) Behavioural diagnosis. In FRANKS, C. M. (ed.) *Behaviour Therapy: Appraisal and Status*. New York: McGraw-Hill.

KANNER, L. (1957) *Child Psychiatry*. (3rd ed.) Springfield, Illinois: Thomas.

KELLEHER, M. J. (1970) *Culture and Obsession: A Comparative Study of Irish and English*. Unpubl. M.D. thesis, University College, Cork.

KELLY, G. A. (1955) *The Psychology of Personal Constructs*. Vols. I and II. New York: Norton.

KENDELL, R. E. (1968) *The Classification of Depressive Illnesses*. London: Oxford University Press.

KENDELL, R. E. & DISCIPIO, W. J. (1970) Obsessional symptoms and obsessional personality traits in patients with depressive illnesses. *Psychol. Med.*, **1**, 65–72.

KENNY, D. T. & GINSBURG, ROSE (1958) The specificity of intolerance of ambiguity measures. *J. Abnorm. Soc. Psychol.*, **56**, 300–304.

KESTENBERG, J. S. (1966) Rhythm and organization in obsessive-compulsive development. *Internat. J. Psychoanal.*, **47**, 151–9.

KIMBLE, G. A. (1955) Shock intensity and avoidance learning. *J. Comp. Physiol. Psychol.*, **48**, 281–4.

KIMBLE, G. A. (1964) *Conditioning and Learning*. London: Methuen.

KIMBLE, G. A. & DUFORT, R. A. (1956) The associative factor in eyelid conditioning. *J. Exp. Psychol.*, **52**, 386–91.

KIMBLE, G. A., MANN, L. I. & DUFORT, R. A. (1955) Classical and instrumental eyelid conditioning. *J. Exp. Psychol.*, **49**, 6, 407–16.

KLERMAN, G. L. (1963) Assessing the influence of the hospital milieu upon the effectiveness of psychiatric drug therapy: Problems of conceptualization and of research methodology. *J. Nerv. Ment. Dis.*, **137**, 143–54.

KLINE, P. (1967) Obsessional traits and emotional instability in a normal population. *Brit. J. Med. Psychol.*, **40**, 153–7.

KLINE, P. (1968a) Obsessional traits, obsessional symptoms and anal erotism. *Brit. J. Med. Psychol.*, **41**, 299–305.

KLINE, P. (1968b) The validity of the Dynamic Personality Inventory. *Brit. J. Med. Psychol.*, **41**, 307–13.

KNIGHT, G. (1964) The orbital cortex as an objective in surgical treatment of mental illness. *Brit. J. Surg.*, **51**, 114–24.

KNIGHT, R. P. (1941) Evaluation of results of psychoanalytic therapy. *Amer. J. Psychiat.*, **98**, 434–46.

KOELLA, W. P. (1966) *Sleep: Its Nature and Physiological Organization*. Springfield, Illinois: Thomas.

KOGAN, N. & WALLACH, M. A. (1964) *Risk Taking: A Study in Cognition and Personality*. New York: Holt, Rinehart & Winston.

KOSTANDOV, E. A. (1963) Role of disturbances of corticofugal influences in the pathology of orienting reflex in schizophrenic patient. *Zh. Vysshei Nerunoie Dyatel'novti*, **13**, 995–1009. (See Stern & McDonald, 1965.)

KRAEPELIN, E. (1921) *Textbook of Psychiatry*. (8th German ed., trans. by BARCLAY) Edinburgh: Livingstone.

KRAKOWSKI, A. J. (1965) Suppression of anxiety with oxazepam in a private psychiatric practice. *Psychosomatics*, **6**, 26–31.

KRAL, V. (1952) Psychiatric observations under severe chronic stress. *Amer. J. Psychiat.*, **108**, 185–92.

KRETSCHMER, E. (1950) *Der sensitive Beziehungswahn*. (3rd ed.) Berlin.

KRINGLEN, E. (1965) Obsessional neurotics: A long-term follow-up. *Brit. J. Psychiat.*, **111**, 709–22.

KRINGLEN, E. (1970) Natural history of obsessional neurosis. *Semin. Psychiat.*, **2**, 403–19.

KROUT, M. H. & TABIN, J. K. (1954) Measuring personality in developmental terms. *Genet. Psychol. Monogr.*, **50**, 289–335.

KUSHNER, M. & SANDLER, J. (1966) Aversion therapy and the concept of punishment. *Beh. Res. & Ther.*, **4**, 179–86.

LABOURCARIE, J., RASCOL, A., JORD, P., GUIRAUD, B. & LEIGNADIER, H. (1967) Perspectives nouvelles de traitment des états melancoliques: Étude therapeutique d'un antidepressif majeur la Chlomipramine (d'après 90 observations). *Revue Med. Toulouse*, **3**, 863–72.

LADER, M. H. (1967) Palmar skin conductance measures in anxiety and phobic states. *J. Psychosom. Res.*, **11**, 271–81.

LADER, M. H., GELDER, M. G. & MARKS, I. M. (1967) Palmar skin conductance measures of predictions of response to desensitization. *J. Psychosom. Res.*, **11**, 283–90. (Reprint 11464.)

LADER, M. H. & MATHEWS, A. M. (1968) A physiological model of phobic anxiety and desensitization. *Beh. Res. & Ther.*, **6**, 411–21.

LADER, M. H. & WING, LORNA (1964) Habituation of the psychogalvanic reflex in patients with anxiety states and in normal subjects. *J. Neurol. Neurosurg. Psychiat.*, **27**, 210–18.

LADER, M. H. & WING, LORNA (1966) Physiological measures, sedative drugs and morbid anxiety. *Maudsley Monogr.*, **14.** London: Oxford University Press.

LANDFIELD, A. W. (1968) The extremity rating revisited within the context of personal construct theory. *Brit. J. Soc. Clin. Psychol.*, **7,** 135–9.

LANE-PETER, W. (ed.) (1963) *Animals for Research.* London: Academic Press.

LANGER, P. (1962) Compulsivity and response set on the Structured Objective Rorschach Test. *J. Clin. Psychol.*, **18,** 299–302.

LANGFELDT, G. (1938) Studiet av tvangsfenomenenes forekomst, genese, klinikk og prognose. *Tidsskr. norske laegef.*, **13,** 16. (Cited by Kringlen, 1965.)

LAT, J. (1963) The spontaneous exploratory reactions as a tool for psychopharmacological studies. A contribution towards a theory of contradictory results in psychopharmacology. *Proc. 2nd Internat. Pharmacological Meeting*, Prague.

LAT, J. (1967) Nutrition, learning and adaptive capacity. In KARE, M. R. & MALLER, O. (eds.) *The Chemical Senses and Nutrition.* Baltimore: Johns Hopkins Press.

LAT, J. (1969) Some mechanisms of the permanent effect of short-term, partial and total, overnutrition in early life upon the behaviour of rats. *Proc. VIII Internat. Congr. of Nutrition*, Prague.

LAT, J., MARTINEK, Z., GOLLOVA-HEMON, E., IRMIS, F. & PRIBIK, V. (1971) *Laboratory of Physiology and Pathophysiology of Behaviour.* Ann Rep. Psychiatric Res. Instit., Prague.

LAWLEY, D. N. & MAXWELL, A. E. (1963) *Factor Analysis as a Statistical Tool.* London: Butterworth.

LAZARUS, A. A. (1958) New methods in psychotherapy: A case study. *S. Afric. Med. J.*, **33,** 660–3.

LAZARUS, A. A. (1963) The results of behaviour therapy in 126 cases of severe neurosis. *Beh. Res. & Ther.*, **1,** 69–79.

LEACH, PENELOPE (1967) A critical study of the literature concerning rigidity. *Brit. J. Soc. Clin. Psychol.*, **6,** 11–22.

LE BEAU, H. (1953) A comparison of the personality changes after i) prefrontal selective surgery for the relief of intractable pain and for the treatment of mental cases, and ii) cingulectomy and topectomy. *J. Ment. Sci.*, **99,** 53.

LEDERHENDLER, I. & BAUM, M. (1970) Mechanical facilitation of the action of response prevention (flooding) in rats. *Beh. Res. & Ther.*, **8,** 43–8.

LEEUW, P. J. VAN DER (1966) Comment on Dr Ritvo's paper. *Internat. J. Psychoanal.*, **47**, 132–5.

LEIBOVICH, F. A. (1959) Changes in biolectrical pattern of the cerebral cortex in depressive states during treatment with iproniazid. *Zh. Neuropatol. Psikhiatr.*, **59**, 1470–9.

LEIBOVICH, F. A. (1961) Changes in the cerebral cortical electrical activity during imizine (Tofranil) treatment of patients with depressive conditions. *Zh. Neuropatol. Psikhiatr.*, **61**, 186–200.

LEITENBERG, H., AGRAS, S., EDWARD, J. A., THOMSON, L. E. & WINCZE, J. P. (1970) Practice as a psychotherapeutic variable: An experimental analysis within single cases. *J. Psychiat. Res.*, **7**, 215–25.

LEVY, D. M. (1952) Animal psychology in its relation to psychiatry. In ALEXANDER, F. (ed.) *Dynamic Psychiatry*. Chicago University Press.

LEVY, R. & MEYER, V. (1971) Ritual prevention in obsessional patients. *Proc. Roy. Soc. Med.*, **64**, 115–20.

LEWIN, W. (1960) Symposium on orbital undercutting: selective leucotomy. *Proc. Roy. Soc. Med.*, **53**, 732–4.

LEWIS, A. J. (1934) Melancholia: A clinical survey of depressive states. *J. Ment. Sci.*, **80**, 277–378.

LEWIS, A. J. (1935–6) Problems of obsessional illness. *Proc. Roy. Soc. Med.*, **29**, 325–36.

LEWIS, A. J. (1938) The diagnosis and treatment of obsessional states. *Practitioner*, **141**, 21–30.

LEWIS, A. J. (1957) Obsessional illness. *Acta neuropsiquiat. argent.*, **3**, 323–35.

LEWIS, A. J. (1965) A note on personality and obsessional illness. *Psychiat. Neurol.*, Basel, **150**, 299–305.

LEWIS, A. J. & MAPOTHER, E. (1941) Obsessional disorder. In PRICE, (ed.) *Textbook of the Practice of Medicine* (pp. 1199–2001). London: Oxford University Press.

LICHTENSTEIN, P. E. (1950) Studies of anxiety. I. The production of a feeding inhibition in dogs. *J. Comp. Physiol. Psychol.*, **43**, 16–29.

LIDDELL, M. A. (1974) *An Investigation of Psychological Mechanisms in Obsessional Patients*. Unpubl. Ph.D. thesis, Univ. of London.

LIN, T-Y. (1953) A study of the incidence of mental disorder in Chinese cultures. *Psychiatry*, **16**, 313–36.

LINDSLEY, D. B. (1960) Attention, consciousness, sleep and wakefulness. In FIELD, J. (ed.) *Handbook of Physiology*, Vol. III. Washington, DC: Amer. Physiol. Soc.

LINDSLEY, D. B., SCHREINER, L. H., KNOWLES, W. B. & MAGOUN, H. W. (1950) Behavioral and EEG changes following chronic brain stem lesions in the cat. *Electroenceph. Clin. Neurophysiol.*, **2**, 483–498.

LO, W. H. (1967) A follow-up study of obsessional neurotics in Hong Kong Chinese. *Brit. J. Psychiat.*, **113**, 823–32.

LOMONT, J. P. (1965) Reciprocal inhibition or extinction? *Beh. Res. & Ther.*, **3**, 209–19.

LORENZ, K. (1966) *On Aggression.* New York: M. K. Wilson; London: Methuen.

LORR, M., RUBINSTEIN, E. & JENKINS, R. L. (1953) A factor analysis of personality ratings of out-patients in psychotherapy. *J. Abnorm. Soc. Psychol.*, **48**, 511–14.

LORR, M. & RUBINSTEIN, E. A. (1956) Personality patterns of neurotic adults in psychotherapy. *J. Consult. Psychol.*, **20**, 257–63.

LOUKAS, K. P. *et al.* (1965) Electronarcosis at Guy's. *Guy's Hospital Reports*, **114**, 223–37.

LUFF, M. C. & GARROD, M. (1935) After-results of psychotherapy in 500 cases. *Brit. Med. J.*, **2**, 54–9.

LUXENBURGER, H. (1930) Herediät u. Familientypus der Zwangsneurotiker. *Arch. Psychiat.*, **91**, 590–4.

LYNN, R. (1963) Russian theory and research on schizophrenia. *Psychol. Bull.*, **60**, 486–98.

LYNN, R. (1966) *Attention, Arousal and the Orientation Reaction.* Oxford: Pergamon Press.

MAATSCH, JACK L. (1959) Learning and fixation after a single shock trial. *J. Comp. Physiol. Psychol.*, **52**, 408–10.

MAIER, N. R. F. (1949) *Frustration: The Study of Behaviour without a Goal.* New York: McGraw-Hill.

MAIER, N. R. F., GLASER, N. M. & KLEE, J. B. (1940) Studies of abnormal behaviour in the rat. III. The development of behaviour fixations through frustration. *J. Exp. Psychol.*, **26**, 521–46.

MAIER, N. R. F. & KLEE, J. B. (1945) Studies of abnormal behaviour in the rat. XVII. Guidance versus trial and error in the alterations of habits and fixations. *J. Psychol.*, **19**, 133–63.

MAIER, N. R. F. & SCHNEIRLA, T. C. (1935) *Principles of Animal Psychology.* New York: McGraw-Hill.

MAILLET-JURQUET, A. *et al.* (1970) La chlorimipramine traitment majeur des états depressifs (à propos de 103 cas, traités par perfusion intraveineuse). *Encephale*, **59**, 180–8.

MAKHLOUF NORRIS, F. (1968) *Concepts of the self and others in obsessional neurosis studied by an adaptation of the Role Construct Repertory Grid.* Ph.D. thesis, University of London.

MAKHLOUF NORRIS, F., JONES, H. G. & NORRIS, H. (1970) Articulation of the conceptual structure in obsessional neurosis. *Brit. J. Soc. Clin. Psychol.*, **9**, 264–74.

MARCIA, J. E., RUBIN, B. M. & EFRAN, J. S. (1969) Systematic desensitization: Expectancy change or counterconditioning? *J. Abnorm. Psychol.*, **74**, 382–7.

MARKS, I. M. (1965) Patterns of meaning in psychiatric patients. *Maudsley Monogr.*, **13**, Oxford University Press.

MARKS, I. M. (1966) Semantic differential uses in psychiatric patients. *Brit. J. Psychiat.*, **112**, 945–51.

MARKS, I. M. (1969) *Fears and Phobias*. London: Heinemann.

MARKS, I. M. (1970a) The classification of phobic disorders. *Brit. J. Psychiat.*, **116**, 377–86.

MARKS, I. M. (1970b) The origins of phobic states. *Amer. J. Psychother.*, **24**, (4).

MARKS, I. M., CROWE, M., DREWE, E., YOUNG, J. & DEWHURST, W. G. (1969) Obsessive–compulsive neurosis in identical twins. *Brit. J. Psychiat.*, **115**, 991–8.

MARQUART, D. I. & ARNOLD, L. P. (1952) A study in the frustration of human adults. *J. Gen. Psychol.*, **47**, 43–63.

MARTIN, B. (1963) Reward and punishment associated with the same goal response: A factor in the learning of motives. *Psychol. Bull.*, **60**, 441–51.

MARTIN, IRENE (1962) GSR conditioning and pseudo-conditioning. *Brit. J. Psychol.*, **53**, 4, 365–71.

MATHER, M. D. (1970) The treatment of an obsessive–compulsive patient by discrimination learning and reinforcement of decision making. *Beh. Res. & Ther.*, **8**, 315–18.

MAUDSLEY, H. (1895) *The Pathology of Mind*. London.

MAYER-GROSS, W., SLATER, E. & ROTH, M. (1955) *Clinical Psychiatry*. (2nd ed., 1960.) London: Cassell.

MELLETT, P. G. (1970) Motive and mechanism in asthma. Communication to the Soc. for Psychosomatic Research, London.

MENNINGER, K. A. (1938) *Man Against Himself*. New York: Harcourt Brace.

METZNER, R. (1963) Some experimental analogues of obsession. *Beh. Res. & Ther.*, **1**, 231–6.

MEYER, V. (1966) Modification of expectancies in cases with obsessional rituals. *Beh. Res. & Ther.*, **4**, 273–80.

MEYER, V. & CHESSER, E. S. (1970) *Behaviour Therapy in Clinical Psychiatry*. Harmondsworth: Penguin.

MEYER, V. & CRISP, A. H. (1966) Some problems in behaviour therapy. *Brit. J. Psychiat.*, **112**, 367–81.

MEYER, V. & GELDER, M. G. (1963) Behaviour therapy and phobic disorders. *Brit. J. Psychiat.*, **109**, 19–28.

MEYER, V. & LEVY, R. (1973) Modification of behavior in obsessive-compulsive disorders. In ADAMS, H. E. & UNIKEL, I. P. (eds.) *Issues and Trends in Behavior Therapy*. Springfield, Illinois: Thomas.

MEYER-HOLZAPFEL, M. (1961) Homosexualität bei Tieren. 'Praxis' Schweiz. *Rdschau. f. Med.*, **50**, 1266–72.

MEYER-HOLZAPFEL, M. (1968) Abnormal behavior in zoo animals. In FOX, M. W. (ed.) *Abnormal Behaviour in Animals*. Philadelphia: W. B. Saunders.

MIKHAIL, A. A. & BROADHURST, P. L. (1965) Stomach ulceration and emotionality in selected strains of rats. *J. Psychosom. Res.*, **8**, 477.

MIKHAIL, A. A. & HOLLAND, H. C. (1966a) A simplified method of inducing stomach ulcers. *J. Psychosom. Res.*, **9**, 343–47.

MIKHAIL, A. A. & HOLLAND, H. C. (1966b) Evaluating and photographing experimentally induced stomach ulcers. *J. Psychosom. Res.*, **9**, 349–53.

MILLAR, T. P. (1969) Who's afraid of Sigmund Freud? *Brit. J. Psychiat.*, **115**, 421–8.

MILLER, H. (1968) Psychiatry and the National Health Service. *Listener*, 29 August.

MILNER, A. D., BEECH, H. R. & WALKER, VALERIE (1971) Decision processes and obsessional behaviour. *Brit. J. Soc. Clin. Psychol.*, **10**, 88–9.

MISCHEL, W. (1968) *Personality and Assessment*. New York: Wiley.

MITCHELL, W. M. (1969) Observations on animal behaviour and its relationship to masochism. *Dis. Nerv. Syst.*, **30**, 124–8.

MITSUDA, H., SAKAI, T. & KOBAYASHI, J. (1967) A clinico-genetic study of the relationship between neurosis and psychosis. *Bull. Osaka Med. School*, Suppl. XII, 27–35.

MOREL, M. (1866) Du Délire Emotif. *Arch. Gen. Med.*, **7**, 385, 530, 700.

MORGAN, M. J. (1968) Negative reinforcement. In WEISKRANTZ, L. (ed.) *Analysis of Behavioural Change*. London: Harper & Row.

MORRIS, D. (1956) The feather postures of birds and the problem of the origins of social signals. *Behaviour*, **9**, 75–114.

MORUZZI, G. (1966) The functional significance of sleep with particular regard to the brain mechanisms underlying consciousness. In ECCLES, J. C. (ed.) *Brain and Conscious Experience*. Berlin: Heidelberg; New York: Springer.

L*

MORUZZI, G. & MAGOUN, H. W. (1949) Brain stem reticular formation and activation of the EEG. *Electroenceph. Clin. Neurophysiol.*, **1**, 455–73.

MOWRER, O. H. (1960) *Learning Theory and Behaviour.* New York: Wiley.

MOWRER, O. H. & LAMOREAUX, R. R. (1942) Avoidance conditioning and signal duration: A study of secondary motivation and reward. *Psychol. Monogr.*, **54**, 5 and whole No. 247.

MÜLLER, C. (1953a) Vorläufige Mitteilung zur langen Katamnese der Zwangskranken. *Nervenarzt.*, **24**, 112–15.

MÜLLER, C. (1953b) Der Übergang von Zwangsneurose in Schizophrenie im Lichte der Katamnese. *Schweiz. Arch. Neurol. Psychiat.*, **72**, 218–25.

MÜLLER, C. (1957) Weitere Beobachtungen zum Velauf der Zwangskrankheit. *Mschr. Psychiat. Neurol.*, **133**, 80–94.

MUNN, N. L. (1950) *Handbook of Psychological Research on the Rat.* Boston: Houghton Mifflin.

MCFARLAND, D. J. (1965) Hunger, thirst and displacement pecking in the Barbary dove. *Anim. Behav.*, **13**, 2–3.

MCKINNEY, W. T. & BUNNEY, W. E. (1969) Animal model of depression. I. Review of evidence: Implications for Research. *Arch. Gen. Psychiat.*, **21**, 240–8.

NACHT, S. (1966) The inter-relationship of phobia and obsessional neurosis. *Internat. J. Psychoanal.*, **47**, 136–8.

NAPALKOV, A. V. (1963) Information process of the brain. In WIENER, N. & SCHADE, J. P. (eds.) *Progress in Brain Research.* Vol. II. Nerve Brain and Memory Models. Amsterdam: Elsevier.

NATURE (1968) Psychiatry is quite respectable. **219**, 1001.

NAUTA, W. J. H. (1958) Hippocampal projection and related neural pathway to the midbrain in cast. *Brain*, **81**, 319–40.

NEKI, J. & KISHORE, A. (1962) Treatment of neurosis. *Indian J. Psychiat.*, **4**, 122.

NISHIZONO, M. (1969) La Pharmaco-psychotherapie anaclitique. *Encephale*, **58**, 289–305.

NOREIK, K. (1970) A follow-up examination of neuroses. *Acta Psychiat. Scand.*, **46**, 81–95.

NORTHFIELD, D. W. C. (1960) Symposium on orbital undercutting: The past and future. *Proc. Roy. Soc. Med.*, **53**, 740.

O'CONNOR, J. P. (1953) A statistical test of psychoneurotic syndromes. *J. Abnorm. Soc. Psychol.*, **48**, 581–4.

ÖDEGÅRD, O. (1966) An official diagnostic classification in actual hospital practice. *Acta Psychiat. Scand.*, **42**, 329–37.

O'DONOVAN, D. (1965) Rating extremity: Pathology or meaningfulness? *Psychol. Rev.*, **72**, 358–72.

O'REILLY, P. B. (1956) The objective Rorschach: A suggested modification of Rorschach technique. *J. Clin. Psychol.*, **12**, 27–31.

ORME, J. E. (1965) The relationship of obsessional traits to general emotional instability. *Brit. J. Med. Psychol.*, **38**, 269–70.

ORME, J. E. (1968) Are obsessionals neurotic, or are neurotics obsessional? *Brit. J. Med. Psychol.*, **41**, 415–16.

ORVIN, G. H. (1967) Treatment of the phobic obsessive compulsive patient with oxazepam, an improved benzodiazepine compound. *Psychosomatics*, **8**, 278–80.

OSWALD, I. (1962) *Sleeping and Waking*. Amsterdam and New York: Elsevier.

PALMER, A. D. & JONES, M. S. (1939) Anorexia Nervosa as the manifestation of compulsion neurosis: A study of psychogeneric factors. *Arch. Neurol. Psychiat.* (Chicago), **41**, 856–960.

PARKER, N. (1964) Close identification in twins discordant for obsessional neurosis. *Brit. J. Psychiat.*, **110**, 496–504.

PARTRIDGE, M. (1949) Some reflections on the nature of affective disorders arising from the results of prefrontal leucotomy. *J. Ment. Sci.*, **95**, 795–825.

PATERSON, A. S. & MILLIGAN, W. L. (1948) The technique and application of electronarcosis. *Proc. Roy. Soc. Med.*, **41**, 575.

PAUL, G. (1969) Behaviour modification research: Design and tactics. In FRANKS, C. M. *Behaviour Therapy: Appraisal and Tactics*. New York: McGraw-Hill.

PAVLOV, I. P. (1927) *Conditioned Reflex*. Oxford: Clarendon Press.

PEARSON, H. A. (1963) Leukemia in identical twins. *New England J. Med.*, **268**, 1151–56.

PERVIN, L. A. (1960) Rigidity in neurosis and general personality functioning. *J. Abnorm. Soc. Psychol.*, **61**, 389–95.

PETTIGREW, T. F. (1958) The measurement and correlates of category width as a cognitive variable. *J. Personality*, **26**, 532–44.

PIAGET, J. (1954) *Construction of Reality in Children*. New York: Basic Books.

PIPPARD, J. (1956) Discussion: Obsessive–compulsive states. *Proc. Roy. Soc. Med.*, **49**, 846.

POLLITT, J. (1956) Discussion: Obsessive–compulsive states. *Proc. Roy. Soc. Med.*, **49**, 842–5.

POLLITT, J. (1957) Natural history of obsessional states. *Brit. Med. J.*, **1**, 194–8.

POLLITT, J. (1960) Natural history studies in mental illness: A discussion based on a pilot study of obsessional states. *J. Ment. Sci.*, **106**, 93–113.

POLLITT, J. (1969) Obsessional states. *Brit. J. Hosp. Med.*, **2**, 1146–50.

POST, F. (1965) *The Clinical Psychiatry of Late Life.* Oxford: Pergamon.

PRABHAKARAN, N. (1970) A case of Gilles de la Tourette's syndrome with some observations of aetiology and treatment. *Brit. J. Psychiat.*, **116**, 539–41.

PROKASY, W. F. & EBEL, H. C. (1964) GSR conditioning and sensitization as a function of inter-trial interval. *J. Exp. Psychol.*, **67**, 113–19.

PROKASY, W. F., HALL, J. F. & FAWCETT, J. T. (1962) Adaptation, sensitization, forward and backward conditioning, and pseudo-conditioning of the GSR. *Psychol. Reports*, **10**, 103–6.

RACHMAN, S. (1966) Treatment in desensitization. No. 3. Flooding. *Beh. Res. & Ther.*, **4**, 1–6.

RACHMAN, S. (1968) *Phobias: Their Nature and Control:* Springfield, Illinois: Thomas.

RACHMAN, S. (1971) *The Effects of Psychotherapy.* Oxford: Pergamon.

RACHMAN, S. (1971) Obsessional ruminations. *Beh. Res. & Ther.*, **9**, 229–35.

RACHMAN, S. & HODGSON, R. (1971) Personal communication.

RACHMAN, S., HODGSON, R. & MARKS, I. M. (1971) The treatment of chronic obsessional–compulsive disorder by modelling. *Beh. Res. & Ther.*, **9**, 237–47.

RACHMAN, S., HODGSON, R. & MARZILLIER, J. (1970) Treatment of an obsessional–compulsive disorder by modelling. *Beh. Res. & Ther.*, **8**, 385–92.

RACHMAN, S. & TEASDALE, J. D. (1969) *Aversion Therapy and Behaviour Disorders: An analysis.* London: Routledge & Kegan Paul.

RADOS, S. (1959) Obsessive behaviour. In ARIETI, (ed.) *American Handbook of Psychiatry*, Vol. I. New York: Basic Books.

RAMZY, I. (1966) Factors and features of early compulsive formation. *Internat. J. Psychoanal.*, **47**, 169–76.

RAPAPORT, D., GILL, M. & SCHAFER, R. (1946) *Diagnostic Psychological Testing*, Vol. I. Chicago: Year Book Medical Publishers.

RAY, S. D. (1964) Obsessional states observed in New Delhi. *Brit. J. Psychiat.*, **110**, 181–2.

RAZRAN, GREGORY (1971) *Mind in Evolution. An East–West Synthesis of Learned Behaviour and Cognition.* Boston: Houghton Mifflin.

REDLICH, F. C. & FREEDMAN, D. (1966) *The Theory and Practice of Psychiatry.* London: Basic Books.

REED, G. F. (1968) Some formal qualities of obsessional thinking. *Psychiat. Clin.*, **1**, 382–92.

REED, G. F. (1969a) Obsessionality and self-appraisal questionnaires. *Brit. J. Psychiat.*, **115**, 205–9.

REED, G. F. (1969b) 'Under-inclusion': A characteristic of obsessional personality disorder. I. *Brit. J. Psychiat.*, **115**, 781–5.

REED, G. F. (1969c) 'Under-inclusion': A characteristic of obsessional personality disorder. II. *Brit. J. Psychiat.*, **115**, 787–90.

REGISTRAR-GENERAL (1953) *Statistical Review of England and Wales, 1949. Supplement on Mental Health, 1953.* London: HMSO.

REITER, P. J. (1969) Erfahrungen mit Luvatren Bei ambulanten, psychiatrischen Patienten. *Schweiz. Arch. Neurol. Neurochir. Psychiat.*, **164**, 169–78.

RESCORLA, R. A. & LOLORDO, V. M. (1965) Inhibition of avoidance behaviour. *J. Comp. Physiol. Psychol.*, **59**, 406–12.

RIMM, D. C. (1970) Comments on: 'Systematic desensitization: Expectancy changes or counterconditioning?' *Beh. Res. & Ther.*, **8**, 105–6.

RIN, H. & LIN, T-Y. (1962) Mental illness among Formosan Aborigines as compared with the Chinese in Taiwan. *J. Ment. Sci.*, **108**, 134–46.

RITTER, B. (1969) Treatment of acrophobia with contact desensitization. *Beh. Res. & Ther.*, **7**, 41–5.

RITVO, S. (1966) Correlation of a childhood and adult neurosis. *Internat. J. Psychoanal.*, **47**, 130–1.

ROHRBAUGH, MICHAEL & RICCIO, DAVID C. (1970) Paradoxical enhancement of learned fear. *J. Abnorm. Psychol.*, **75**, No. 2, 210–16.

ROITBAK, A. I. (1960) Electrical phenomena in the cerebral cortex during the extinction of orientation and conditioned reflexes. In JASPER, H. H. & SMIRNOV, G. D. (eds.) *Moscow Colloquium on Electroencephalography of Higher Nervous Activity. EEG. Clin. Neurophysiol.*, Suppl. 13, 91–100.

ROSEN, I. (1957) The clinical significance of obsessions in schizophrenia. *J. Ment. Sci.*, **103**, 773–86.

ROSENBERG, B. G. (1953) Compulsiveness as a determinant in selected cognitive-perceptual performances. *J. Pers.*, **21**, 506–16.

ROSENBERG, C. M. (1967a) *Obsessional Neurosis.* M.D. thesis, University of Witwatersrand.

ROSENBERG, C. M. (1967b) Familial aspects of obsessional neurosis. *Brit. J. Psychiat.*, **113**, 405–13.

ROSENBERG, C. M. (1967c) Personality and obsessional neurosis. *Brit. J. Psychiat.*, **113**, 471–7.

ROSENBERG, C. M. (1968a) Obsessional neurosis. *Austr. N.Z. J. Psychiat.*, **2**, 33–8.

ROSENBERG, C. M. (1968b) Complications of obsessional neurosis. *Brit. J. Psychiat.*, **114**, 477–8.

ROSENTHAL, D. (1970) *Genetic Theory and Abnormal Behavior*. New York: McGraw-Hill.

ROTH, M. (1959) The phenomenology of depressive states. *Can. Psychiat. Ass. J.*, **4** (Suppl.), S32–S53.

ROTH, M. (1965) Physical methods of treatment in mental disease. *Practitioner*, **194**, 613–20.

ROUTTENBERG, A. (1966) Neural mechanisms of sleep: Changing view of reticular formation function. *Psychol. Rev.*, **73**, 481–499.

ROUTTENBERG, A. (1968) The two-arousal hypothesis: Reticular formation and limbic system. *Psychol. Rev.*, **75**, (1).

ROWELL, C. H. F. (1961) Displacement grooming in the chaffinch. *Anim. Behav.*, **9**, 38–63.

RÜDIN, E. (1953) Ein Beitrag zur Frage der Zwangskrankheit, insobesondere ihrere hereditären Beziehungen. *Arch. Psychiat Nervenk.*, **191**, 14–54.

RUSSELL, G. F. M. (1965) Metabolic aspects of Anorexia Nervosa. *Proc. Roy. Soc. Med.*, **58**, (10).

RUTTER, M. (1971) Normal psychosexual development. *J. Child Psychol. Psychiat.*, **11**, 259–83.

RYCROFT, C. (1966) *Psychoanalysis Observed*. London: Constable.

SAKAI, T. (1967) Clinico-genetic study on obsessive compulsive neurosis. *Bull. Osaka Med. Sch.*, Suppl. XII, 323–31.

SALZMAN, L. (1966) Therapy of obsessional states. *Amer. J. Psychiat.*, **122**, 1139–46.

SANDLER, J. (1954) Studies in psychopathology using a self-assessment inventory. 1. The development and construction of the inventory. *Brit. J. Med. Psychol.*, **27**, 142–5.

SANDLER, J. (1964) Masochism: An empirical analysis. *Psychol. Bull.*, **62**, 197–204.

SANDLER, J. & HAZARI, A. (1960) The obsessional: On the psychological classification of obsessional character traits and symptoms. *Brit. J. Med. Psychol.*, **33**, 113–22.

SANDLER, J. & JOFFE, W. G. (1965) Notes on obsessional manifestations in children. *Psychoanal. Study of the Child*, **20**, 428–38.

SARGANT, W. (1952) Anxiety states and their treatment by intravenous acetylchlorine. *Proc. Roy. Soc. Med.*, **45**, 515–16.

SARGANT, W. (1957) *Battle for the Mind*. London: Heinemann.

SARGANT, W. (1962) The present indications for leucotomy. *Lancet*, **1**, 1197.

SARGANT, W. & SLATER, E. (1950) Discussion on the treatment of obsessional neuroses. *Proc. Roy. Soc. Med.*, **43**, 1007–10.

SARGANT, W. & SLATER, E. (1954) *An Introduction to Physical Methods of Treatment in Psychiatry*. London.

SCHACHTEL, E. G. (1969) On attention, selective inattention and experience: An inquiry into attention as an attitude. *Bull. Menninger Clinic*, **33**, No. 2, 65–91.

SCHAPIRO, S. & SALAS, M. (1970) Behavioral response of infant rats to maternal odor. *Physiol. & Behav.*, **5**, 815–17.

SCHMIDT, J. P. (1968) Psychosomatics in veterinary medicine. In FOX, M. W. (ed.) *Abnormal Behaviour in Animals*. Philadelphia: W. B. Saunders.

SCHNEIDER, K. (1925) Schwangs zus Tände un Schizophrenie. *Arch. Psychiat. Nervenk.*, **74**, 93–107.

SCHNEIRLA, T. C. (1968) Instinct and aggression. In MONTAGU, M. F. A. (ed.) *Man and Aggression*. London:

SCHOENFELD, W. N. (1950) An experimental approach to anxiety, escape and avoidance behaviour. In HOCH, P. R. & ZUBIN, J. (eds.) *Anxiety*. New York: Grune & Stratton. (1964, New York: Hafner.)

SCOVILLE, W. B. (1960) Late results of orbital undercutting. *Proc. Roy. Soc. Med.*, **53**, 721.

SEARS, ROBERT R. (1934) Effect of optic lobe ablation on the visuomotor behavior of goldfish. *J. Comp. Psychol.*, **17**, 233–65.

SHANNON, C. E. & WEAVER, W. (1949) *The Mathematical Theory of Communication*. Illinois: University of Illinois Press.

SHARPLESS, S. & JASPER, H. (1956) Habituation of the arousal reaction. *Brain*, **79**, 655–80.

SHELDON, B. L., RENDEL, J. M. & FINLAY, D. E. (1964) The effect of homozygosity on developmental stability. *Genetics*, **49**, (3).

SHIELDS, J. (1962) *Monozygotic Twins Brought Up Apart and Brought Up Together*. London: Oxford University Press.

SHORVON, H. (1946) The depersonalization syndrome. *Proc. Roy. Soc. Med.*, **39**, 779–92.

SIDMAN, M. (1953) Avoidance conditioning with brief shock and no exteroceptive warning signal. *Science*, **118**, 157–8.

SIDMAN, M. (1955) Some properties of the warning stimulus in avoidance behaviour. *J. Comp. Physiol. Psychol.*, **48**, 444–50.

SIDMAN, M. (1966) Avoidance behaviour. In HONIG, W. K. (ed.) *Operant Behaviour: Areas of Research and Application.* New York: Appleton-Century-Crofts.

SIDMAN, M., HERRNSTEIN, R. J. & CONRAD, D. C. (1967) The maintenance of avoidance behaviour by unavoidable shock. *J. Comp. Physiol. Psychol.*, **50**, 533–57.

SIGAL, J. J., STARR, K. H. & FRANKS, O. M. (1958) Hysterics and dysthymics as criterion groups in the study of introversion–extraversion. *J. Abnorm. Soc. Psychol.*, **57**, 143–8.

SINES, J. O. (1959) Selective breeding for development of stomach lesions following stress in the rat. *J. Comp. Physiol. Psychol.*, **52**, 615–17.

SKOOG, G. (1959) The anancastic conditions: A clinical study. *Acta Psychiat. Neurol. Scand.*, Suppl. 134.

SKOOG, G. (1965) Onset of anancastic conditions: A clinical study. *Acta Psychiat. Scand.*, Suppl. 184.

SLADE, P. D. (1971) Rate of information processing in a schizophrenic and a control group: The effect of increasing task complexity. *Brit. J. Soc. Clin. Psychol.*, **10**, 152–9.

SLATER, E. (1943) The neurotic constitution. *J. Neurol. Neurosurg. Psychiat.*, **6**, 1.

SLATER, E. (1964) Genetical factors in neurosis. *Brit. J. Psychol.*, **55**, 265–9.

SLATER, E. & COWIE, V. (1971) *The Genetics of Mental Disorders.* London: Oxford University Press.

SLATER, E. & ROTH, M. (1969) In MAYER-GROSS, W., SLATER, E. & ROTH, M. *Clinical Psychiatry*, 3rd ed. London: Baillière, Tindall & Cassell.

SLATER, E. & SLATER, P. (1944) A heuristic theory of neurosis. *J. Neurol. Psychiat.*, **7**, 49–55.

SLATER, P. (1945) Scores of different types of neurotics on tests of intelligence. *Brit. J. Psychol.*, **35**, 40–2.

SNYDER, B. (1967) Creative students in science and engineering. *Universities Quarterly*, **21** (2), 205–18.

SOKOLOV, Y. N. (1963) *Perception and the Conditioned Reflex.* Oxford: Pergamon Press.

SOLOMON, R. L. (1964) Punishment. *Amer. Psychologist*, **19**, 239–53.

SOLOMON, R. L. & BRUSH, E. S. (1956) Experimentally derived conceptions of anxiety and aversion. In JONES, M. R. (ed.) *Nebraska Symposium on Motivation.* Lincoln: University of Nebraska Press.

SOLOMON, R. L., KAMIN, L. J. & WYNNE, L. C. (1953) Traumatic avoidance learning; the outcomes of several extinction procedures with dogs. *J. Abnorm. Soc. Psychol.*, **48**, 291.

SOLOMON, R. L. & WYNNE, L. C. (1953) Traumatic avoidance learning: Acquisition in normal dogs. *Psychol. Monogr.*, **67**, (4, whole No. 354).

SOLYOM, L. (1969) A case of obsessive neurosis treated by aversion relief. *Can. Psychiat. Ass. J.*, **14**, 623–6.

SOLYOM, L., ZAMANZADEH, D., LEDWIDGE, B. & KENNY, F. (1971) Aversion relief treatment of obsessive neurosis. In RUBIN *et al.* (eds.) *Advances in Behavior Therapy*. London: Academic Press.

SPERLING, B. & BROFFKA, A. (1954) Erfahrungen mit der Leukotomie bei den sogenannten Zwangsneurosen. *Arch. Psychiat. Nervenk.*, **192**, 143–56.

STADDON, J. E. R. & SIMMELHAG, V. L. (1971) The 'superstition' experiment: A re-examination of its implications for the principles of adaptive behaviour. *Psychol. Rev.*, **78**, (1).

STAFFORD-CLARK, D. (1954) Electronarcosis at Guy's. *Guy's Hospital Report*, **103**, 306.

STAFFORD-CLARK, D. (1965) Electronarcosis at Guy's. *Guy's Hospital Report*, **114**, 223.

STAFFORD-CLARK, D. (1967) *Psychiatry for Students*. London: Allen & Unwin.

STAMPFL, T. G. (1968) Implosive therapy: The theory, the subhuman analogue, the strategy and the technique. In ARMITAGE, S. G. (ed.) *Behavior Modification Techniques in the Treatment of Mental Disorders*. Battle Creek, Mich.: V.A. Publication.

STEINER, J., JARVIS, M. & PARRISH, J. (1970) Risk-taking and arousal regulation. *Brit. J. Med. Psychol.*, **43**, 333.

STENGEL, E. (1945) A study on some clinical aspects of the relationship between obsessional neurosis and psychotic reaction types. *J. Ment. Sci.*, **91**, 166–87.

STENGEL, E. (1948) Some clinical observations on the psychodynamic relationship between depression and obsessive compulsive symptoms. *J. Ment. Sci.*, **94**, 650–2.

STENGEL, E. (1956) Discussion: Obsessive compulsive states. *Proc. Roy. Soc. Med.*, **849**.

STERN, J. A. & MCDONALD, D. G. (1965) Physiological correlates of mental disease. *Ann. Rev. Psychol.*, **16**, 225–64.

STERN, J. A., SURPHLIS, W. & KOFF, E. (1965) Electrodermal responsiveness as related to psychiatric diagnosis and prognosis. *Psychophysiol.*, **2**, 1, 57–61.

STERN, R. (1970) Treatment of a case of obsessional neurosis using thought-stopping technique. *Brit. J. Psychiat.*, **117**, (539).

STEWART, M. A., WINOKUR, G., STERN, J. A., GUZE, S. B., PFEIFFEN, E. & NORNUNG, F. (1959) Adaptation and conditioning of the galvanic skin response in psychiatric patients. *J. Ment. Sci.*, **105**, 1102–11.

STINNETT, J. L. & HOLLENDER, M. H. (1970) Compulsive self-mutilation. *J. Nerv. Ment. Dis.*, **150**, (5).

STOLZ, STEPHANIE B. (1965) Vasomotor response in human subjects. Conditioning and pseudo-conditioning. *Psychom. Sci.*, **2**, 181–2.

STRAUS, E. (1948) On obsession: A clinical and methodological study. *Nerv. Ment. Dis. Monogr.* No. 73.

STRELTSOVA, N. L. (1955) The characteristics of some unconditioned reflexes in schizophrenics. In *Proc. of the All Union Theoretical–Practical Conference.* Moscow: Medgiz. (See Lynn, 1966.)

STRUPP, H. H. & BERGIN, A. E. (1969) Some empirical and conceptual bases for co-ordinated research in psychotherapy. *Internat. J. Psychiat.*, **7**, 18–90.

SYKES, K. & TREDGOLD, R. F. (1964) Restricted orbital undercutting. A study of its effects on 350 patients over ten years, 1951–60. *Brit. J. Psychiat.*, **110**, 609–40.

SZILARD, J. & STUTTE, E. (1968) Enzephalitis mit Stammhirn-symptomatik bei Kindern und Jugendlichen. *Schweiz. Arch. Neurol. Neurochir. Psychiat.*, **101**, 212–16.

TAYLOR, J. G. (1963) A behavioural interpretation of obsessive–compulsive neurosis. *Beh. Res. & Ther.*, **1**, 237–44.

TECCE, J. J. (1971) Contingent negative variation and individual differences. *Arch. Gen. Psychiat.*, **24**, 1–6.

TEITELBAUM, P. (1966) The use of operant methods in the assessment and control of motivational states. In HONIG, W. K. (ed.) *Operant Behaviour: Areas of Research and Application.* New York: Appleton-Century-Crofts.

THOMPSON, RICHARD F. & SPENCER, A. (1966) Habituation: A model phenomenon for the study of substrates of behaviour. *Psychol. Rev.*, **73**, 1, 16–43.

THORPE, J. G., SCHMIDT, E., BROWN, P. T. & CASTELL, D. (1966) Aversion-relief therapy: A new method for general application. *Beh. Res. & Ther.*, **2**, 71–82.

TIENARI, P. (1963) Psychiatric illnesses in identical twins. *Acta Psychiat. Scand.*, **39**, Suppl. 171.

TINBERGEN, N. (1949) *Social Behaviour in Animals.* London: Methuen.

TINBERGEN, N. (1951) *The Study of Instinct*. Oxford: Clarendon Press.

TINBERGEN, N. (1959) Comparative studies of the behaviour of gulls (Laridae): A progress report. *Behaviour*, **15**, 1–70.

TINBERGEN, N. & VAN IERSEL, J. J. A. (1947) Displacement reactions in the three-spined stickleback. *Behaviour*, **1**, 56–63.

TITAEVA, M. A. (1962) EEG investigations of the reactivity of the central nervous system in patients with a catatonic form of schizophrenia. In ROKHLIN, L. L. (ed.) *Problemy Schizophrenii*. Vol. II. *Voprosy Pastogeneza i Lecheniya*. Moscow: The Ministry of Health, The RSFFR. (See Stern & McDonald, 1965.)

TIZARD, BARBARA (1968) Habituation of EEG and skin potential changes in normal and severely subnormal children. *Amer. J. Ment. Defic.*, **73**, 1, 34–40.

TRAUGOTT, N. H. & BALONOV, L. YA. (1961) A neurophysiological analysis of certain depressive syndromes. *Zh. Neuropatol. Psikhiatr.*, **61**, 91–8.

TRUAX, C. B. & CARKHUFF, R. R. (1967) *Towards Effective Counselling and Psychotherapy*. Chicago: Aldine Press.

TRYON, R. C. (1940) Genetic differences in maze-learning in rats. *39th Yearbook, Nat. Soc. for the Study of Education*. Part 1, 111–19.

TYSON, R. L. & SANDLER, J. (1971) Problems in the selection of patients for psychoanalysis: Comments on the application of the concepts of 'indications', 'suitability', and 'analysability'. *Brit. J. Med. Psychol.*, **44**, 211–28.

ULRICH, R., HUTCHINSON, R. & AZRIN, N. H. (1965) Pain-elicited aggression. *Psychol. Record.*, **15**, 111–26.

VAN RENYNGHE DE VOXVRIE, G. (1968) L'anafranil (G34586) dans l'obsession. *Acta Neurol. Belg.*, 787–92.

VAUGHAN, M. (1971) *A Retrospective Study of the Relationships between Obsessional Personality, the Occurrence of Obsessions in Depression, and the Symptoms of Depression*. Unpubl. M.Phil. dissertation. Instit. of Psychiatry, University of London.

VENABLES, P. H. (1958) Stimulus complexity as a determinant of the reaction time of schizophrenics. *Can. J. Psychol.*, **12**, 187–90.

VENDETEVA, R. A. (1961) Inhibition of vascular reactions in depressive conditions. *Zh. Neuropatol. Psikhiatr.*, **61**, 99–103. (See Stern & McDonald, 1965.)

VENKOBA, R. A. (1964) A controlled trial with 'valium' in obsessive compulsive state. *J. Indian Med. Assoc.*, **42**, 564–7.

VERNON, W. M. (1969) Animal aggression: Review of research. *Genet. Psychol. Monogr.*, **80**, 3–28.

VINOGRADOVA, O. S. (1961) The orientation reaction and its neurophysiological mechanisms. Moscow Acad. Pedag. Sciences, RSFSR. (See Lynn, 1966.)

WALKER, V. J. (1967) *An Investigation of Ritualistic Behaviour in Obsessional Patients.* Unpubl. Ph.D. thesis, Instit. of Psychiatry, University of London.

WALKER, V. J. & BEECH, H. R. (1969) Mood states and the ritualistic behaviour of obsessional patients. *Brit. J. Psychiat.*, **115**, 1261–8.

WALLERSTEIN, R. S. (1969) The relationship of psychoanalysis to psychotherapy: Current issues. *Internat. J. Psychoanal.*, **50**, 117–26.

WALTER, W. G. (1966) Electrophysiologic contributions to psychiatric therapy. In MASSERMAN, J. H. (ed.) *Current Psychiatric Therapies*, Vol. 6. New York: Grune & Stratton.

WALTON, D. (1960) The relevance of learning theory to the treatment of an obsessive–compulsive state. In EYSENCK, H. J. (ed.) *Behaviour Therapy and Neuroses.* Oxford: Pergamon Press.

WALTON, D. & MATHER, M. D. (1963) The application of learning principles to the treatment of obsessive–compulsive states in the acute and chronic phases of illness. *Beh. Res. & Ther.*, **1**, 163–74.

WARR, P. B. & COFFMAN, T. L. (1970) Personality, involvement and extremity of judgement. *Brit. J. Soc. Clin. Psychol.*, **9**, 108–21.

WARREN, W. (1960) Some relationships between the psychiatry of children and of adults. *J. Ment. Sci.*, **106**, 815–26.

WATTS, F. (1971) *An Investigation of Imaginal Desensitization as an Habituation Process.* Unpubl. Ph.D. thesis, University of London.

WECHSLER, D. (1965) *The Measurement and Appraisal of Adult Intelligence.* (4th ed.) Baltimore: Williams & Wilkins.

WEINER, I. B. (1967) Behaviour therapy in obsessive–compulsive neurosis: Treatment of an adolescent boy. *Psychotherapy: Res. & Prac.*, **4**, 27–9.

WELFORD, A. T. (1962) Arousal, channel-capacity and decision. *Nature*, **194**, 365–6.

WESTPHAL, C. (1878) Zwangsvorstellungen. *Arch. Psychiat. Nervenk.*, **8**, 734–50.

WETZEL, R. (1966) Use of behavioural technique in a case of compulsive stealing. *J. Consult. Psychol.*, **30**, 367–73.

WHITELEY, R. H. & WATTS, W. A. (1969) Information cost, decision consequences, and selected personality variables as factors in predecision information seeking. *J. Pers.*, **37**, 325–41.

WHITTY, C. W. M. (1955) Effects of anterior cingulectomy in man. *Proc. Roy. Soc. Med.*, **48,** 463.

WICKENS, DELOS D. & WICKENS, CAROL (1940) A study of conditioning in the neonate. *J. Exp. Psychol.*, **26,** 94–102.

WILLETT, R. A. (1960) Chapter 15, pp. 566, 601, 602. In EYSENCK, H. J. (ed.) *Handbook of Abnormal Psychology*. London: Pitman Med. Publishing Co.

WILSON, W. P. & WILSON, N. J. (1961) Observations on the duration of photically elicited arousal responses in depressive psychoses. *J. Nerv. Ment. Dis.*, **133,** 438–40.

WINOKUR, G., GUZE, S., STEWART, M., PFEIFFER, E., STERN, J. & HORNUNG, F. (1959) Association of conditionability with degree of reactivity in psychiatric patients. *Science*, **129,** 1423–24.

WISOCKI, PATRICIA A. (1970) Treatment of obsessive–compulsive behaviour by covert sensitization and covert reinforcement: A case report. *J. Beh. Ther. & Exp. Psychiat.*, **1,** 233–9.

WITTKOWER, E. D. (1968) Transcultural psychiatry. In HOWELLS, J. G. (ed.) *Modern Perspectives in World Psychiatry*, pp. 697–712. London: Oliver & Boyd.

WOLFENSBERGER, WOLF & O'CONNOR, NEIL (1965) Stimulus intensity and duration effects on EEG and GSR responses of normals and retardates. *Amer. J. Ment. Defic.*, **70,** 21–37.

WOLFENSBERGER, WOLF & O'CONNOR, NEIL (1967) Relative effectiveness of galvanic skin response latency, amplitude and duration scores as measures of arousal and habituation in normal and retarded adults. *Psychophysiol.*, **3,** 4, 345–50.

WOLFF, H. H. (1970) *The Place of Dynamic Psychiatry in Medicine*. Soc. of Clinical Psychiatrists.

WOLFF, H. H. (1971a) Basic psychosomatic concepts. *Postgrad. Med. J.*, **47,** 530.

WOLFF, H. H. (1971b) The therapeutic and developmental functions of psychotherapy. *Brit. J. Med. Psychol.*, **44,** 117–30.

WOLPE, J. (1953) Learning theory and abnormal fixations. *Psychol. Rev.*, **60,** 111–16.

WOLPE, J. (1958) *Psychotherapy by Reciprocal Inhibition*. Stanford: Stanford University Press.

WOLPE, J. (1964) Behaviour therapy in complex neurotic states. *Brit. J. Psychiat.*, **110,** 28–34.

WOLPE, J. & LAZARUS, A. A. (1966) *Behaviour Therapy and Techniques*. Oxford: Pergamon Press.

WOODRUFF, R. & PITTS, F. N. (1964) Monozygotic twins with obsessional neurosis. *Amer. J. Psychiat.*, **120**, 1075–80.

WORSLEY, J. L. (1968) Behaviour and obsessionality. In FREEMAN, H. (ed.) *Progress in Behaviour Therapy*. Bristol: John Wright.

WORSLEY, J. L. (1970) The causation and treatment of obsessionality. In BURNS, L. E. & WORSLEY, J. L. (eds.) *Behaviour Therapy in the 1970's* (Proceedings of a Symposium). Bristol: John Wright.

YATES, A. J. (1962) *Frustration and Conflict*. London: Methuen.

ZEIGLER, H. P. (1964) Displacement activity and motivation theory. A case study in the history of ethology. *Psychol. Bull.*, **61**, 363–76.

ZETZEL E. R. (1966) 1965: Additional notes upon a case of obsessional neurosis: Freud 1909. *Internat. J. Psychoanal.*, **47**, 123–9.

Author Index

Subject Index